HOMEOPATHIC CARE
for CATS & DOGS

HOMEOPATHIC CARE
for CATS & DOGS

Small Doses for Small Animals

DON HAMILTON, DVM

Foreword by Richard H. Pitcairn, DVM, PhD

Homeopathic Educational Services
Berkeley, California

North Atlantic Books
Berkeley, California

Published by   and
North Atlantic Books   Homeopathic Educational Services
P.O. Box 12327   2124 Kittredge Street
Berkeley, California 94712   Berkeley, California 94712

Cover photos: Puppy: © Pieter Bregman/istockphoto.com.
     Kittens: © stefan1234/istockphoto.com
Cover and book design by Suzanne Albertson
Printed in the United States of America

Homeopathic Care for Cats & Dogs: Small Doses for Small Animals is sponsored by the Society for the Study of Native Arts and Sciences, a nonprofit educational corporation whose goals are to develop an educational and cross-cultural perspective linking various scientific, social, and artistic fields; to nurture a holistic view of arts, sciences, humanities, and healing; and to publish and distribute literature on the relationship of mind, body, and nature.

This book is intended to supplement the advice of a veterinarian who can examine your companion animal. Many conditions are very amenable to home care, but other situations warrant veterinary assistance. I recommend that you as the animal guardian seek as much information as possible to assist you in making an informed decision on proper health care. If you have any concerns about your companion's safety or health, please obtain a veterinary examination before attempting home treatment. But do remember that you are ultimately in charge of your companion animals, so make your own decision after obtaining all the information you need.

North Atlantic Books' publications are available through most bookstores. For further information, visit our Web site at www.northatlanticbooks.com or call 800-733-3000.

Library of Congress Cataloging-in-Publication Data
Hamilton, Donald, 1954–
    Homeopathic care for cats & dogs : small doses for small animals / Don Hamilton ; foreword to the second edition by Richard H. Pitcairn. —2nd ed.
        p. cm.
    Summary: "A revision of the Homeopathic Care for Cats and Dogs published in 1999, this manual brings homeopathic pet care current while providing the same guidance on basic symptoms, treatment options, and home care"—Provided by publisher.
    1. Cats—Diseases—Homeopathic treatment. 2. Dogs—Diseases—Homeopathic treatment. I. Title. II. Title: Homeopathic care for cats and dogs.
    SF985.H35 2010
    636.8'0895532—dc22
                                                    2010018814
       1 2 3 4 5 6 7 8 9 SHERIDAN 14 13 12 11 10

ACKNOWLEDGMENTS

TO KD FOR HER SUPPORT, ENCOURAGEMENT, proofreading, and patience during these long projects (book-writing and marriage!). To Dana Ullman for starting me on the writing path by asking for this book. To Richard Pitcairn for starting me on the right foot with homeopathy. To all of my clients and patients, from whom I have learned so much about medicine and healing, and who still teach me every day. To Thich Nhat Hanh, His Holiness the Dalai Lama, Pema Chödrön, Eckhart Tolle, and the many other spiritual teachers who have guided me through this life, whether directly or through their recorded material. Last but not least, to all the wild animals, plants, and places. I pray for you every moment.

Special thanks to Kathleen Dudley of Fine Feline Photography for the wonderful images throughout the book.

In memory of my father, Phil, for instilling integrity as well as the belief that one can do whatever one wishes. And in memory of my mother, Barbara, for proofreading and support (first edition), and for a lifetime of support and encouragement, especially for encouraging me to be different. Also in memory of Edward C. Whitmont, MD—one of the bright lights.

CONTENTS

Part Two
HOMEOPATHIC TREATMENT

APPENDIX 545

FOREWORD

PERSISTENT AND CHRONIC DISEASE IS ONE of the greatest frustrations for those who love animals. It is equally so for the doctors who care for them. It is a tribute to the growing and dedicated group of veterinarians that are willing to look at new ways to heal disease that they are aware of the limitations of conventional medicine *and are unwilling to accept them.* Don Hamilton is one of these pioneers, a brave and dedicated healer who has made the study of homeopathy his life's passion.

In this book, he carefully and clearly lays down the essential knowledge needed to use homeopathy successfully. To read this book is to prepare you to help your animal with the many day-to-day vicissitudes of life. But more than this, it will make you a knowledgeable and cooperative client.

The greatest challenge to the homeopathic practitioner is to communicate the more accurate deeper perspective of health and disease necessary for them to do their good work. So many people in our busy modern times want the problem solved quickly and easily. Yet, the sad reality is that they would not be at the doorstep of a different kind of vet if they had not already tried everything that conventional medicine could offer. For many clients this is their "last hope." Yet it is extraordinarily sad to see the animal that *could* be cured with patience and persistence, only to have that not happen because of the wrong expectations.

Perhaps the greatest lesson for all of us is seeing the differences between the familiar effects of conventional allopathic medicine with its rapid drug effects and that of the true healing of homeopathy. The latter works with the natural healing abilities of the body and allows the time needed for the body to repair itself. A good comparison is the healing of an injury. We *know* it takes time for the wound to shrink, fill in, and scab over. We would be astonished if all this happened in a couple of hours. Yet, strangely, we have become accustomed and even *expectant* of this kind of rapid change in the treatment of chronic diseases. All would be fine if this resulted in healing, but it does not. More and more drugs are needed as the poor animal languishes and waits for his life to be restored.

Dr. Hamilton carefully makes it clear that this satisfaction with drug effects is based on an unrealistic picture of health and disease. He takes you step by step into a clarity that will serve you well, a perspective that will enable you to be a real partner in helping your animal recover his health.

This understanding is not something peculiar to homeopathy. It applies to all true methods of healing, and it happens that homeopathy is one of these. So, take some time, read this book carefully, and learn of one of the greatest discoveries in the history of medicine. We are fortunate to have a healer of Dr. Hamilton's stature take us on this journey.

Richard H. Pitcairn, DVM, PhD

PREFACE TO THE SECOND EDITION

THE MOST GRATIFYING OUTCOME OF WRITING this book has been the stories I have heard, from both clients and nonclients, of how they have helped their animals with this information. In some cases, even animals whose veterinarians had run out of options turned around with suggestions from the book. Each story fills me with joy, for that was the driving purpose for the book all along, to help animals and their guardians and to reach far more people than I possibly can in one-on-one consultations.

During the decade since the book was first published, I have kept notes on information and issues I wanted to add, some small and some large. This book, like veterinary practice, is a lifelong unfolding. With time I see more that needs inclusion in the book as well as areas I've overlooked. I constantly strive to learn, and I pass on all that I can in this book in hopes that people and animals benefit.

To that end, I have added recommendations and many remedies to a large number of sections. Some sections I have completely reworked. I now use remedies mostly in liquid form, even diluting with water, so the section on remedy administration is essentially new. I have greatly expanded the vaccine chapter, with new information on vaccine damage, titers, and nosodes. And finally, my favorite addition is an entirely new chapter on our relationship to and our understanding of animals. I am passionate about animals, both those with whom I live and those wild ones whom I only occasionally observe. In Chapter Seventeen, titled "The Bigger Picture," I examine our Western cultural beliefs and our interactions with animals, wild and domestic. It is a work in progress and a work that will ultimately result in an entire book on these topics. This chapter is necessarily introductory regarding such a broad

Don Hamilton, DVM

topic, and I am certain some concepts will be new and possibly difficult. I am still processing these ideas, which represent a significant passion for me and a significant portion of my life's work to come.

In short, while this is an updated version of the 1999 edition, I have striven to enhance it substantially so that it provides valuable new information, not only for those who do not own the first edition but also for those who do. I am especially grateful for the support my book has had, as well as for the benefit it has been to so many. I am honored to continue to share this journey with you—not only the journey we share as those whose lives intertwine with animals, but also this larger journey on planet earth, where we discover who we really are.

July 4, 2009

PREFACE TO THE FIRST EDITION

I GRADUATED FROM VETERINARY SCHOOL IN 1979, full of knowledge and hope for success in veterinary medicine. I desired not only financial success but also to use my skills to help reduce suffering among our companion animals. Naturally I had some trepidation about my ability to utilize my newly acquired education to its fullest, but I had the confidence of having attained the degree of Doctor of Veterinary Medicine.

I quickly saw that my new tools gave me an opportunity to help in many situations. I worked in an emergency clinic during some of my early years, and the rewards were great even though the work was hard. When I went back to a "normal" clinic in 1984, I felt that my skills were well honed from three years of experience in general practice followed by two years in emergency medicine. It was not long, however, before I became frustrated at a large group of patients—the ones I had not seen at the emergency clinic. These cases were primarily cats and dogs with skin diseases, although they included other illnesses as well. The essential feature in each case was that the patient's symptoms could not be eliminated; they could only be minimized. These animals were not necessarily very sick, but they returned over and over, or their guardians called again and again looking for relief for their companions. Prednisone (a synthetic steroid, often inappropriately called "cortisone") was the drug of choice for most of these conditions, and I knew it was too dangerous to keep these animals on the drug, yet whenever I tried to wean them off the medicine, their symptoms returned. Not only did the symptoms recur quickly, but they also seemingly increased in intensity each time the drug was stopped.

I don't know who was more frustrated—my clients or I. As guardians of their companion animals, they often did not understand why I refused to let them have as much prednisone as they needed. On the other hand, I could not seem to convey the danger inherent in keeping an animal on the drug. And these animals did suffer, itching day and night, keeping themselves and their guardians awake. I wondered at times if I really had the necessary skill to heal animals. Then one day, a colleague whom I respected remarked to me in *his* frustration that all we really had to treat with were "fluids, antibiotics, and steroids." Bells rang in my head at that statement— I knew it was not *my* limitation that was keeping me from giving more than temporary relief; it was a limitation of conventional medicine.

I began to search for other methods, for something to help these animals and to help me not feel so hopeless. I first studied acupuncture in 1986, and I became certified in veterinary acupuncture in 1987. Acupuncture was rather well accepted and understandable, but as much as I loved and still love the beauty of traditional Chinese medicine, this modality did not give me what I sought. It is a great healing practice in the right hands, but it did not stick with me. It was not my calling.

In 1986 I had also begun to investigate homeopathy. The more I learned, the more intrigued I became, and by 1990 homeopathy had become a significant part of my practice. I was fascinated by homeopathic principles, and I was drawn to homeopathy's gentle, noninvasive method of treatment. My "environmentalist" side was equally impressed with the eco-friendly nature of homeopathic medicines: no toxic chemicals, very small doses needed, remedies can last virtually forever. No need for constant consumption and garbage production.

I also began to see the power of these small doses, as illnesses that I had previously thought incurable (from a conventional perspective) began to improve. And the more I studied homeopathic theory, the more it made sense. Homeopathic theory, like conventional theory, is just a *model* of health and disease. But *this system converged with my practice experience.* On the other hand, the conventional medicine that I had learned in school and in postgraduate study fell short. I could not fully explain disease *as I observed it* with conventional theory. With homeopathic principles, however, not only did I understand what was happening in my patients, but I could also begin to predict what would happen.

Homeopathic medicine had become my vocation. By 1993 I was ready to leave conventional medicine and devote my practice fully to homeopathy. While no method is perfect, I find homeopathic practice satisfying, and I find that I am able to help many of those cases that formerly frustrated me. Additionally, while homeopathy provides the tools to treat very serious illness successfully under the care of an experienced practitioner, it is also very user-friendly for less serious conditions. Many trips to the clinic can be avoided by prompt at-home treatment. With this awareness, I decided to write this book in the hope that I can help even more animals and people than I could possibly touch in person. I have tried to distill my years of experience into the pages of this book, and I believe that it will guide you to better care for your companions.

When I approached the book, my main obstacle was the difficulty, indeed the seeming impossibility, of creating a book that is at once a reference for home use of homeopathic medicine yet true to the principles upon which we practice this medicine. A how-to resource typically takes the form of "if this condition, use these treatments." Yet this form immediately betrays the most fundamental homeopathic tenet: the assertion that individuals are different and thus we must tailor treatment to each individual. As it is unfeasible to take individuality into account to any degree in a resource book, I reached a quandary almost before I began. To do justice to homeopathy, therapy must be unique to the patient and so cannot be readily selected without taking the case of the patient. This idea, however, limits the treatment section of the book to one statement, that is, "See your homeopathic prescriber for all health problems." I had to find a compromise, one that encourages some home treatment but with an understanding of homeopathic principles and not simply rote prescribing.

A second concern involves how we homeopaths understand disease and how this affects treatment interpretation. Homeopathic practitioners evaluate cure by much more rigorous standards than conventional practitioners. The latter may see symptom improvement or cessation as signs of cure regardless of other factors, such as overall patient health. Additionally, conventional practitioners consider the disappearance of one disease followed by the onset of another disease to be unrelated events, assuming that they had cured the first disease, only to have a second disease arise later. By contrast, homeopathic practitioners consider *all* symptoms and conditions affecting a patient as pertinent to the success of treatment, and we evaluate seemingly unconnected symptoms together to ascertain the general status of health as well as to determine the best homeopathic medicines for the patient. In essence, one patient only has one illness, even if her illness has many different symptoms. Furthermore, we only use the word *cure* when all levels of the patient's condition improve, including (most importantly) her mental health. If only certain symptoms—even one "disease" (by conventional standards)—improve without overall improvement, we do not say we have cured the patient. In fact, in some cases, we may see this as a worsening.

Attempting to use homeopathy without applying these guidelines of cure may prove no more helpful than conventional therapy. The only gain will be absence of toxicity. This does not, however, mean complete absence of danger. Homeopathic treatment is not without side effects or risks, contrary to common thought. While this risk is immensely less than that inherent in conventional drug therapy, some risk is present if we improperly administer homeopathic medicines, especially those with higher potencies (see Chapter Three, "The Nature of Cure"). Homeopathy is indeed quite safe, but serious or nonresponsive conditions should be under the care of a qualified homeopathic prescriber.

The solution is not to substitute homeopathy for allopathy as treatment for specific conditions. *(Homeopathy,* from the Greek for "like" and "suffering," means the use of medicines that act in a similar manner as the disease to encourage the healing forces of the body. *Allopathy,* from the Greek for "other" and "suffering," means the use of medicines that oppose the disease, thereby blocking healing forces.) Using "homeopathic medicines" in an allopathic manner, that is, treating specific conditions rather than specific individuals, is fraught with many of the same problems as using conventional drugs. Strictly by definition, a homeopathic medicine is not simply a medicine that has been prepared according to homeopathic methods. The medicine is truly homeopathic only when it is correctly prescribed. This is one of the problems with using most combination homeopathic remedies repetitively for serious conditions, as this approach does not apply homeopathic principles. Results are therefore usually poor, although they may afford temporary relief. For minor self-limiting problems, combination remedies may help if you simply cannot determine the correct single remedy. I know of at least one case, however, where aggressive administration of a combination remedy to an arthritic dog may have pushed the dog into kidney failure.[1] (Since publication of the first edition, I saw a case in my practice where a guardian had used a combination remedy long term, which appeared to cause a liver problem.) This type of situation is extremely rare and even somewhat uncertain, so you need not be afraid to use the medicines. Just don't hesitate to seek help if you don't see timely improvement. And don't continue to administer remedies that are not working appropriately. The first section of the book will help with this understanding.

Supplanting allopathy with homeopathy involves a much deeper, more fundamental change (a paradigm shift). One's basic understanding of life, health, and disease must shift in order to allow treatment to proceed most effectively. Transformation on this level often occurs with some difficulty and at a slow pace, at least in the beginning. I believe that the principles of homeopathy will make sense in a way that allopathy does not, though. With most people the new ideas slowly take hold until a shift in understanding suddenly occurs and the *old* concepts seem foreign.

What I hope to accomplish with this work, then, is to aid this shift in your thinking process so that you understand homeopathy on its own ground. I hope to explain health and disease in a way that makes sense and helps you to understand how and why your companion animal becomes ill. I will show you how disease changes its appearance over time in an individual. This is in contrast to the concept of different diseases affecting that individual over time. You will see that all symptoms of illness in one individual (two- or four-legged) are intimately interconnected. Obtaining this understanding will not only allow better use of the treatment section for simple problems, but should guide you in knowing when and how to work with an experienced practitioner. Hopefully, you will be more able to assess the response to any type of therapy (not just homeopathy) by perceiving the meaning of symptom progression in your companion animals. Additionally, your grasp of disease principles will encourage better observation and thus facilitate learning on all levels. This includes recognition of individuality among animals and adaptation of treatment as needed in honor of that individuality.

The book is divided into five main sections. The first section covers health and disease theory and how homeopathic medicine affects this balance. The second section gives ideas for treatment of more specific conditions, grouped by body system. In the third part, the *"Materia Medica,"* I have given overall descriptions of individual medicines. The fourth section presents information about vaccination, a practice that has become overused in modern medicine; I believe it has gone way beyond disease prevention and is often a disease cause. The last part has appendices of resources and a glossary. I tried to define words as I introduced them, but the glossary may help if you are unclear about the meaning of a medical or homeopathic term.

As I suggested above, Section Two is of necessity somewhat of a compromise to ideal homeopathic prescribing. I have tried, however, to encourage classical homeopathic thinking in this section by showing you how to view these illnesses from this perspective, rather than simply listing remedies that may apply. While you are certainly at liberty to skip the section on homeopathic principles and go straight to the treatment section, I strongly suggest you refrain from doing so. Grasping the theory and principles will greatly enhance your success with treatment and will improve your ability to assess your companion's health in a way that you may have thought impossible. This should improve your communication with your veterinarian, particularly if she is trained in homeopathy. And this will result in better teamwork when you need a veterinarian's assistance.

I do recommend that you consult a veterinarian for any problem that does not rapidly respond to treatment. Obviously, any problem that appears serious warrants immediate consultation so that you accurately comprehend the severity of the situation. It is within your rights, however, to participate in the decisions regarding treatment, so be firm and keep asking questions until you understand. Seek a second opinion if you have any doubts about a diagnosis or about treatment plans. Consult a homeopathic or other holistic practitioner for alternate suggestions.

Conventional therapy has a place and can be a lifesaver, so don't be rigid in refusing treatment. Use this medicine when it is needed. In my opinion, however, most conventional methods should be reserved for *life saving* situations. Unfortunately, in current practice, drugs are often readily prescribed without an assessment of true need. This is especially true with antibiotics and steroids. Use these drugs when necessary, but only when necessary. Living organisms are amazingly adept at healing most illnesses if given a chance. We would all have died out long ago if this were not the case.

A note about word usage: many situations arise when a pronoun could apply to either a male or female. In these situations, I have chosen to randomly use one or the other rather than he/she, s/he, her/him, and so on. If I need to be specific, I have endeavored to be clear.

Finally, I wish to address ethics as they apply to our companion animals. As a veterinarian, I am an advocate for the rights of these wonderful beings who inhabit the earth and our homes, sharing this journey with us. It is my conviction that these animals and all plants and animals, domesticated or wild, have inherent rights that are *separate from their ability to benefit humans.* I believe them to be of equal value, or at least I cannot determine relative value, and I don't believe that any human has the capability to do so.

Furthermore, just because we learn from animals does not mean they exist only to teach us or to help us. They exist and we exist, side by side. They have the same right to exist as we do. I therefore avoid the use of the term

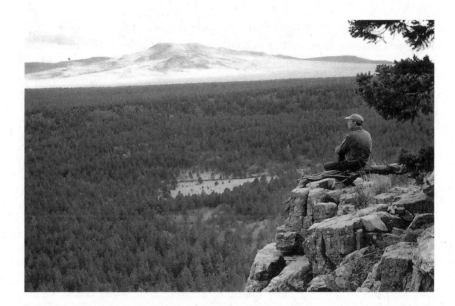

owner, even though our cultures define the human-animal relationship in this manner. I prefer the term *guardian,* and I prefer *companion* to *pet,* although the latter does not necessarily convey a demeaning relationship.

I have also developed a strong opposition to animal research for these reasons. I simply cannot abide the torture of other beings for the sake of humans. We do not learn that much anyway, at least not in the big picture. For that matter, I do not agree with research on dogs to save other dogs, or cats for cats. If we cannot learn from clinical experience, we need to find other methods. It is true that we all depend upon taking the lives of others (plants are living beings also) for survival; it is a characteristic of nature. But it should be done with sanctity and with respect. Abuse and lonely death in a stainless steel cage is far from either concept.

As an extension, I do not use products such as shark cartilage or TriSnake (a Chinese herbal medicine that contains just what it says—three snakes). I cannot justify killing sharks or snakes to save mammals.

I ask that you begin to cultivate an "I-thou" relationship with your companion animals, with wilderness, with strangers. We simply cannot guess their value to us, a value that in some ways parallels their independence from us. Domestication has arguably benefited humans and nonhumans greatly and may always do so, at least to some degree. But we must see these creatures who live in our midst not as a replacement for their wild cousins but as a connection to the wild. Let us never forget our roots—not just the long-ago ancestors we call prehistoric humans but the wilderness from whence we arose. If we ever cut ourselves apart from wilderness, we will no longer be human.

Part One
HOMEOPATHIC PRINCIPLES

Chapter One
INTRODUCTION TO HOMEOPATHY

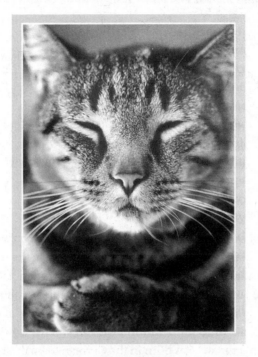

Historical Development of Homeopathy

The physician's highest and only calling is to make the sick healthy, to cure, as it is called. The highest ideal of cure is the rapid, gentle and permanent restoration of health; that is, the lifting and annihilation of the disease in its entire extent in the shortest, most reliable, and least disadvantageous way, according to clearly realizable principles.

—Dr. Samuel Hahnemann[1]

It is the sole duty of the physician to heal the sick. It is not his sole duty to heal the results of sickness, but the sickness itself.

—James Tyler Kent, MD[2]

Samuel Hahnemann: The Founding of Homeopathy

An introduction to homeopathic medical history must begin with its founder, Samuel Hahnemann. As one of the greatest thinkers in the history of medicine, Hahnemann stands alongside individuals such as Hippocrates, Paracelsus, and Huang Di (known as the Yellow Emperor and author of *The Yellow Emperor's Classic of Medicine,* a synopsis of traditional Chinese medicine written in the third millennium BCE and still used today).

Samuel Hahnemann[3] was born in the German town of Meissen in 1755 to a family of porcelain painters and designers. They were very poor, but as he was an excellent student, he was able to obtain his education through the beneficence of educators who waived schooling fees. By the age of twelve, young Samuel was tutoring his classmates in Greek and Latin, and he went on to become fluent in French and English as well. His father, although somewhat opposed to Samuel's education, preferring that Samuel obtain work to help support the family, nevertheless was instrumental in inspiring creative thinking in his son. The elder Hahnemann would give Samuel a problem to consider and lock the boy in a room, and upon the father's return from work he would require an answer. Although this treatment seems harsh, it instilled great conceptual skill in Samuel, who remembered his father with great respect and admiration.

Samuel entered medical school in 1775 and obtained his degree in 1779. During the early years of his career he studied foreign languages as well as chemistry and became a chemist of good reputation. He published several papers in both chemistry and medicine as well as translating various texts in both fields into German from English, French, Italian, and Latin.

The medical practice of the time was rather crude and harsh. Strong chemicals induced agonizing episodes of vomiting and diarrhea in an attempt to purge the body of supposed poisons; bloodletting was employed to rid the body of supposed excesses of blood; cautery and other painful methods were utilized in order to treat various skin ailments. By current standards, most of these treatments created more damage than help. Many patients died from treatment rather than from their illness.

Hahnemann rapidly became disillusioned with medicine, especially when he could not help his own children. He wrote,

> It was painful for me to grope in the dark, guided only by our books in the treatment of the sick—to prescribe according to this or that (fanciful) view of the nature of diseases, substances that only owed to mere opinion their place in the *materia medica* ... substances [that] may ... easily change life into death. ... To become in this way a murderer or aggravator of the sufferings of my brethren of mankind was to me a fearful thought.

Furthermore he wrote that

> children were born to me, several children, and in course of time serious diseases occurred, which, because they afflicted and endangered the lives of my children—my flesh and blood—caused my conscience to reproach me still more loudly, that I had no means on which I could rely for affording them relief.[4]

This conundrum eventually led Hahnemann to abandon practice and rely upon chemistry and his translations for a living. This period, however, laid the groundwork for his later discoveries, as it afforded him the opportunity to study medical and chemical texts of the masters. As an expert in both fields, Hahnemann was well qualified to critique these texts, and he often added translator's footnotes that were critical of the original author, gaining him quite a reputation in the field of chemistry.

Provings and the Law of Similars

Hahnemann eventually translated a text on *materia medica* by the noted Scottish physician William Cullen; the German translation appeared in

1790. Where Cullen attributed the curative power of *China* in intermittent fever (malaria) to its bitter and astringent properties, Hahnemann added a critical footnote. (*China* is pronounced "keena," and it is phonetically the same as the Peruvian word for bark. It comes from the tree called the *kina-kina* tree, or "bark of barks," and the primary ingredient is quinine.) Hahnemann had tested *China* on himself to understand its effects, as he reported in his footnote:

> I took, for several days, as an experiment, four drams of good *China* twice daily. My feet and finger tips, etc. at first became cold; I became languid and drowsy; then my heart began to palpitate; my pulse became hard and quick . . . then pulsation in the head, redness of the cheeks, thirst . . . to sum it up: all those symptoms which to me are typical of intermittent fever . . . all made their appearance. This . . . recurred when I repeated the dose and not otherwise. I discontinued the medicine, and I was once more in good health.[5]

In essence, Hahnemann had uncovered a stunning clue to understanding medicinal properties: first, that their effects on the body are not due to speculated characteristics such as bitterness or astringency. Rather, each drug's impact is different from all other drugs and is thus unique. Secondly, and more importantly, he established a scientific method of ascertaining their true properties—testing the substance on a healthy person who could diligently record the effects on the body. Hahnemann thus founded an objective system of pharmaceutical study, one that allowed investigators to know exactly what effects each drug caused when introduced into the human body. He called this method a *"pruefung"*—a test or trial. The word has been loosely adapted and translated into English as a "proving."

As a chemist, Hahnemann was also concerned with the practice of polypharmacy, that is, mixing several substances together according to their theoretical properties to achieve a combined effect. He felt that it was impossible to predict the response of combining drugs and that only by administering one medicine at a time could a physician interpret its effects, whether during a proving or during treatment. Using one medicine at a time was to remain a standard in his therapeutic recommendations throughout his life, though he briefly experimented with alternating medicines.

Because of the similarity of *China's* effects to the symptoms of intermittent fever, Hahnemann proposed that it was this similarity that enabled

China to treat intermittent fever effectively, in contrast to Cullen's theory. Taking this idea further, Hahnemann eventually proposed that all medicines work by this action, curing diseases that have symptoms similar to the drug's effects. He called this principle the "law of similars."

This idea was not entirely new when Hahnemann proposed it. Similar ideas exist in the Hippocratic writings as well as in those of Paracelsus, who wrote that "Never a hot illness has been cured by something cold, nor a cold one by something hot. But it has happened that like has cured like."[6] Whether Hahnemann was familiar with his predecessors' writings is unclear, but even if he was, his contribution stands upon its own merit, for he crystallized the concept into a rational system of medicine. This system has existed for nearly two hundred years, and the principles remain essentially unchanged, though there are now considerably more medicines in use and there are computer programs to help find the correct homeopathic medicine for a sick individual. The immensity of his contribution simply cannot be overstated.

Compassionate Treatment and Seeing the Patient as an Individual

Another area where Samuel Hahnemann broke new ground was his compassionate treatment of the mentally ill. As with much of medicine during his time, violence was the rule in treatment of the insane. In 1796, Hahnemann published an article describing his successful treatment of such a patient in 1791–1792. In a footnote to this article he wrote, "I never allow any insane person to be punished by blows or other painful corporeal inflictions, since there can be no punishment where there is no sense of responsibility, and since such patients only deserve our pity and cannot be improved, but must be rendered worse, by such rough treatment."[7] Hahnemann was a kind, caring physician, and as such he stressed gentle methods for all cases, as indicated by the quotes at the beginning of this chapter; these quotes begin his major work, the *Organon of the Medical Art*. His call for rapid, gentle methods and the least disadvantage to his patients signify his emphasis upon compassionate medicine.

A corollary to this concern is his insistence upon individual treatment. Rather than trying to lump people into disease categories, Hahnemann recognized that each person was unique and thus deserved individual attention.

Although he contributed much more, these concepts provide an essence of Hahnemannian medicine and form the backbone of homeopathic medicine even to this day: testing of medicines on healthy humans (provings), the single medicine, the law of similars, treatment of the individual rather than the disease, and compassionate medicine.

Constantine Hering: The Father of American Homeopathy

Constantine Hering, another German physician and a correspondent of Hahnemann, was one of the next major figures in homeopathy. As a student, Hering was selected to write a book denouncing homeopathic theory. During his research, he naturally read some of Hahnemann's writings and became intrigued. Rather than simply attacking Hahnemann, as was the original intent of the book, Hering decided to test Hahnemann's theories and ultimately became convinced of their truth. He then continued his medical studies and graduated in 1826 with a thesis that acknowledged the value of homeopathy—a most difficult task in the face of stiff opposition from the "old school" (homeopathic practitioners in the last century often referred to their orthodox colleagues as the "old school").[8]

Shortly after graduation, Hering traveled to South America, where he practiced as a botanist and zoologist for the German government. During this time he conducted a proving on the venom of the bushmaster snake (*Trigonocephalous lachesis*). The remedy, known as *Lachesis,* has become one of the major remedies in our homeopathic medicine chest. (Incidentally, Lachesis was one of the three sisters of fate in Greek mythology—the one responsible for cutting the thread of life. Thus a fitting name for such a deadly snake.)

After a few years in South America, Hering sailed for Philadelphia, where he lived until his death in 1880 and where he established the Hahnemann Medical College. This institution still exists, though homeopathic medicine has not been taught there for many years, and recently the school has opted to change its name, presumably to distance itself from homeopathy. Because of his many contributions, Hering is generally known as the "father of American homeopathy."

Hering's Rule of Cure

Hering authored one of the most comprehensive books on the homeopathic *materia medica.* It comprises ten volumes and is still in use today. He also contributed another major principle of healing—now known as Hering's Rule of Cure:

> In all chronic and lingering cases the symptoms appearing last,
> even though they may appear insignificant, are always the most
> important in regard to the selection of a drug; the oldest are the
> least important. . . . Only such patients remain well and are really
> cured who have been rid of their symptoms in the reverse order
> of their development.[9]

This concept was extended to state that cure proceeded from inside to outside, from above downward, and from most vital to least vital organs. In practice, the reverse order of appearance may be the most important of these guidelines, as there can be conflict among the four tenets of Hering's Rule. (We often say "Hering's Law of Cure," but since *law* suggests something unbreakable, *rule* is a better word.)

The Rise and Fall of Homeopathy in the Nineteenth Century

Despite strong resistance from the allopathic school, homeopathy flourished in the United States during the latter half of the nineteenth century, with as many as twenty-two homeopathic medical schools and around fourteen thousand doctors calling themselves homeopaths. Many of these physicians were not classical (Hahnemannian) homeopaths and in fact may have contributed to the ultimate decline of homeopathic medicine, but at the time these numbers accurately represented the importance of homeopathy in the medical community—at least in the public eye.

Following dramatic successes of homeopathy in the face of epidemics, such as cholera outbreaks in the late 1830s and early 1840s and a yellow fever outbreak in 1878, the public as well as many physicians became homeopathic converts. Many of these physicians, however, simply tried to use homeopathic medicines in an allopathic manner—without proper case-taking or individual prescribing—and they eventually obtained poor results. They then blamed homeopathic theory rather than their failure to adhere to the theory for the lack of success.

These practitioners tended to use low potencies, even material doses, rather than the higher dilutions advocated by Hahnemannian practitioners of the time. This was partly because low potencies can have a temporary impact even if they are not prescribed correctly according to homeopathic principles. These repeated low-potency prescriptions could sometimes alleviate symptoms, but often they would not cure illness. The allopathic converts' failure was not due to their use of low potencies, however. It was because they did not understand homeopathic principles and therefore they generally chose an incorrect remedy. The correct remedy will work in most cases regardless of the potency, whereas the wrong remedy will not work at all.

A second reason for low potency usage was that conventional medical training was becoming increasingly materialistic (materialism is the theory that physical matter is the only reality and that everything, including thought, feeling, mind, and will, can be explained in terms of matter and physical phenomena[10]). As a consequence, many of the converts simply did not believe that high dilutions could have any impact.

A rift opened between the classical homeopaths (generally high-potency prescribers) and the allopathic converts (who used homeopathic medicines—generally low potencies—incorrectly, but often called themselves homeopathic physicians). This conflict badly damaged the morale and the standing of homeopathic practitioners around the turn of the nineteenth century.

James Kent: Preparing the Way for Homeopathy's Future

James Kent was one of the last great torchbearers for homeopathy before its decline in the United States early in the twentieth century. Kent, who coined the phrase "Hering's Law," was a great medical doctor in his own right and made numerous contributions to homeopathy that continue to influence the discipline to this day. A prominent high-potency advocate, Kent authored books on theory and *materia medica* as well as a repertory that still serves as a basis for modern repertories. His *Lectures on Homeopathic Philosophy* is arguably one of the clearest, most important books ever published on disease and is simply wonderful reading. While he intended the book as a supplement to Hahnemann's *Organon* and thus owes a great debt to Hahnemann, Kent wrote with a clarity and understanding that was unmatched by English translations of the *Organon* until very recently. Modern editions only recently supplanted his repertory, and a great many practitioners still use Kent's *Repertory*. And Kent's *Lectures on Materia Medica* stands equally tall as a source for understanding the scope of homeopathic medicines. (Today we use many more remedies than in Kent's day, remedies that are not included in these books—although probably 90 to 95 percent of the time these original remedies will suffice.)

Kent comes the closest of anyone to rivaling Hahnemann's influence and possibly has had even more influence in the twentieth century. His guidance spawned several generations of doctors who kept the practice of homeopathy alive in the United States during its dark ages from the 1920s until the 1970s. These courageous doctors followed their own hearts and their own wisdom in the face of tremendous changes in medicine. The great push toward materialistic science as a basis for medicine all but drove other schools of thought out of existence, except for those individuals willing to practice according to their experience rather than according to the fashion of the time.

The heavy emphasis toward reductionistic or materialistic thinking created a great struggle in the minds of many conventional doctors. They simply could not accept that homeopathic medicines could be effective since these medicines were so highly diluted. This issue remains at the crux of the struggle between homeopathic and allopathic practitioners to this day. During the mid-nineteenth century, the assertion by homeopaths that highly diluted medicines could have an impact, let alone cure illness, was simply too much for their "old school" counterparts to accept.

The seeds were sown for the waning of homeopathy's initial flourish. Theoretical struggles, combined with competition for business, induced great resistance within the allopathic community. In 1894, *Life* magazine wrote that, "The effect of a red flag on a bull is that of a lullaby compared with the fury of the 'regular physician' when you flaunt the banner of homeopathy at him."[11] In 1844 the American Institute of Homeopathy was formed and was our country's first national medical association. The conventional physicians formed the American Medical Association (AMA) in 1846, in large part as an attempt to combat the inroads that homeopathic physicians were making into medicine. This resistance, along with growth in the patent drug industry (the Eli Lilly company, for example, began with patent medicines), led to financial and legal support for conventional medicine. For example, legal action instigated via conventional medical associations began to limit the ability of homeopathic physicians to practice in some states. And when the split occurred between the various groups of homeopaths, it was simply too much for the homeopathic community to resist. By the early years of the twentieth century, the discipline of homeopathy had all but disappeared.[12] This had been accurately predicted by Hering, who said, "If our school ever gives up the strict inductive method of Hahnemann, we are lost and deserve only to be mentioned as a caricature in the history of medicine."[13]

The Resurgence of Homeopathy in the Twentieth Century

Homeopathy was not to be only a caricature, however. While its presence in the United States virtually vanished during much of the twentieth century, many countries continued to support homeopathy. European nations such as France, Germany, the United Kingdom, and the Netherlands maintained bases of support, as did many Latin American countries. And India maintained large numbers of homeopathic doctors and a rich legacy that never really diminished as in the West. Indian culture is not so rationalistic and materialistic as that of the United States, which may explain why homeopathy as a concept never challenged the Indians like it did in other parts of the world. Today, both the European practitioners and the so-called Indian school provide great stimulus to furthering homeopathic thought and practice.

In the United States, the resurgence of homeopathic medicine began in the early 1970s, thanks in large part to the force of George Vithoulkas, a well-known Greek homeopath who trained many of the new generation of homeopathic physicians. Vithoulkas's books also greatly impacted our understanding of disease and homeopathy. Today, homeopathic medicine has nearly the influence it did in the 1800s and is widely practiced throughout the world. This resurgence has brought many new ideas and many new leaders, such as Rajan Sankaran, Massimo Mangialavori, Jan Scholten, and many others too numerous to mention. These practitioners bring fresh ideas to an old medicine, often enriching without diluting its efficacy, even its beauty. There is some disagreement again between those who wish to stick to Kent and Hahnemann and those who utilize the "new thinking," but this debate seems to strengthen rather than weaken homeopathy's place in medicine. Even more broadly, holistic therapies, including homeopathy, have once again become a major voice in medical thought throughout the world. These "alternative" movements have also begun to challenge some conventional tenets such as vaccination and antibiotic use, especially as we recognize how damaging these latter practices can be. Today, people everywhere realize that health is more about supporting our bodies rather than trying to kill or stop "invaders" from causing illness, recognizing that these "invaders" are more symptom than cause of illness. In the human body, for example, only 10 percent of our cells are human cells; the rest are bacteria and other organisms, without which we cannot survive. In other words, we are not separate beings from the world around us, and we depend upon bacteria to live. In our intestines, for example, bacteria produce many of the B vitamins, which we then absorb; they also digest much of our food for us. Without these bacteria, we would not survive well. So the idea that we can kill "bad" bacteria is fraught with danger and misunderstanding. The bacteria are not the problem; rather they overgrow when we get out of balance. Further, attempting to kill the ones that have overgrown will also kill the others that help to keep the balance. Becoming aware of these issues has led many people to seek more gentle, holistic methods, including homeopathy, as their first choice for treatment.

Veterinary Homeopathy

Veterinary homeopathy dates almost to the time of its first use for human disease. Johan Joseph Lux, a German veterinarian, was using homeopathy by the early 1830s, and Georg Adolph Weber, also a German veterinarian, joined Lux's ranks by the mid-1830s. Lux was an early supporter of isopathy, an outgrowth of homeopathy, in which potentized (homeopathically prepared—see below in this chapter) products of disease are used to treat that same disease. For example, blood from a cow affected with anthrax was potentized for use on other cattle with anthrax. This idea eventually proved fruitless in most cases, as only a similar substance rather than an identical one seems to have the power to cure. (Although sometimes, potentized drugs or vaccines can reverse damage from the original—conventional—use of the same drug or vaccine.) Sometimes prevention is possible, however, and the concept of isopathy led to the use of nosodes as preventives (see Chapter Sixteen, "Vaccination," for more information on nosodes).

Current use of homeopathic medicines in animals has had three primary forces: in the United Kingdom, veterinarians George MacLeod and Christopher Day have been at the forefront, publishing books as well as teaching others how to use homeopathic medicines with success in large as well as small animals. Dr. Richard Pitcairn has done the same in the United States and is personally responsible for introducing homeopathy to scores of veterinarians; he has provided for the North American veterinary community what Vithoulkas gave to the field of human medicine. And as in human medicine, today veterinary homeopathy is widespread, and many practitioners guide and invigorate this medicine to new heights.

Those of us in homeopathy owe a great debt of gratitude to these individuals in human and veterinary medicine, along with a great many others too numerous to list—in particular, to those who carried the torch during the "homeopathic dark ages," for without them this beautiful method of treatment might have indeed been relegated to caricature status as Hering feared.

General Introduction to Homeopathic Medicine

Hahnemann's frustration with the medicine of his time included not only its ineffectiveness but also its harsh methods. His search for a different approach stemmed from this frustration as well as his strong scientific mind. The development of homeopathic medicine blended these facets into one model of healing.

Provings and the Law of Similars: Understanding Our Medicines

The use of provings marked a major step forward in medicine by providing a rational, scientific, reproducible method of studying the actions of drugs through testing them upon healthy humans. Prior theories of the working actions of drugs were primarily speculative, based upon properties such as bitterness or astringency and the hypothetical implications of these properties. Hahnemann's decision to give minute, potentized doses of drugs to willing provers gave the medical profession the chance to understand exactly what impact these drugs had upon the body. This test method uncovered not only the physical effect but also the changes to the mental state. This was a giant leap forward in its recognition that disease is not limited to physical symptoms but includes the mental state as well. Hahnemann further deduced that the available, observable symptoms are not the disease but are only representative of the disease—and that the true disease is unknowable by the human mind. Additionally, the symptoms only guide us to appropriate medicines and to prognosis, but we cannot understand the extent or the mechanism of the true disease.

The way the symptoms direct us to the best homeopathic medications ultimately materialized as the Law of Similars, in that the appropriate medicine for an illness is the one that can create the same (actually a very close similar) symptom picture as that of the natural disease. Each substance has the capability of inducing a set of symptoms in a healthy individual; this symptom group is known as a drug disease or medicinal disease, and it is this that stimulates the curative response in the sick individual. The proving gives the symptoms of the medicinal disease. These symptoms are compiled into an orderly description that lists mental symptoms, physical symptoms, and general symptoms. General symptoms affect the whole body and include such conditions as the side of the body more likely to be affected and situations that improve or worsen the symptoms. For example, someone in a *Pulsatilla* state tends to have symptoms on the right side of the body and is worse in a stuffy room and worse from eating fatty foods.

Finding the Remedy with the *Materia Medica* and the Repertory

Once the various remedy pictures are compiled, they are grouped into a *materia medica*—a list of homeopathic medications and their respective medicinal diseases (symptom pictures). From this list of medicines, we choose the one that most closely fits the symptom picture of the illness in the individual we wish to treat.

As the number of remedies grows, it becomes harder to remember the different remedy pictures at all times, so another text was created to assist the process. A repertory is sort of the opposite approach to that of the *materia medica*. In the repertory, symptoms are listed with the various medicines that may have the symptom. Typically, the symptoms are arranged in sections according to parts of the body; each section is alphabetized. In Kent's *Repertory*, for example, the sections start with mind, vertigo, head, eye, vision, ear, hearing, and so on—and end with perspiration, skin, and generalities. The listing is more or less from head down, as in the *materia medica*. Let's look at a symptom as an example.

Perhaps your puppy always has diarrhea in the house when he is left alone. A rubric (defined as a symptom as listed in the repertory) from Kent's *Repertory* that might be helpful is "Rectum: diarrhea: alone, when." In this case only one remedy is listed—*Stramonium*. Often, many remedies will be in a given rubric. *Stramonium* is not necessarily the correct remedy in this case—it must be confirmed by reading the *materia medica* description of *Stramonium* to see if other characteristics of your puppy fit *Stramonium*. This is an essential part of homeopathy: each individual is treated as such; we do not prescribe on one symptom only. We always try to elicit a few characteristic symptoms and find a remedy that has a similar complex of symptoms. On the other hand, each homeopathic remedy picture is vast, so we will never find all of the known symptoms of *Stramonium*, for example, in a dog that needs *Stramonium*. It is not necessary that the individual has all the symptoms of the remedy, but it is essential that the remedy have all of the primary symptoms of the individual.

Furthermore, the repertory is not a final guide to the correct remedy. The remedy must be studied in the *materia medica* to confirm the choice. The repertory is only used to lead to possible choices. For experienced practitioners the repertory is a reminder—we look at possible rubrics and see the remedies, and if we know our remedies, we can quickly narrow the list to a few choices, or even the correct remedy, with a perusal of appropriate rubrics. The trick is choosing the right symptoms to emphasize. This will be covered in more detail in Chapter Five, "Using Homeopathy at Home"— although the process for using this book is simplified, as there is no true repertory section.

To summarize the process of finding a remedy: we know the symptom pictures of available remedies because of provings and their representation in the *materia medica*. We then "take the case" of the ill individual to ascertain the most important symptoms. The unusual symptoms are the most important, as these provide the best differentiation between remedies. We often speak of the "strange, rare, and peculiar" symptoms as those most likely to guide us to the correct remedy. Once we obtain the characteristic symptoms—those that best represent the illness as it expresses in the individual—we look them up in the repertory to find which medicines can have each symptom. By comparing rubrics to see which remedies cover most or all of the symptoms, we narrow the choices of remedies down to a small number. We can then read the *materia medica* to determine which of these provides the best fit to the case.

In this book, however, there is no true repertory, since this work is meant to cover primarily acute diseases (see Chapter Two, "The Nature of Disease"). In Part Two you will find sections on different body systems, but each section gives a description of that system in health and disease, then lists remedies that may be useful, with a brief description of how to use that remedy for that specific condition. You will then use the *materia medica* (Part Four, Chapter Eighteen) to see if the remedy also fits the overall picture of your animal's illness. This is sort of a shortcut approach, listing the remedies I have found most commonly needed.

What Is a Homeopathic Medicine?

Once we choose a remedy, we then must give the remedy to the sick animal or person—so a description of remedies is in order. First, just what is a remedy, and how do remedies differ from drugs? Although we call them homeopathic medicines as well as homeopathic remedies, the latter name is more commonly applied, as they are said to remedy the situation. Conventional drugs, on the other hand, generally mask symptoms but do not cure the person. This difference is because of the different mode of action within the two systems. Medicines generally have two basic phases of impact, which we call their primary and secondary effects. These are action-reaction effects. The primary effect is the direct action of the drug upon the body, and the secondary effect is the body's reaction to the primary drug effect. A good example is that of stimulant drugs like caffeine. The primary effect of caffeine is obviously stimulation—it gets a lot of people going in the morning. But the secondary effect is drowsiness, which begins as the drug effect of caffeine wears off—and this drowsiness is generally greater than had the person not had the coffee.

Allopathy (conventional medicine; treatment by opposites) depends upon the primary effect for its therapeutic drug use. To a large degree this is based upon treatment by contraries. If we have a fever, we take aspirin to bring down the fever. The underlying assumption is that the symptoms are the illness and that these symptoms are of no benefit to the body. By contrast, homeopathy works from the assumption that the body generally knows best how to respond to illness and that it only needs assistance in its efforts, not resistance to those efforts. The similar remedy, called the simillimum, reinforces the body in its direction of healing. This is accomplished via the secondary effect of the medicine.

Since the primary effect of the simillimum is so similar to the disease in existence, the secondary effect will be similar to the body's attempt to rid itself of the original illness. The net result is to strengthen the body in this attempt. A fever is seen not as a problem but as the best method of eliminating the disease at hand. Fever is the first stage of inflammation, which is the initial reaction of the immune system. The simillimum will not necessarily increase the fever if it is already high, but it may initiate a fever in an animal that has been too sick to mount a fever. Another way of explaining this is that often a sick animal cannot react fully to illness and cannot engage all parts of the inflammatory process. The correct homeopathic remedy will guide the body to respond fully to the illness, thus bringing about a cure. If a fever is already present prior to administration of the simillimum, the fever will drop, often rapidly, but due to the body's own efforts (and the secondary remedy effect) and not the drug's primary effect.

Potentization: Dilution and Succussion

Hahnemann found that the secondary effect occurred even as very small amounts of the drug were given, so he continued to dilute the drugs to use smaller and smaller amounts. Initially, this was to minimize the drastic impact of the crude drugs in existence at the time. But once again this man of genius and great fortune uncovered a startling phenomenon. It turned out that the more he diluted the medicines, as long as they were shaken vigorously at each step, the more powerful they became: the secondary effect grew as the primary effect was diminished by dilution. Hahnemann called this process potentization[14]—it produces more and more potent medicines at each step. (Hahnemann also used the term "dynamization," as the process releases the dynamis, or vital force—the dynamic power—of the medicine, "even those substances which, in their crude state do not manifest the least medicinal power in the human body.") The vigorous shaking he called succussion, so potentization consists of sequential dilution and succussion. The paradoxical impact of potentization contributes to the strong allopathic resistance to homeopathic medicine.

As a point of comparison, the allopathic approach to minimizing harsh drug effects was to refine the drugs down to the "active ingredients" and eliminate those ingredients responsible for side effects—primary but unwanted drug effects. This approach also created more powerful medicines with fewer undesired effects, but these still depend upon primary drug effects to suppress symptoms. The outcome has meant that allopathy has become more proficient at thwarting the body's attempts to heal itself. This can result in poorer health in the long run, although dramatic impact is possible with modern drugs—impact that may be helpful in dramatic situations that need urgent stabilization.

Remedies are potentized according to two main dilution scales: C potencies and X potencies. The letters stand for their Roman numerical values and reflect the method of dilution during preparation. Centesimal (C) potencies are diluted by a factor of one hundred at each step, while decimal (X) potencies are diluted by a factor of ten at each step. Remember that after each dilution the solution is shaken vigorously.

Suppose a pharmacist needed to prepare a remedy from table salt in the C scale (this is the remedy *Natrum muriaticum*). She would take one part of the salt and dilute (dissolve) it in ninety-nine parts of liquid (typically a water-alcohol mix), shake it vigorously, and this becomes a 1C potency (one part plus ninety-nine parts equals one hundred parts, thus the dilution factor is one hundred). She would then take one part of this 1C stock and dilute it in ninety-nine parts liquid; once this is succussed it becomes a 2C potency. One part of 2C to ninety-nine parts liquid becomes a 3C, and so on. Thus, a 1C has 1/100th of the original concentration, a 2C has 1/10,000, and a 3C has 1/1,000,000 of the original concentration. We commonly use potencies up to 10,000C—the dilution is quite staggering to think about, even to those of us who are dedicated homeopaths.

In a similar vein, we prepare an X potency using one part of the original substance, in this case salt, to nine parts liquid, and this becomes a 1X. One part of the 1X diluted with nine parts liquid becomes a 2X, and so on. The dilutions are not so great with the X potencies, thus these are not as potent as the C potencies and are rarely used above 200X.

If a substance is not dissolvable in water, the first three potencies may be done using lactose (milk sugar). If we needed to prepare a remedy from sulfur, for example, we could take one part of sulfur and ninety-nine parts of lactose and grind it for one hour in a mortar and pestle to produce a 1C. One part of the 1C with ninety-nine parts of lactose produces a 2C after another hour of grinding; one more repeat makes a 3C. From the 3C the process is converted to liquid dilution. Similarly, with plant materials, lactose may be used, or sometimes the plant is macerated and allowed to steep in an alcohol solution to produce a "mother tincture," and further dilution proceeds in liquid as usual.

Once the stock solutions are produced in the desired potencies, the remedies for consumption are made from these stock solutions. Thus the laborious process need not be repeated for each prescription. Lactose pellets are coated with a few drops of an 87 percent alcohol stock solution of the desired potency, and this produces a vial of pellets of the same potency.

For humans, the dose of pellets is generally dissolved under the tongue. With animals, we either simply drop the pellets in their mouth, dissolve them in a small amount of water, or grind them into a powder that is poured into the mouth. It is best to avoid handling the pellets as they are easily neutralized, so use a spoon or the cap of the vial to hold the pellets to drop them into your companion's mouth. Don't mix remedies into foods, as the foods may also neutralize the remedy. Remedies may also be dispensed as a liquid, usually 20 percent alcohol. I find this easier for administration to dogs and cats, and I use this method when I dispense remedies. Furthermore, with another decade of practice since the first edition of this book, I have found liquid dosing to be much better in most cases, so I rarely give dry potencies (see Chapter Five, "Using Homeopathy at Home").

Summary

We test homeopathic medicines through provings on healthy humans to determine their activity—their medicinal effect, or remedy picture. We look for both mental and physical effects.

We choose medicines based upon the law of similars—the medicine that can create a transient set of symptoms that most closely matches the symptoms of illness is the one that can stimulate a cure. The *materia medica* lists medicines and their symptom pictures, and the repertory lists symptoms and remedies that may have those symptoms as part of the symptom picture, or drug disease, of that remedy. These books assist us in our search for the correct remedy, which we call the simillimum.

When a cure happens, it usually follows Hering's Rule of Cure (this is most apparent with chronic illness). That is, improvement occurs in an orderly manner, with most recent symptoms disappearing first. Additionally, the most severe symptoms and those affecting the most important organs will improve early in the curative reaction. Finally, the direction of cure is often from inside out and from top to bottom, although these are not always consistent.

We utilize the secondary effect of a medicine for the curative impulse. In other words, it is the body's reaction and not the drug itself that ultimately cures illness. This is why cures are so complete.

Homeopathic medicines are prepared through potentization—dilution and succussion. This may be through tenfold (X potencies) or hundredfold (C potencies) dilution steps. The more dilute the potency, the stronger the medicine becomes; this is due to succussion—vigorous shaking after each dilution.

Medicines may be dispensed as pellets, tablets, or liquid, and these are administered directly into the mouth. They should not be handled nor placed in foods.

Chapter Two
THE NATURE OF DISEASE

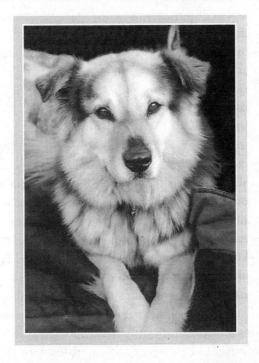

Conventional Medicine and the Rationalist School

Holistic Medicine and the Empirical School

Acute Disease versus Chronic Disease

Disease as Individual Phenomenon

Symptoms Are Not Disease; They Only Represent the Illness

Symptoms Are Actually the Healing Process

What Is Disease?

How Does Disease Arise?

What Is a Healthy Animal?

Summary

UNDERSTANDING DISEASE IS ESSENTIAL TO successful treatment. Whether you are treating minor problems at home or working with a practitioner on serious conditions, the more informed you are, the better your choices will be in treating your animals. In this chapter, I hope to help you see how disease affects the body, so you will better understand how the body can heal.

Conventional Medicine and the Rationalist School

When I studied disease in veterinary school in the late 1970s, we focused upon pathology (damage to body tissues) and upon external causes such as bacteria and viruses. While our study of pathology indicated how the body responds when ill, I do not remember much emphasis upon healthy processes. Nor did we make connections concerning illnesses that affect the body at different times or in different manners. We learned numerous conditions that might affect the body, but we studied them all as separate entities. By contrast, as a homeopath I now see that different outbreaks of disease are often expressions of one illness rather than different illnesses (see below).

Additionally, we sought a cause *outside the body* in almost all situations. If we could associate an organism with a pattern of symptoms, then we considered that organism to be the sole cause of this symptom complex. We then gave the symptom complex a name associated with the "causative organism" and considered another mystery solved.

Feline leukemia virus disease is an example. In the late 1950s and early 1960s, veterinarians had observed cats with immune suppression, anemia, and leukemia—elevated numbers of white blood cells (cells involved in immune response to disease)—without understanding why these cats were ill. In 1964, researchers in Scotland found a virus in cats with lymphosarcoma, a cancer of the lymph nodes. Other researchers later identified the same virus in cats with the immune-suppressive and leukemia disorders. They called the virus the "feline leukemia virus" and claimed that it caused these symptom complexes. Modern veterinary virologists still deem this causal relationship correct, and many people simply say that cats with these symptoms have "feline leukemia," in spite of the existence of many cats with identical symptoms that do not have the virus. Some cats with these symptoms have the feline immunodeficiency virus, a related virus discovered in the 1980s. And some cats have neither virus but the same symptoms.

Conventional medical practitioners view disease in the same manner—seeking outside organisms (bacteria, viruses, fungi, fleas, worms, and so on) to account for illness when possible. If a disease seems unlikely to be infectious, then the cause is sought at the most elemental level. Researchers employ microscopes and other tools to look for abnormalities. If the abnormalities fit into a pattern, they will be implicated as the cause of disease. For example, inadequate insulin production by the pancreas is said to cause diabetes mellitus. Or in some cases insulin is present, but the "cause" of disease is attributed to the body's inability to respond to insulin.

This type of reasoning has its roots in the philosophical heritage commonly called the rationalist school of thought. It applies logic to understand how disease affects the body at the most basic physical level. Rationalist practitioners propose theories about the inner workings of the body and then attempt to fit their observations to the theories. The physician with the most impact upon this approach was Galen, a second-century Roman. Galen postulated that four humors circulated in the body, and that imbalances in these humors resulted in illness. He based his humoral theory of disease upon speculation or a priori knowledge (based upon theory rather than experiment or experience) more than upon observation of patients. Galen's influence continued almost unopposed for over a thousand years, and even today many consider him the father of modern medicine.

While Galen's theory was rather holistic in some ways, his inception of the theory embraced the notion that understanding the cause of disease was possible through abstract philosophical conjecture.

René Descartes, perhaps the epitome of the rationalist genre, strongly espoused the view of the body as a machine. He did not believe animals experienced pain or emotion, and thus he felt that cries of animals undergoing vivisection (surgery on live animals, without anesthesia or analgesia) were reflexes only, not evidence of pain.

While we may wish to dismiss this as the poor understanding of a seventeenth-century thinker, this thinking persists today among "scientists" involved with much animal research. Rationalist investigators, seeking physical understanding of disease, subject many millions of animals to torture every day in the United States and the rest of the world. These researchers may grudgingly admit that animals experience pain, but many dismiss concern for the welfare of laboratory animals. Furthermore, when others assert that not only do animals experience physical pain but that they also have emotions and thus may experience mental suffering, researchers respond with a cry of anthropomorphism (projecting human traits onto animals).

If we accept the idea that animals have emotions, research becomes even harder to justify. As the backbone of conventional (rationalist) medicine, research must be justified (rationalized) by the medical community. When we question researchers about the moral implications of research, the most common response is, "But it saves lives." "Whose lives?" we might query.

Animals are surgically, chemically, and physically inflicted with terrible pain in an attempt to mimic known, named diseases. Studying the physical impact of these conditions hypothetically leads to better understanding of possible therapies. The rationalist assumption is that we can logically deduce causes of illness through the study of pathology. Thus, cadavers are autopsied to assess damage. From this perspective, once these physical causes are understood, treatment is simple; these processes need only to be reversed or opposed. The body is treated much like a machine, and it is not even considered capable of repairing itself once disease begins. This provides a method of approaching disease that simplifies the understanding of a truly formidable body of knowledge. But for holistic practitioners, this system falls short, as we believe the body to be much more than machinelike.

One study that inadvertently supported holistic thinking involved several groups of rabbits. These rabbits were injured and various treatments tested for effectiveness. One group of rabbits consistently recovered faster than other groups with the same treatment. Investigation by puzzled researchers finally uncovered the reason: the caretaker for that group treated them with much kindness and petting, thus their (relative) emotional well-being led to faster healing. Mechanistic (rationalistic, reductionist) theories cannot explain such a phenomenon.

The rationalist school also defines illness by the symptoms shared among different individuals, thus emphasizing commonality and minimizing individuality. With diabetes, for example, any individual with sugar (glucose) in the urine, increased thirst, and increased urine output is considered to be diabetic. Standard therapy involves dietary changes (the same for everyone) plus either oral glucose-lowering medicine or injected doses of insulin. Thus, when a person or animal has a set of signs that correlate with a pattern of a known disease, that individual is said to have the same disease. Once this diagnosis is established, treatment is already decided, as all individuals with a given disease receive virtually the same treatment. This greatly simplifies the practice of medicine.

For several years, I practiced according to this philosophy and its methods, having learned them in veterinary school as the best, most modern ways to aid the sick. In many cases, animals did seem to be greatly helped. Some situations, however, proved resistant to these techniques. And the longer I was in practice, the more of the resistant cases I encountered. Many animals that seemed responsive at first eventually stopped responding. I became frustrated, as I often found no answers to help these suffering creatures. I could give higher doses of drugs or use stronger drugs, but ultimately the body would produce symptoms of illness no matter what I tried to do. What I ultimately saw was that *attempts to oppose the expression of illness were of necessity destined to fail.*

A classic example, one that frustrates veterinarians everywhere, is the dog or cat with skin disease. The poor animal itches constantly unless some kind of medicine is given. Steroids ("cortisone") will stop the itch, but each time they are administered, relief is less complete. As these animals kept coming back every year, needing more and more drugs, I realized I was only helping these animals in a limited sense. My medicine could help provide relief, but it could not eliminate the problem.

Meanwhile, the illnesses continued to worsen, even during periods of remission. Thus, the dog with an allergy to fleas may be symptom-free during the winter, but when spring comes and the flea population emerges, the itching returns. Typically, the dose of steroid that worked the prior year proves inadequate and must be increased. *Even though we could not see the progression during the symptom-free winter season, the allergy has worsened.* The patient must therefore be sicker than he was the year before, despite the body's continual attempts to heal. Broadening my observation to all diseases, I saw that we rarely cured anything, even by conventional standards. We merely bought time. This awareness—that my medical knowledge was limited—disturbed me, and I sought answers elsewhere.

Holistic Medicine and the Empirical School

In 1985 I began to look into holistic healing methods to see if other modalities provided hope for these situations. I studied acupuncture first, as this was familiar and had the most credibility. Traditional Chinese medicine (TCM), which underlies acupuncture theory, provided an entirely new way of looking at disease. TCM has thousands of years of history and success using an empirical understanding of health and disease. (Empirical systems rely upon observation of patients and practical application of treatment. Observation comes first, and theory second. Remember that rational systems place theory first.)

Because they have great respect for their ancestors, the Chinese never considered dissecting human bodies to understand disease. Observing living patients became the basis of their medical practice. This observation quite naturally led to the understanding that some nonphysical energy lies at the heart of life and health. (As well-known veterinarian Allen Schoen asks, "What is the difference between a cadaver and a live person?") This energizing quality, or life essence, they call Qi (pronounced "chee"). TCM practitioners focus upon the somewhat subtle concept of Qi rather than upon the relatively concrete body (as compared to rationalists' dissection-centered focus):

> The concept of Qi is at the heart of Chinese medicine. Qi defines life, even though it is impossible to grasp, measure, quantify, see, or isolate Qi. An invisible force known only by its effects, Qi is recognized indirectly by what it fosters, generates, and protects.... Qi begets movement and heat.... Life cannot be separated from the way it manifests. When the heart beats and the breath is warm ... life exists within the body. When the heart stops beating and the body becomes cold, the life force, or Qi, is no longer present.[1]

Health is not perceived in a physical way only. Rather, health exists when bodily energies remain in balance, when the Qi flows evenly throughout the physical body.

My acupuncture teachers even suggested that our intent as we administered treatment might affect the outcome. What a beautiful idea! And yet it is a sobering one. Without conscious goodwill, we might do more harm than good, even with technically correct methods. I began to realize that something more was involved than the physical, rational world alone, something we might not fully comprehend. Qi, life force, intent—these terms represent something almost beyond our ken. Yet that something may be essential to healing, to wholeness.

The empirical school of thought, as exemplified in TCM and homeopathy, is the other major force in medicine, and it is often at odds with the rational school. Empirical medicine generally begins with the premise that we cannot know ultimate causes of disease (such as exactly why we get cancer), and that any attempt to do so will end in failure—thus treatments based upon this approach will fail as well. Empirical approaches maintain their basis in what is directly visible and confirmable. Conditions that influence disease generation *can* be known (such as stress, exposure to cold wind, and so on) by observation and experience of how illness occurs in many individuals. Thus, while one may not know everything about a disease state affecting an individual, *what one knows is certain* because it has been directly observed or reported by the patient.

In contrast, much of rational medicine is based upon speculation and theory, as evidenced by the constant change in concepts and treatment seen in this medicine. New drugs and treatments come and go with regularity, and many discarded ones having been found harmful along the way, leaving numerous injured people in their wake. Homeopathy and acupuncture, as examples of empirical medicine, have remained constant throughout their history (two hundred years for homeopathy and over five thousand years for acupuncture).

I first heard of homeopathy at about the same time that I began my acupuncture studies. The homeopathic medical system seemed far-fetched and confusing as I first heard it explained. And yet I found it intriguing, even compelling. I began to study in earnest, and this path produced dramatic changes not only in my understanding of healing, but more importantly, in my comprehension of health.

My practical experience up to this point did not accord with my allopathic training in disease theory. No matter how I applied my knowledge of pathology to living animals, things often did not mesh. As I transited into a more empirical mode of thinking, my observations of illness began to more closely match my understanding of disease. Since homeopathic and TCM theories are based upon empirical observation of the living body, these systems clarified what I saw in animals under my care. This proved to be a welcome relief after years of confusion in my attempt to apply rational, pathology-based methods. (My use of the word *rational* in connection with conventional medicine does not imply that holistic modalities are not rational or logical. In fact, in many ways homeopathy and acupuncture proceed much more logically than allopathy. I am simply referring to the rationalist school in this case.)

At first, my questions continued to reflect my allopathic background, so I found myself constantly frustrated. I remember asking a colleague, "What homeopathic medicines do you suggest for a cat with feline leukemia virus infection?" She answered with the question, "What is wrong with the cat?"

I said to myself, "Didn't I just tell her it had feline leukemia virus?" So it went until I just let the question drop. It was a long time before I realized that it was the difference in how an individual expressed symptoms that was important. The name we gave a disease was just that—an externally applied label that really did not reflect the cat's illness. *Whereas I learned in veterinary school to diagnose and treat diseases, I was now learning to diagnose and treat individuals who have disease.* While this may seem only a semantic differentiation, the gap between these ideas is vast.

It is this emphasis that begins to demarcate the boundary between rational and empirical approaches to healing. Whereas conventional medicine focuses upon the illness, holistic therapies, such as TCM and homeopathy, center upon the individual who is ill. The latter systems assert that disease symptoms represent the predisposition of the individual as much as that of the disease.

Another distinction between empirical medicine and rationalist medicine is that most empirical modes see that, since symptoms of illness reflect the individual, different outbreaks of disease within an individual must be connected. Thus a person who has a bladder infection one year and pneumonia the next year has not had two discrete diseases. Rather, she has had two different expressions of one illness. Most of the disease symptoms she has during her life are representations of an internal chronic disease (see the next section for a definition of chronic disease), which is individual to her. Just as no two snowflakes are the same, no two people have identical illnesses, though there are similarities. This understanding applies to chronic disease, which today comprises the vast majority of illness. The principle does not always include episodes of acute (contagious) illness.

Acute Disease versus Chronic Disease

Acute (generally contagious) diseases, such as childhood illnesses in humans, are an exception in that symptoms remain mostly constant among different individuals. This is because the symptoms are primarily associated with the infectious organism rather than the host. Individual expression still occurs, however, and for homeopathy it is this individual expression that provides the key to successful remedy selection. With influenza in humans, for example, all infected people tend to have fever, weakness, headaches, and so on. But one person may vomit severely, another have watery diarrhea, another have unquenchable thirst, and still another have no thirst.

Acute illnesses are less individual than chronic disease. These diseases tend to affect young individuals, regardless of the species, and most individuals in the species are susceptible to these infectious organisms. In dogs, acute diseases include distemper, infectious hepatitis, and parvovirus disease. In cats, panleukopenia (feline distemper) and the upper respiratory viruses are acute disease organisms. Since acute illnesses are infectious, they generally affect the individual for a short time, though the disease is often intense, even life-threatening. Once the person recovers, however, the disease is gone. There is no reinfection and usually no lingering disease, though there may be residual symptoms that do not progress. This is in sharp contrast to chronic illness (see below).

A further characteristic of contagious diseases is that these often have beneficial effects. These diseases provide normal means of strengthening the individual as well as the population. Individually, they seem to enhance the functioning of the immune system so that over time one becomes more able to heal. Within a population, acute diseases help cull out weaker individuals, thus enhancing survival of the herd (pack, pride, flock) and of the species. This places vaccination into question as possibly counter to these forces (see Chapter Sixteen, "Vaccination").

I'll give two quotes from empirical physicians to further elucidate these two categories of illness. James Kent, the famous homeopath, differentiated acute and chronic illness as follows:

> An acute miasm is one that comes upon the economy, passes through its regular prodromal [incubation] period, longer or shorter, has its period of progress and period of decline, and in which there is a tendency to recovery. A chronic miasm is one that has its period of prodrome, period of progress and no period of decline; it is never ending, except with the death of the patient.[2]

Philip Incao, a contemporary anthroposophical physician, put it more simply: "*Acute* is a fire that burns strongly, then burns itself out. *Chronic* is a fire that smolders on and on and never really burns out" [Incao's italics].[3]

Chronic disease encompasses everything except the acute, contagious illnesses. In essence, chronic illness can be understood as an inability of the body (or of the body's immune system) to heal whatever malady with which it is afflicted. An individual with chronic disease never completely recovers from the illness, and instead he worsens over time. The gradual deterioration that we associate with aging is really chronic disease. Healthy individuals remain relatively strong throughout their lives and deteriorate rapidly as they near death.

Almost all adult diseases (and many juvenile illnesses) fall into the chronic disease category, including such syndromes as hypothyroidism, hyperthyroidism, skin disease (including "flea allergy dermatitis"), diabetes, cancer, inflammatory bowel disease, arthritis, lupus—in short, the vast majority of illness. Even such organism-associated illnesses as the feline leukemia virus complex, the feline immunodeficiency virus, the feline infectious peritonitis complex, and probably Lyme disease are chronic illnesses, since the organisms associated with these illnesses do not usually cause problems unless the host individual has a weakened immune system. The same holds true for HIV/AIDS in humans.

Furthermore, in a given individual with multiple diagnoses, we see that they are different expressions of the same illness, as only *one* disease can occur in a body, and that disease continues over the life of the individual. This one disease is an inability to cope with the stresses of life, whether physiological or mental, and it creates a fundamental weakness in the body (more accurately, a weakness of the vital force, a malfunction of the immune system).

Disease as Individual Phenomenon

Variation is the raw material of evolutionary change. It represents the fundamental reality of nature, not an accident about a created norm. Variation is primary, essences are illusory. Species must be defined as ranges of irreducible variation.

—Steven Jay Gould[4]

As an evolutionary biologist, Gould developed his perspective from close study of many members of different species. He observed presumably healthy individuals rather than studying disease, and he saw that individuality, rather than commonality, stands foremost in natural systems. His conclusion strongly supports the assertion by homeopathic practitioners that each individual is different from all others in some ways and deserves individual treatment.

If each individual is different when healthy, it is to be expected that each individual must react differently when sick. This reaction depends upon how and where each individual has weaknesses. No two individuals have just the same areas of handicap, though there may be similarities. As a result, two people may have the same conventional diagnosis, but their total symptom picture will look much different.

Let's look at some cats with hyperthyroidism (overactivity of the thyroid gland) to see how this works. All three cats in the following table are fairly classic cases from a conventional perspective, as can be seen in Table 2-1.

Table 2-1

GEORGE	LENAI	E.C.
Thyroid hormones increased (T 4 = 17.4)	Thyroid hormones increased (T 4 = 13.2)	Thyroid hormones increased (T 4 = 14.5)
Rapid heart rate and restless	Rapid heart rate and heart palpitation	Rapid heart rate and heart palpitation
Emaciation	Emaciation	Weight loss
Vomiting and diarrhea	Vomiting	Vomiting

But now take a look at Table 2-2 and see how different the symptoms look in the same three cats.

Table 2-2

GEORGE	LENAI	E.C.
Overheated easily, ears hot	Chilly, sleeps under stove	Neither hot nor cold
Fearful and angry	Demands attention	Wants to be alone
Yawns with panting	Dry coat, thirsty	Constipation
Picky appetite	Liver inflammation	Easily gets abscesses
Respiratory distress with panting	Flatulence when picked up	Licks kitty litter, rocks, walls

If we only judge by the shared symptoms, as listed in Table 1, it is easy to say these cats have the same illness. Comparing the symptoms in Table 2, however, things look very different. The individual nature of illness becomes clear, and we see that each cat really has a different illness, with some common symptoms.

Symptoms Are Not Disease;
They Only Represent the Illness

These symptom patterns are not the disease, however. Rather, they provide a glimpse of the disease, a visible representation. The actual disease is invisible and mysterious. We may only speculate as to its true nature, using these discernible clues as our guides. Perhaps a useful analogy is our understanding of gravity. We cannot directly observe the force itself, but we learn about it through its effects upon our physical world. Similarly, with our vital force and diseases we observe how the body responds to try to comprehend the nature of health and illness. The apple falling from the tree is not gravity; it merely shows the existence of gravity. Similarly, diarrhea is not the disease, but it shows something about the nature of disease in the individual.

The word *symptom* means "a condition arising from and accompanying a disease and constituting evidence of it."[5] Even by definition, something deeper is implied. While this is understood by conventional medicine at some level, therapeutics have focused not upon the "something deeper" but upon the superficial. Treatment by contraries, the backbone of allopathy (treatment by other, as opposed to homeopathy's treatment by likes), aspires simply to minimize the symptoms. By so doing, the true disease is merely obscured and thus allowed to increase without detection. This is the case when we give drugs such as prednisone for skin allergies, and even antibiotics for most conditions, since rarely is the organism the real cause of illness. As homeopaths, our goal with skin allergies is to stop the allergy from occurring rather than just to minimize the symptoms. We are trying to return the body function to the normal state of not being allergic.

Viewing the body mechanistically, allopaths equate the symptoms with the disease. The aim of allopathic therapy is thus elimination of these signs of illness as the goal and as the only necessary standard for cure. To an allopath, removal of these symptoms constitutes removal of the disease. Giving antibiotics for a bladder inflammation (cystitis) is thought to cure the cystitis; surgical excision of a tumor is believed to (potentially) cure the body of cancer.

But does tumor removal really cure cancer? Scientists now can detect substances in the blood associated with certain cancers. Interestingly, removal of the cancerous growth has no impact upon the levels of these substances. This kind of evidence confirms what empirical practitioners have asserted for centuries: *the physical symptom is not the disease, but only an indication of disease.*

Symptoms Are Actually the Healing Process

Not only is this physical symptom not the disease, it is really the body's *healing process.* What we see as symptoms are actually the body's attempts to rid itself of disease. We now understand, for example, that fever has a function. The elevated body temperature makes it hard for bacteria and viruses to survive. Artificially reducing the fever with drugs may make the animal feel better for a time, but the immune system is thereby inhibited, possibly leading to worsening of the condition overall. A perfect example is the onset of Reye's syndrome in children with influenza following aspirin administration to reduce fevers. Allopaths believe this condition is a side effect of aspirin; to a homeopath this is a result of thwarting the body's effort to heal, and we call this "suppression" (see Chapter Three, "The Nature of Cure").

Similarly, diarrhea and other discharges are methods to cleanse the body of toxins or organisms. As such, these are part of the body's healing process rather than diseases. In food poisoning, for example, bacteria or bacterial poisons are ingested with spoiled food. Quite naturally, the body responds with vomiting and/or diarrhea to purge the gastrointestinal tract of these dangerous substances. Using medications to stop the discharges limits this action.

I remember a puppy with parvovirus (a severe, often life-threatening, intestinal viral infection) that I saw years ago. The pup had made it through the most intense phase of his illness. He had stopped vomiting and was able to hold down some broth and water. He still had relatively intense diarrhea, though his energy was improving. I administered some Lomotil to slow the diarrhea, but within a couple of hours his condition worsened dramatically. As I watched his decline, I realized that I had interfered with his ability to discharge the excess bacterial growth and the resultant toxins from his intestines. These toxins then were being absorbed through his damaged intestinal lining, making him much sicker. I saw much too clearly the potential damage of treatment by contraries—the backbone of allopathic medicine.

Use of "cold medicines" has a similar effect; you may feel better but the cold will generally last twice as long. Any time drugs are used to modify the response to disease (i.e. symptoms) there is a possibility of worsening the disease.

What Is Disease?

If the symptoms themselves are not the disease, just what is disease? To the best of our understanding, the malfunction we see as disease originates on a prephysical level. It is not exactly psychosomatic, yet it is closer to this idea than to physical, mechanistic theories. Hahnemann stated that "In the state of health the spirit-like vital force animat[es] the material ... organism [and] reigns in supreme sovereignty."[6] Disorder of this vital force, or spiritual essence, thus constitutes disease at its most basic level. From the vital force the disease may progress (worsen) into the mental/emotional plane and finally into the material (physical) body. The vital force, like Qi, is perhaps best understood as a concept rather than something concrete. Like Qi, we cannot directly experience the vital force any more than we can directly experience disease, but we use these ideas to aid our understanding.

What exactly does this mean? I will explain using the onset of influenza in a human, as we can understand the subtle differences better from our own experience. Try to remember a time when you had the flu. You may recall that it did not just arrive at once, but rather it came on gradually, though you may not have recognized it right away.

According to homeopathic theory, the influenza first impacted your vital force. A disorder of the vital force might not be perceptible, but perhaps it was that first sign of unease you felt just before the flu emerged. As it progressed into the mental realm, the disturbance became stronger, but your mental state remained basically stable. As the influenza strengthened, you probably began to develop some emotional changes (though emotional changes are often better seen by someone other than the affected person, so you may not have recognized these changes). If you were deeply affected, you may have become fearful that you might die—even though influenza is a minor illness. Or perhaps irritability emerged; haven't we all been around friends (never ourselves!) who become irritable when sick? At this stage the illness manifested as emotional (fear) or behavioral (irritability) changes, yet you may not have been visibly sick. The transition from mental and emotional illness to physical symptoms is variable—in some people the distinction is clear, while in others the physical changes arise along with the psychological changes. At some point, however, the physical changes emerge (malaise, fever, sore throat, vomiting, diarrhea, muscle aches, etc.), and we understand the previous unease.

What might we see in our animals? I remember many times having a guardian bring her companion into my clinic with a vague complaint such as, "He is just not acting like he normally does." I would examine the animal, and everything usually appeared normal. If the guardian was concerned, we would submit blood for analysis. The results would typically be normal. We would all be reassured that nothing was wrong, but a couple of months later the guardian would return with a very sick companion. Sadly, this frequently happens with cancer onset and occurs in people as well. Even with sophisticated diagnostic techniques, disease in its early stage often cannot be identified by physical methods, as it exists in these nonphysical arenas.

Thankfully, we usually have much earlier signs of disease. Let's look at the more typical progression of disease to understand how the body reacts to illness. Once disorder affects the physical body, the vital force follows some patterns so that damage is minimized. The nature of the reaction is that outer regions and less critical organs take the brunt of disease as long as possible. Additionally, whenever possible, functional disorders occur rather than pathological changes. Functional disorders include fever, discharges (vomiting, diarrhea, mucus production), even convulsions—bodily responses that can be accomplished *through increased activity of normal bodily processes*. By contrast, pathological disease involves altering the physical structure of the body—for example, the intestinal thickening of inflammatory bowel disease, calcium deposits in arthritis, or the formation of tumors when cancer arises. These physical changes consume greater energy during their formation as well as during repair, thus reversal of pathology is much more difficult than reversal of functional disorders.

The first signs of illness in young, relatively healthy animals are functional—generally fever and discharges. Think of children with their common symptoms of runny noses, diarrhea, and fevers. The stronger the vital force (overall health), the greater the portion of disease force that can be diverted into functional symptoms. (I use the term *disease force* to represent the intensity or quantity of illness occurring in the body). This is why children and young animals often run such high fevers, and generally without damage unless we interfere. It is this interference that leads to Reye's syndrome when we give aspirin to feverish children—we compel the vital force to retreat to a deeper level of illness (pathology). (See Chapter Three, "The Nature of Cure.")

The ability to tolerate intense *functional* disorder is actually a sign of health. As long as the body can utilize functional changes to heal illness, the disease can move more swiftly through the body. By contrast, an individual with a weak vital force (i.e. poorer immune system) may not be able to tolerate a high fever. In this case, he would resort to pathology to absorb the disease force.

Once pathological change becomes necessary, the vital force tries to localize the disease and restrict the illness to less vital organs. The most obvious choice is the skin—a necessary organ, but one that can tolerate a lot of damage and still provide basic functions. After dogs and cats pass through the age of functional disease—and as their disease force increases— they begin showing illness on their skin. The appearance of skin ailments is pathetic, and watching our beloved companions' constant scratching is a difficult task in itself. But this skin disease has the capability of absorbing a lot of disease force.

Suppression of these skin symptoms by administration of drugs will be followed by deeper illness unless the vital force can return the focus of disease to the skin once the drugs are stopped. We often refer to these deeper symptoms, like Reye's syndrome following aspirin, or like liver damage from antibiotic or prednisone use, as side effects of drugs. To a homeopath, however, these "side effects" represent this disease movement as it progresses more deeply into the body. The following case is a good example of this disease progression. While this unfortunate dog had more symptoms than most dogs, his case is not that unusual, and it shows rather clearly the body's response to disease and treatment.

Max, a standard poodle, was brought to my clinic at seven years of age with a multitude of problems. Max's guardian had done everything she knew to do for him, but he just kept getting sicker. Max's previous veterinarians had taken all the proper steps to diagnose and treat him, yet I imagine they found his case puzzling and frustrating. When I listed his symptoms on a time line, however, the progression was clear from a homeopathic perspective. As a puppy, he had the normal schedule of vaccinations. At five months, when he was taken in for a rabies vaccination, he had begun to have some ear problems and mild bronchitis. Three weeks following the rabies vaccine, his guardian took him back because he had developed a skin rash. Treatment with antibiotics cleared the rash, but three months later it had returned. The veterinarian prescribed stronger antibiotics. Additionally, for the next two years he required bathing with strong medicated shampoos to control the skin disease, though it never disappeared entirely. He also received regular vaccinations during this time.

At age two and a half, Max had his first convulsion. The seizures continued sporadically over the next two years, then worsened, so he was put on phenobarbital (an anticonvulsant) at age four and a half. Twelve days after starting the phenobarbital, Max had his first bout of pancreatitis. He had several flare-ups of the pancreatitis over the ensuing months. Later that year, two weeks after a vaccination, he developed a bronchial inflammation, diagnosed as kennel cough. When Max was six, his veterinarian diagnosed him as hypothyroid and prescribed thyroid hormone. Two months later he had general anesthesia and a dental cleaning. Two weeks after the dental cleaning, Max developed a weakness in his hips followed by a head tilt. Despite all of his health problems, Max was vaccinated a month after the head tilt and hip problems, and shortly thereafter he had his worst convulsion ever.

Reviewing Max's disease, we can see that the progression follows a pattern, moving from one organ system to another. As disease intensity grows, this progression follows a general hierarchy of least to most critical systems. Empirical practitioners have noted this pattern over centuries of observation. The order varies with individual tendency, but is basically: (1) skin, ears, nose, eyes, mouth, lung mucous membrane surfaces (superficial involvement, as with bronchitis); (2) stomach, intestines, urinary bladder; (3) glands (including pancreas, reproductive, thyroid, adrenals, pituitary), lungs (deeper in the lungs, as with pneumonia); (4) kidneys, liver; (5) heart, brain. Internalization often stays within organ systems; for example, urinary bladder diseases may progress to kidney disease, and nose and sinus disease may lead to asthma or other lung disease. Other relationships may exist as well: ear diseases tend to move to brain disorders (at first functional, later pathological) if suppressed with steroids and antibiotics.

In Max's case, the progression was as follows: first he developed skin and mucous membrane symptoms—exterior, relatively innocuous. As the disease force grew, these skin symptoms increased. Max's veterinarians attempted to eliminate the skin symptoms, however, and the disease moved internally, to the seizural disorder. While this sounds like a big leap, it is not—mild convulsions are often unaccompanied by tissue changes, thus this is a functional symptom, not pathological.

The phenobarbital, prescribed for the convulsions, interfered with the body's use of seizures as a means to "discharge" some of the disease force. The disease thus sought another outlet, and pancreatitis ensued. Now the disease had entered a serious pathological form, one that is potentially life-threatening. During this same time span, Max developed thyroid problems and deeper lung disease, both representing approximately the same level of illness as the pancreas involvement (group 3 above). After starting the thyroid hormone, and with the stress of general anesthesia, Max's problems shifted again. The head tilt, weakness in the rear legs, and the severe convulsion all suggest some development of pathological changes in the brain and spinal cord, indicating that the disease was touching critical organ systems.

As you can see in Max's case, as his overall health deteriorated, he began to have more and more symptoms. The body has a limited capacity to absorb disease force in any one area. Thus, as it contends with an ever greater disease burden, it must create symptoms in more places—involving more organ systems. Homeopaths believe suppressive treatment (therapy that opposes the body's healing attempts) contributes to this worsening. We often see animals with several allopathic diagnoses: hypothyroidism, kidney failure, liver failure, epilepsy. When we see multifocal illness in animals—no matter the age—we know the vital force is weak and the animal is quite ill.

Imagine a community living along a river. In an especially wet year, with heavy rainfall, these rains may begin to produce flooding. At first, when flooding is minimal, people spread out and reinforce levees all along the river, protecting farmland and outlying houses as well as the town. If the rains continue and the floods worsen, the townspeople must retreat and concentrate upon levees guarding the center of town where most people and structures reside. Breaks will appear at many places in the levees where resources are insufficient to maintain them. These many breaks are like the many symptoms of disease in older or weaker animals. Once the disease force—the flooding in our metaphor—overwhelms the immune system, the immune system must retreat, allowing symptoms in less critical organs while protecting critical organs to the best of its ability.

How Does Disease Arise?

While this example works well for understanding the body's resistance, the metaphor does not accurately suggest cause. Homeopaths believe disease to be not the result of an outside force like a flood so much as of the inner disorder or disruption of the vital force. As Louis Pasteur, the "father of bacteriology," said, "the microbe is nothing, the terrain everything."[7] Terrain refers to the body and its susceptibility to disease, including infectious agents. This susceptibility is specific to each individual. From where does this susceptibility derive? It may either be transmitted from parent to offspring or acquired through exposure to some stress. Parent-to-offspring transmission may be genetic, or it may be on another level that homeopaths understand as transference of a weak vital force. (This concept is expressed in traditional Chinese medicine as a deficiency of *jing* in the offspring. Jing is the Qi that is inherited from the parent.)

The nature of this susceptibility is chronic disease. Although such stresses as drugs and vaccines add tremendously to the level of chronic disease, these have come late in the game. How did this susceptibility arise in the first place? Generations of poor diet, pollution, and damaging medical treatment have certainly been a large factor. The major success of agriculture in supporting large numbers of humans is likely another culprit, as the Darwinian concept of survival of the fittest is not a factor when strong individuals provide support for the weaker members of a community. This applies to the domestic animals of the community as well.

I believe another factor in the development of chronic diseases is our movement away from integration with the natural world. This paralleled our transition into an agricultural state. Hunter-gatherer people tend to operate within nature, while agricultural people attempt to separate themselves from nature. The further we feel from others—any other beings, not just humans—the greater the threat we perceive them to be. I think this generated fear, and that the fear itself has engendered much illness. It also has driven the allopathic approach of looking outside the body for causes of disease, in contrast to the holistic tendency to look inward.

I have heard this fear expressed from many sources, but I wish to list two that I found poignant. I heard an interview with a Native American (I apologize that I do not know his name), who said that members of his tribe never felt afraid of the woods and the wilderness in which they lived; rather, they felt embraced by and intimately connected to the wilderness.

They were astonished when white men came and expressed fear of the wilderness.

Einstein conveyed a similar feeling in a quote that was given to me by a friend. I have been unable to locate the specific source, so I do not know if the quote is exact or a paraphrase, but from other similar passages in Einstein's writings, I believe the quote is a fair representation: "We often suffer from a sort of optical delusion. We act as if we are not connected to everything and everybody. . . . We think that we are not connected to life in all its forms. It is the most painful delusion in the world today."

It is this delusion, I believe, that indeed allows us to treat other people, other species, and our home, the earth, with such disrespect. Operating under this delusion allows us to experiment on animals, for example. While we may gain some knowledge in the short term, we lose in the end, since we will ultimately suffer from all that we do to those we presume to be lower than ourselves. We cannot separate ourselves from these others in the end, and the suffering probably adds to the chronic disease in the world by increasing fear and pain. As Chief Seattle said (this one is certainly a paraphrase), "Whatever befalls the earth befalls the sons of the earth. Man did not weave the web of life; he is merely a strand in it. Whatever he does to the web, he does to himself."

Whatever the nature of the origin of chronic disease, it impacts all of us greatly. Cancer and autoimmune diseases occur at ever increasing levels as the overall population health diminishes. Virus infections, like colds and influenzas, impact us to a much greater extent than even twenty or thirty years ago. These various manifestations of illness are visible effects of disease, but they are not the disease itself. The disease itself is a weakened immune system—another way of describing chronic disease. When the signs of disease become more serious, more frequent, and more widespread, they tell us that we harbor more disease force than ever before. We see this in our companion animals in the same way; severe illnesses like cancer arise in much younger animals than when I graduated from veterinary school. Autoimmune disease was rare then, though today it is quite common. We have damaged our earth so deeply, and continue to damage her with chemical, nuclear, and electromagnetic pollution. Cell phones and cell towers broadcast damaging radiation widely; wireless Internet, so common today, is mostly unrecognized as a disease cause, but I have seen it induce illness in a friend, and we are creating a subclass of humans who cannot live in our cities anymore because of wireless Internet. Just last year a woman in the Santa Fe, New Mexico, area committed suicide because she ran out of places to live, as she could not be around wireless Internet. Such forces as these make it harder and harder to stay healthy, and they also make it harder and harder to treat illness.

The goal of homeopathic treatment is to touch disease at its deepest level—that of the vital force—thereby affecting change in the *fundamental* health of the sick individual, two-legged or four-legged. We hope to reinstate the vigor of the vital force so the immune system can regain health. With a correct homeopathic remedy, the external symptoms will diminish along with alleviation of disease, but this is not by masking of symptoms. In fact, sometimes the visible signs of illness increase under homeopathic therapy in the early stages of treatment. This phenomenon is called an aggravation or a healing crisis. This is partly explained as the resonance of the remedy with the body—the correct medicine vibrates at a harmonious frequency to the disease, and the resultant harmonic vibration releases energy.

Another way to explain an aggravation is that previously thwarted healing responses are now able to occur. An animal with a poor vital force may be unable to mount a proper response to influenza or to a bacterial overgrowth. (I use the term "overgrowth" rather than "infection" to suggest that, as per the Pasteur quote above, the bacteria grow in response to a poor immune system. They have been present all along, but in balance until the body weakened; then they grew to fill a created niche.) After a well-chosen remedy, one might see a development of fever, inflammation, and discharges. The vital force is now resisting disease and beginning the healing process. (Remember that symptoms are methods of healing.) Providing that the patient feels better overall, these are excellent signs that improvement is imminent. You might wonder how an animal could feel better with this inflammation occurring. If you remember a time when you had the flu, you might remember a point where your mental state shifted and you felt the disease lifting. This lift is usually prior to the shift in the physical symptoms. In an animal, you might see that she watches you as you walk by, for example, rather than remaining in a state of indifference.

Additionally, since the symptoms move inward as the disease worsens, they will move outward as it heals. More visible and more superficial signs indicate this exteriorization of disease. This is especially so when combined with reduction in signs of deeper disorder. Disappearance of chronic diarrhea in conjunction with appearance of skin inflammation is a nice progression. If the same skin inflammation had been treated with drugs (with consequent disappearance) prior to development of the diarrhea, reversal of illness is almost certain.

You will only be treating more acute, simple illnesses on your own, so this healing response may not be as evident. If your companion is chronically ill, however, you may be working with a homeopathic practitioner, and this will assist your understanding of how disease occurs and how it heals. See Chapter Three, "The Nature of Cure," for more information on the curative response to treatment.

What Is a Healthy Animal?

As a final examination of disease, I will briefly discuss healthy animals. My perception of health and disease has changed considerably since I began to study and practice holistically, and particularly through homeopathy. My veterinary education did not include a sense of how a truly healthy animal should appear. Many conditions we considered to be normal in dogs and cats I now understand to be early signs of illness. Over time, our standards have deteriorated as the health of the population has deteriorated. Evidence for this in humans can be gleaned from comparison of average weight tables from the insurance industry. Accepted weights have increased with each revision of the tables, reflecting the obesity of modern North Americans.

I don't believe we really know what a healthy dog or cat looks like these days. We can only speculate. Virtually the entire population of domestic animals (as well as humans) has chronic illness. In animals, we have come to accept many abnormal symptoms as normal. For example, a common perception about dogs is that they have a strong smell (doggy odor). Many dogs do have a strong smell, but healthy dogs do not have much odor, even without regular bathing. Some other symptoms that we accept as normal include eye discharge (tearing) in poodles and other small dogs, tartar buildup on teeth (which need to be cleaned regularly), wax buildup in ears, strong breath in animals, cats vomiting hair balls, oily or flaky skin, anal sacs needing regular emptying, and so on. Other abnormal conditions include excessive fleas and worms as well as behavior problems. The list is endless, and none of these are normal in healthy animals. They are signs of chronic illness and signs that these animals are in a weakened condition. They are thus at risk for more obvious and more serious symptoms of chronic disease, such as autoimmune illness (the bulk of current illness, including such diagnoses as thyroid diseases, diabetes, arthritis, lupus, inflammatory bowel disease, and degenerative myelopathy) and cancer.

From my perspective as a homeopath, the suppressive nature of most therapy contributes directly to this deterioration. We have traded the risks associated with acute illnesses for ever-increasing levels of chronic illness. We have done this through the use of vaccinations and much of modern medicine. Treatments to eliminate symptoms, without removing the under-lying disease state, tend to make the body more ill. The disease is not allowed to express itself in its natural way due to strong drugs or surgery. Thus the disease seeks a different outlet. As the drugs, vaccinations, and surgery have weakened the vital force, the "new" condition is more severe than the orig-inal complaint. Vaccinations not only induce chronic disease as a means to prevent acute disease, they also keep some individuals alive who would otherwise succumb to the acute forms of these diseases. While this may seem humane, it perpetuates chronic illness by thwarting Darwin's "sur-vival of the fittest," which serves to strengthen populations.

Over time and generations, the vitality of the population diminishes by these forces. Homeopathic practitioners believe that the amount of chronic illness present in parents at the time of conception is passed to the offspring at a comparable level. Thus, each generation is less healthy than the last if nothing is done to remove the disease in a given generation. Consider pure-bred animals: without the use of careful breeding practices, these lines of animals may become progressively more prone to illness. This genetic (and nongenetic but inherited) transmission of weakness is transmission of chronic disease.

It is possible to reduce this chronic disease accumulation, however. Simply stopping vaccination and drug use, along with proper diet, can begin to have an impact. Introducing modern processed foods to native popula-tions caused deterioration of population health within one generation. Three to four generations were required to *completely* reverse this damage with nutrition alone.[8] When suppression or vaccine-induced damage is involved, some form of therapy such as homeopathy is necessary to shift the balance. And two to three generations may still be required to return to *total* health, even with homeopathic treatment, although vast improvement is attainable even in the first generation. See Chapter Three, "The Nature of Cure," and Chapter Sixteen, "Vaccination," for more information.

Dorothy Shepherd, a London homeopathic physician during the first half of the 1900s, felt it was even possible to remove karmic sin with homeopathy.[9] While this may seem a stupendous claim, it is really just another way of saying that chronic disease can be eliminated, as they are perhaps only different terms for the same idea. If disease begins at the spiritual level, that is the same locus of karmic sin, and thus karmic sin is the nidus of disease. Spiritual illness leads naturally to psychic disease. Continuing this line of reasoning, the epidemic of psychological illness in the world today in animals (human as well as nonhuman) is nothing more than chronic disease, and perhaps nothing more than karma. The vast numbers of humans *and animals* taking Prozac and similar drugs is evidence of this epidemic. As such, it is imminently curable, although a paradigm shift is necessary, which is no easy task. This idea has been proposed by many, including James Kent, George Vithoulkas, Harris Coulter, and Martin Miles.[10]

Summary

Conventional (allopathic) medicine is rooted in the rationalist school of thought. Rationalist practitioners believe it is possible to theoretically understand disease and that this understanding leads to ways to counteract disease. The rationalist system equates symptoms with the disease itself, thus the belief that the disease can be fully understood. Allopathic medicine (a rationalist system) thus uses treatment by contraries (drugs that oppose symptoms) as the basis of its therapeutics. Additionally, most illness is thought to come from an outside agent.

Holistic disciplines such as homeopathy and traditional Chinese medicine have their roots in the empirical school of thought. Empirical practitioners believe that the cause of illness is unknowable, but that disease originates from within the individual. The individual is thus the only agent capable of healing disease, and practitioners thus attempt to encourage healing by the body. The following observations come from homeopathic principles:

Each individual's disease expresses uniquely (since it arises within the individual), although common symptoms may exist among different individuals.

Symptoms represent clues to the nature of illness, but these symptoms are not the total disease, which remains invisible.

Disease names are only external labels and do not represent the full extent of illness in an individual.

Acute illness has a relatively rapid duration, leaving the affected individual relatively disease-free and immune to further impact from that acute illness. Acute illnesses are generally infectious diseases; they are usually only a threat in young animals. Acute illness may strengthen a population by eliminating weaker individuals.

Chronic disease is slow and insidious, and no immunity develops, as the primary disorder is immune suppression, not infection. *Organisms associated with chronic illness* (such as feline leukemia virus and feline infectious peritonitis virus) *require this preexisting weakness in order to infect an animal.*

The first responses to illness are generally functional, such as fevers and discharges. As illness worsens, physical changes begin to appear.

Physical symptoms of illness begin on the surface of the body, and as illness worsens, the symptoms move more deeply into the body.

Stopping symptoms from manifesting where the body first puts them forces the body to move the disease inward in response. For example, treating skin disease with prednisone may result in liver or kidney disease.

Over time, using strong drugs or vaccination to alter disease weakens a population. This occurs because disease moves deeper among all members due to inheritance of illness by progeny. Offspring enter the world with approximately the same level of chronic disease as their parents, then add to that level through exposures to pollutants and stressors. This may be minimized with proper diet and holistic medicine.

Vast improvement can be attained in one generation with many types of holistic medicines, including homeopathy, but it may take as long as three to four generations to *completely* restore health.

Chapter Three
THE NATURE OF CURE

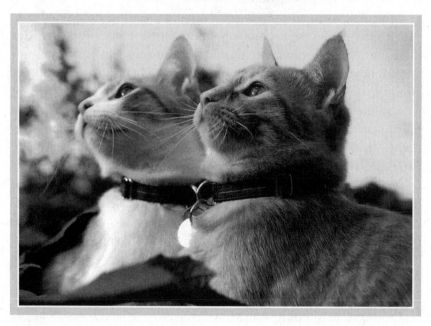

Cure

Partial Cure

Palliation

Suppression

Noncurative Aggravation

No Effect

Natural Disease Cycles

Summary

ONE OF THE PROBLEMS WITH ASSESSING the response to treatment, whether conventional or holistic, is a lack of definition or understanding of what constitutes a cure. In this chapter, I will define not only cure but also several other possible responses to treatment. These categories are based upon homeopathic principles, but you can apply them to any therapy to better understand its effectiveness. Once you understand disease and cure, you will better understand just how various therapeutic methods impact your companion's health. This should assist you with any decisions you must make regarding his or her health care. The information in this chapter builds upon an understanding of disease, so it is imperative that you first read Chapter Two, "The Nature of Disease."

General usage assumes that disappearance of symptoms means a cure has taken place. This is not necessarily the case, as it may be only a remission, or it may mean the disease has been pushed to a deeper level. The difference is very important. Intertwined with this confusion is the conventional viewpoint that the body is afflicted with different diseases at different times, and that these diseases are unrelated. From this perspective, the disappearance of one set of symptoms, followed by the onset of a new set of symptoms, are two discrete events. One disease is said to be cured, only to be replaced by another disease, usually more severe than the first, and the patient is felt to be unfortunate to be so unlucky as to come down with the second disease "right after the first one was cured." If we take the perspective that these are not separate diseases, but rather separate manifestations of one disease, the events become clearer and more logical.

From this alternate perspective, the body has several possible responses to treatment. Conventional practitioners consider many of these to be curative, but in fact they have very different implications. The types of response are cure, partial cure, palliation, suppression, noncurative aggravation (with or without worsening of symptoms), and no response. It is the first four categories that allopaths may deem curative responses, as all include improvement in at least one symptom, and that symptom may be the only one monitored. In a cat with hyperthyroidism (overactive thyroid gland), for example, thyroid hormone level is the conventional basis for evaluation. Conventional practitioners may accept a reduction in hormone levels as evidence that therapy is effective, sometimes even in the face of worsening symptoms. To a holistic practitioner, improvement in symptoms is the most important guideline and may outweigh a contradictory laboratory finding.

With homeopathic treatment, lab findings may normalize well after the animal clinically improves.

As with most categorization attempts, these divisions are not black and white, so some overlap may occur between them. Furthermore, reading all descriptions will help you understand them individually, as the contrasts in part define the categories. Interpreting remedy response is one of the more difficult tasks of a homeopath. It is most important and most difficult in chronic disease, so you will not need to be proficient with all of the subtleties. If your companion has chronic disease, you should be working with an experienced homeopathic practitioner. In that case, she will be able to interpret the remedy response. (See Chapter Two, "The Nature of Disease," for definitions of acute and chronic disease.)

The more you understand the possible responses, however, the more comfortable you should be with the progress. This will help you with patience as well, and patience is sometimes the most difficult aspect of holistic therapy. Curing chronic disease according to homeopathic guidelines takes time—sometimes a long time. The time it takes to cure chronic disease is in relation to the time that it took for the animal to develop the disease. A serious skin disease, for example, may require two or three years before the animal returns to health. Many other chronic ailments take a year or longer as well.

With acute diseases, you may not see all of the gradations of response. The most important principle is that you see improvement in your companion's mental and emotional state as well as in his physical symptoms. Additionally, you should not need to repeat the (correct) remedy too frequently or for an inordinately long time. See Chapter Five, "Using Homeopathy at Home," for more information on remedy administration.

Even though you will only be treating acute problems, it is still important to read and understand how the body can respond to treatment, as this will greatly assist your interpretation, even with relatively simple conditions. It is especially important to understand the difference between palliation and cure, as these are the responses you will most often see and which are hard to differentiate. As you begin to see how the body responds in acute illness, you will more quickly be able to see if a chosen remedy is appropriate. And if you face a chronic disease in your companion at some later time, this will help you understand that condition as well.

Cure

Cure includes improvement in symptoms along with improvement in the underlying disease state. Homeopathic practitioners use a system of guidelines to assess response to treatment rather than simple subjective evaluation. The bases of the guidelines were established by Constantine Hering, MD, in the last century, and are known as Hering's Rule of Cure. (Actually, Paracelsus and the Hippocratic writings preceded Hering in this, although Hering's formula is more complete and formal.) These tenets assert that when a cure is happening, the symptoms of disease will disappear in a predictable and orderly manner. The directions of removal of symptoms are from head to feet and internal to external. More serious symptoms and afflictions of more critical organs should abate prior to less serious symptoms and less critical organ troubles, and recent symptoms will subside before older conditions improve.

A corollary to Hering's Rule is that often an old symptom that has gone away, either on its own or through inappropriate (suppressive) treatment, may return when a curative reaction to a remedy occurs. This return of an old symptom is hailed as an excellent sign, as it means the vital force is able to shift the focus of disease back to the prior condition, which is typically less severe than the more recent malady. Usually the return is transient, and the old symptom will disappear without further treatment as the healing process continues. Occasionally, the old symptom returns but does not resolve under the influence of the medicine that restored its appearance, and this is evidence that a new remedy is needed to continue the cure.

Other evidence for cure includes mental and emotional improvement, *gradual* lessening of symptoms, and moving of symptom patterns from more important to less important organ systems. Mental and emotional improvement is critical and must accompany any curative response. The disease may also move from a pathological level to a functional level (for example, ulcerated, infected skin heals, but the dog still has itchy skin with no visible skin damage—see Chapter Two, "The Nature of Disease"). Often confusing is that the disease may be more visible and appears worse for a time, such as elimination of convulsions followed by eruption of a bad "ear infection." While I as the practitioner would delight in the outward movement, my client as the guardian of the dog may be unhappy at the visible evidence of discomfort. Additionally, the local symptoms may actually worsen for a time, although the patient feels better mentally. A cat with an upper respiratory disease, for example, may produce more nasal discharge and cough more often, yet is more playful and hungrier. This is known as a curative aggravation (some call it a healing crisis) and generally indicates a favorable response.

Finally, with cure there is no need for constant repetition of medicine, and once a condition heals it does not return. This may take months or years for chronic diseases, however, and often is cyclic, with periods of improvement alternating with periods of worsening, but with overall improvement over time. We often see this pattern in acute illness as well, though the time span is in hours or days rather than months to years. I refer to this as the "two steps forward and one back" pattern of improvement. Obviously, "one step forward and two back" would have quite a different implication, and is usually indicative of palliation (see below).

Partial Cure

A partial cure occurs when a remedy acts curatively but does not improve *all* symptoms of illness. In this case, Hering's laws would apply to the symptoms that did improve. Most importantly, disappearance of these symptoms would *not* be followed by appearance of more serious symptoms. If other symptoms appeared, they would be less serious and more external. An improved sense of well-being and better vitality will accompany the moderation of symptoms, and frequent repetition of remedies is not required. Suppose your cat had a bladder "infection" and a chronic sinus discharge. The first remedy may clear the cystitis, leaving the cat feeling better, but not affect the sinus condition. This would be a partially curative response as long as no deeper symptom arose following disappearance of the bladder problem. Another remedy would now be needed to continue the cure, focusing upon the sinus inflammation but still directed toward the entire cat.

Another partially curative reaction occurs when, as with cure, a recent problem disappears and an older or more superficial problem resurfaces. In a partially curative reaction, the resurfaced problem does not respond to the remedy that brought the patient to this state, and a new remedy is needed to continue the cure. Sometimes guardians (or even human patients) don't remember the superficial problem having occurred previously, but since the direction of cure follows Hering's Rule, we still know the response is a curative one (partially or fully curative). It may be that the person has forgotten the old condition—sometimes they remember when it resurfaces—or maybe the body sort of bypassed that layer as their disease developed.

Palliation

Palliation means alleviation of symptoms (often rapid) *without affecting the course of the underlying disease.* The patient feels better for a time, but the body is still affected and continues to deteriorate, in contrast to the *apparent* improvement. Typically, the state of well-being does not last, the symptoms return, and ever stronger treatments or doses of medicine (or more frequent dose repetition) are required to maintain the palliated state, until finally the treatment is no longer effective or the condition deteriorates. Often only some symptoms improve, while other symptoms remain the same or worsen. Upon stopping treatment, the condition returns essentially unchanged, except in intensity. Often the intensity is much greater when the palliative treatment is stopped, particularly if the treatment has been administered for a long time. (This is in contrast to partial cure, wherein those symptoms that do not improve will not worsen, and when treatment is stopped, this improvement does not reverse.)

An example of palliation is the use of prednisone to alleviate skin itching. Each year more and more of the drug is needed, until finally it stops working or the condition is suppressed. (Most allopathic medicines are palliative according to homeopathic principles of healing. They can become suppressive—see below—if repeated too often or over a long time.) Palliation may be compared to the state of a pressure cooker with constant heat under it. With time, more and more weight (repetition of the palliating agent) is required on the spout to keep the steam inside. Eventually, the weight will blow off, returning the symptoms of disease (the steam) to a visible level and at much greater intensity than if the steam had released all along. Symptoms are in a similar way a means of "releasing steam" so that the disease does not increase as rapidly.

Palliation, then, is deceptive due to the apparent improvement in symptoms initiated by the medicine. It is ultimately of no benefit, possibly even harmful, in most cases—especially in chronic disease. A possible exception would be with diseases that are acute and truly self-limiting. In this case, a medicine might palliate symptoms without affecting the body deeply enough to interfere with return to health. The medicine could thus provide the benefit of relief from symptoms while the body heals. You may see palliation when you give antibiotics, or even homeopathic remedies, for acute conditions like abscesses, for example. In this case, the abscess may improve as long as you give the antibiotic or the palliating remedy, but when you stop the medicine, the abscess recurs. If you see this with homeopathic treatment, you need to choose a different remedy. It is important for you to understand the difference between this response and a curative reaction. In the latter case, a few remedy doses will stimulate the body in such a manner that the abscess heals completely. Sometimes only one dose is sufficient.

A second exception wherein palliation is helpful is with older patients with terminal conditions, when cure may not be possible, other than death, which is actually a form of cure in certain situations (an easier death may result with curative remedies). A curative remedy in an animal with terminal illness provides relief as it helps the animal leave more gracefully, without as much struggle as often ensues at death's door. But from the perspective that cure means getting better and staying alive, we can only palliate in these terminal states, meaning we can relieve symptoms but cannot return the animal to living health, though this can be a tremendous gift to animals or humans at this time.

Let's look at Dolly's case to further understand palliation and cure. Though this is a chronic disease, the same principles apply as for acute diseases. Dolly is a female cocker spaniel who was nine years old when her guardian first consulted me about her condition. She had a severe brain disorder manifesting as convulsions, mental confusion, and a poor ability to relate to her guardians. She would frequently get "stuck" in corners— that is, she would get her head into a corner or into a small space such as between a chair and an end table, and she simply could not find her way out. She also had a palsy involving the facial nerves on one side, so that drinking and eating were difficult. Prior to this, when she was vaccinated, she became very hyperactive for a few days, and even jumped off an eight-foot-high deck in a frenzy on one occasion. Although I did not make the connection at the time, I now believe Dolly was suffering from a type of autism/hyperactivity/attention-deficit disorder syndrome, the same condition that afflicts so many children these days.

The first remedy I chose (*Helleborus* 10M) produced fairly quick improvement after an intensification of symptoms, so it seemed curative. The improvement lasted about three weeks, a little short for a 10M potency, but the response was good so I gave a 1M to boost the action. The 1M lasted about two weeks, so I repeated it and got about one and a half weeks. At this time, I was suspicious that the *Helleborus* was only palliating but wanted to give it a little longer, so I repeated the 1M once more. The response this time was a dramatic worsening ("the weight blew off the pressure cooker"), a sure sign that the remedy had indeed been only palliative.

A key to the interpretation (of course, this is easy to see in hindsight) was the rapid improvement with short duration of action, *especially when the duration of response grew shorter upon repetition.* Additionally, while some of Dolly's symptoms were better, others were not, and when the remedy wore off she was the same as prior to the remedy. If the remedy had been curative or partially curative, she would have improved overall without dropping back to her original level when it was time to redose. The body will tell us more definitively what the reaction is if we keep giving the remedy, however. Either the vital force will stop reacting, or, as in Dolly's case, the symptom picture will dramatically worsen, both responses indicating that the remedy has been palliative. Continually repeating a noncurative remedy also has the potential to cause suppression, a dangerous situation (see below). For these reasons, you should not repeat remedies indiscriminately, especially higher potencies (30C and over). Experienced practitioners may repeat these remedies, but we understand remedy response and how and when to repeat.

Dolly's next remedy (Nux moschata 1M) resulted in a different response. On the day after the remedy she was listless; then she was better for three days. This was followed by two days of severe incoordination, then ten days of nearly normal behavior. She then had three days of depression and some incoordination, a week of "fairly normal" activity, five days of mild inco-ordination, then improvement. This pattern continued for about a month, followed by continual improvement in all mental symptoms over a seven-month period. After six to seven months, she developed a return of an old ear "infection" (discharge), a vaginal discharge, and some crusty skin on her nose and the pads of her feet. Her guardian put some antibiotic-steroid ointment in the ears for a couple of days, only to have the brain problems recur mildly. She immediately stopped the ointment, and the brain-related symptoms regressed without treatment. The ear problem cleared up over the next few months, also without additional treatment except a repeat of the *Nux moschata* 1M.

This response, clearly curative, had several hallmarks of a curative reaction: (1) an aggravation followed by slow, steady improvement, (2) long duration of response, (3) return of old symptoms, (4) interior to exterior movement of disease, (5) more severe to less severe symptoms, and (6) permanent restoration of health without need for constant medication. The improvement in this case followed the "two steps forward, one back" pattern for the first six weeks as the body shifted into improved health. As noted above, this is a common healing process, so too-rapid assessment of response may lead to errant decisions. It is not necessary for all of these stages to be present in a curative reaction, however. Often, especially with acute illness, the animal simply begins to improve, though it is generally slow and steady improvement. Immediate improvement is always a sign to pay close attention, as this often portends a palliative response.

Suppression

Suppression, in contrast to palliation, involves a much more serious impact upon the body, as the result is rapid deterioration in the condition. When symptoms are suppressed, treatment (often aggressive) eliminates some of the symptom picture, with temporary improvement followed by sudden decline, often with eruption of an entirely new, more serious pattern of symptoms. Using the example of the pressure cooker, palliation becomes suppression when the spout of the cooker is permanently sealed. In this instance the pressure (disease) will increase with no visible signs (symptoms) until finally the lid blows off, resulting in vastly more damage than release of steam through the spout.

Suppression can occur as a result of any type of treatment, including homeopathy (rarely), although strong drugs and surgery are the most common causes. The vital force, in attempting to maintain health in a manner that is the least threatening to life, will place the focus of disease in a given location and with appropriate symptoms. Any method that forces the removal of these symptoms has the potential to also force the locus of disease to a more dangerous location or organ, or to a more serious affection of the same organ system. For example, medical doctors of the past century recognized that aggressive (suppressive) treatment of colds often resulted in asthma. Another possible consequence of suppression is development of severe mental problems, as in Dolly's case when the ear ointment was applied and the mental symptoms returned. Fortunately for Dolly, in her case the guardian stopped the ointment before suppression (a more permanent condition) resulted.

I remember a case from my conventional practice, when I performed a radical mastectomy on a dog with cancer of multiple breasts on one side of her body. Recovery from surgery was normal but was shortly followed by rapid deterioration. Blood testing revealed acute kidney failure, which, at the time, I attributed to anesthesia complications. Looking back and evaluating this case using homeopathic principles led me to the conclusion that removal of the tumor caused a suppression of the disease. Since the body could no longer maintain the disease in the breast, the disease manifested in the kidneys, which are much more vital organs. The result was then sudden deterioration, ending in death.

Stopping the treatment (if possible) in these suppression situations does not typically result in a return to prior conditions. Deep treatment such as homeopathy can in some cases restore the balance by returning the prior condition. Many cases are not treatable, however, as with surgical removal of a mammary tumor such that the body cannot return the old symptom.

Suppression is very rare with acute illness, as the disease force is generally not massive enough to move deeply. The body can usually keep the disease in more superficial symptoms. If symptoms do move more deeply, as with Reye's syndrome (following aspirin in fever), generally they return to the superficial level once we stop treatment, though it may take some time. The most common responses to homeopathic remedies in acute illness are cure, palliation, and no reaction. Conventional medicines usually palliate in acute illness.

The main risk of suppression from homeopathic medicines is with overzealous repetition of high-potency incorrect (but close) remedies in chronic diseases. While the correct homeopathic medicine has great power to induce a curative reaction, most of the time an incorrect remedy has minimal impact. In some cases, however, a remedy is close enough to impact the body even though it will not induce a cure. With minimal repetition this remedy will palliate, but with heavy repetition it may suppress the symptoms.

Suppression is more common with conventional medicines because of the power of these drugs. Since these drugs usually oppose symptoms, they interfere with the body's attempts to heal. They also have the power to override the immune system in almost every individual and almost every situation.

Noncurative Aggravation

In a noncurative aggravation, symptoms intensify following administration of a medicine. While this is similar to the response with a curative aggravation, no improvement follows the aggravation of disease. No increase of well-being follows, and when the aggravation ends, the animal returns to the state that existed prior to administering the medicine, or even worsens. Additionally, with noncurative aggravations the aggravated state often lasts much longer than when the medicine is curative. In rare cases (almost always in chronic rather than acute illnesses), administration of a remedy is followed by a worsening that does not abate. This is more likely with higher potencies (over 30C), or in an animal with a very weak vital force. Noncurative aggravations are said to sometimes occur when a remedy is close to correct although not on the mark. Its energy disturbs the vital force in a disharmonious fashion, while a correct (homeopathic) prescription will resonate harmoniously with the vital force. In a sense, this is like the aggravations we can see when we repeat palliative remedies, as with Dolly, but here the aggravation occurs shortly following the remedy, without intervening improvement. It is an example of the gray zones (overlap) between these various categories.

A noncurative reaction is usually self-limiting, and by the time we have waited to see if it is a curative or noncurative reaction, no steps are needed to counteract the reaction. In some cases, however, it is necessary to give another remedy to change the response. This is rare in acute illness, so you will not likely see this with home treatment. If your companion has a long aggravation that is weakening her, change the remedy. You might even consider contacting an experienced practitioner or a friend with more experience than you. If you cannot find an appropriate remedy, *Nux vomica* will often counter an aggravation. This step is only necessary if the aggravation is weakening the patient, and once again this is very rare in the conditions you will treat at home. Books on remedy relationships help here, and some *materia medicas* (Boericke, Vermeulen's Concordant MM, and Phatak) list these relationships as well.

No Effect

Finally, if a medicine is far removed from the correct one, we will see no response, as the remedy does not resonate with the patient. In these situations, you need to rethink your patient's illness and try to choose a better remedy. Perhaps you focused upon common symptoms of her illness rather than upon her individual response to disease.

We may also see no apparent response with an appropriate remedy and simply need a higher potency or some repetition, but in these cases you must watch closely. You should see some indication, even if only subtle mental improvement, within a reasonable time following a remedy if the remedy is curative. If not, it's best to move on to another remedy or consult someone with more experience. You may see your patient worsen here, but if you observe carefully you will see that the worsening is simply the natural course of disease, as if you had not administered a remedy.

It is important to understand that any of the above categories can occur with any alternative modalities as well as with conventional treatment. Since holistic therapies tend to use more gentle methods, however, suppression occurs rarely with these modalities. The percentage of cases that respond via each category will vary according to the modality and the practitioner as well as the patient and client. Accurate interpretation of treatment response, no matter what treatment modality, will aid in assessing the value of that treatment.

Natural Disease Cycles

Disease symptoms rarely remain fixed; most conditions tend to cycle from better to worse to better, at least in the short term. This makes interpretation more difficult, as sometimes what we think is remedy response is merely normal cycling. Studies show, for example, that people tend to consult health care practitioners when their symptoms (or those of their companion animals) are most intense. The healer administers some treatment, her patient improves, and everyone is happy. But soon the symptoms recur, and the cycle repeats. You probably experience this with the flu, wherein you may feel better for a time, hoping you are coming out of your illness, only to worsen again. Keep this in mind as you interpret your remedies and your patients. If you just keep seeing up and down movement, you may only be seeing the disease on its own. Unless you can definitely tie this movement to your remedy administration, it's likely natural cycling. Time will tell.

If you see a pattern, however, in the times when your patient is better or worse, this may be helpful in choosing a good remedy. Many remedy states show such patterns. *Lycopodium* patients, for example, tend to worsen between 4 and 8 p.m., so if your companion's condition seems to fit *Lycopodium* and he also worsens around this time, this can confirm it as a good choice. But remember, never rely upon only one parameter to choose a remedy. See Chapter Five, "Using Homeopathy at Home," for more information on remedy selection.

Summary

Cure

There is increased well-being and a return of normal behavior. The patient shows signs of appropriate response to disease, such as fever and discharges. An aggravation may occur three to fourteen days (sometimes longer) after a remedy in a chronic illness. Aggravations are less common in acute illness and usually occur and disappear within a number of hours. There is gradual disappearance of symptoms of illness, often cyclic. Occasionally (in chronic disease) we see a return of previously treated (usually suppressed) symptoms. Movement of symptoms is from more to less important systems, from internal to external, from recent to older symptoms, from head to toe, and from pathological to functional. If there is movement through old or external symptoms, it is usually fairly rapid, although skin (including ear) symptoms may be slow to resolve.

Partial Cure

This is essentially the same process as cure, but all symptoms may not disappear, necessitating use of another remedy. There is an increase in well-being and no worsening, in contrast to palliation and suppression. The improved symptoms are deeper and/or newer symptoms, while those that remain are less serious and/or older symptoms. There is overall improvement.

Palliation

One or more symptoms disappear or improve, often rapidly. Other symptoms remain the same or worsen. New symptoms may appear ("side effects"). There is no overall improvement, though there may be temporary alleviation of symptoms. Stopping treatment may result in return of (temporarily improved) symptoms, usually more intense, especially in chronic diseases. Continuation of treatment sometimes results in deterioration of condition. In acute, self-limiting conditions, healing may occur while the condition is being palliated. In this case, palliation may alleviate symptoms while the animal heals on its own. In chronic illness (and sometimes acute illness), palliation masks symptoms, but the disease continues to worsen, thus the animal appears worse upon stopping the palliative medicine.

Suppression

One or more symptoms disappear completely. The patient deteriorates mentally and emotionally. Although the major symptoms are gone, the patient is not in optimum health, even though the previous "disease" may be considered "cured." After a period of time, a crisis occurs with eruption of a "new disease," more serious than the original condition. The new condition involves more serious organs or systems.

Noncurative Aggravation

The patient suffers an intensification of existing symptoms. This may be temporary, or it may persist. Once the worsening abates, the patient returns to the same condition that existed prior to administration of the medicine. Whether the worsening does or does not abate, another medicine will be needed to improve the condition. This is most common in chronic diseases in weak individuals.

Natural Disease Cycles

Remember that most diseases have their intrinsic cycles, with times of improvement alternating with worsening. This may confuse your interpretation, but if you notice a pattern, it can help choose the best remedy.

Part Two
HOMEOPATHIC TREATMENT

Chapter Four
WHERE TO START WHEN YOU HAVE A SICK COMPANION

When to Seek Veterinary Help

Working with a Homeopathic Veterinarian

Aids and Obstacles to Cure

Other Treatment Methods

Summary

I RECOMMEND THAT YOU READ THIS CHAPTER before beginning treatment. This should help you decide whether or not you should use home treatment on your own, or if you should seek outside care. It will also help you make a transition to holistic care, and it will show you some situations that might limit your companion's healing. If your home treatment is not working, one of these "obstacles to cure" may be part of the problem.

Once you decide to proceed with home treatment, go to Chapter Five, as it gives specific information on using homeopathic medicines. There is also a guide to using the treatment chapters. You then should read the appropriate chapter and section that deals specifically with your companion's current problem. These sections give detailed information about treatment as well as situations that are beyond home care.

Many conditions are very amenable to home care, and this is the primary purpose for this book. In some cases, however, it is unwise to attempt home treatment. In the treatment chapters, I indicate when you should seek veterinary care in specific situations. In this chapter I list general conditions that warrant assistance. If you have an experienced homeopath within a reasonable driving distance, that is your best option if you need help. If you do not have a veterinarian in your community who does homeopathy, perhaps a veterinarian there is holistic or is at least sympathetic to your desire for holistic care. If you have a veterinarian who will work with you on local support, many homeopathic veterinarians will consult by telephone and assist you with complicated homeopathic prescribing.

The local support is essential, however. Through the years that I have consulted in these types of situations, I have found most veterinarians very willing to help in any way they can. Most veterinarians truly do care and want to help, but we get limited information on holistic methods in veterinary school (though this is changing dramatically as many schools open their doors to holistic therapies). Having an outside veterinarian consult over the telephone is rather unusual and difficult to accept at first. I struggled with this concept when I first met people who practiced this way, though I now find that it can be very successful. As more veterinarians learn holistic and homeopathic methods, this will become less necessary; until then, it is sometimes the best solution.

Have patience with your local veterinarian. She does care but may find your needs difficult because she does not have the training to help you directly. With time, however, she will probably see that you are not rejecting her help; rather you simply want the best for your companion, and you want to work with her rather than against her. And it is in your companion's best interests to work with her. She has many skills that you need. You should not try to go it alone in many cases.

It is also very important to develop a working relationship with your veterinarian even if you treat most problems at home. Sometimes you simply need the guidance of someone with more experience, and you will sometimes have problems that you cannot treat at home. As with all relationships, good honest communication and an open heart will assure that you have the support when it is needed.

In addition to providing guidelines for working with homeopathic and conventional veterinarians, this chapter gives information about conditions that may interfere with healing. This includes such items as diet, household stress, vaccinations, and conventional medicine. There is also a section on working with other modalities in conjunction with homeopathic treatment. Some conditions may warrant simultaneous treatment, at least for a time. Additionally, some guardians are more comfortable making a slow transition to holistic treatment. This section gives some guidelines for the transition.

When to Seek Veterinary Help

If your companion's illness is interfering with his eating (for more than a day or two) or is in any other way serious or life threatening, have a veterinarian examine him to help you with monitoring and/or treatment. Don't let your determination to succeed or your fear of conventional medicine keep you away from help. It is not worth allowing the situation to get out of hand. Many veterinarians are very understanding about holistic care, and this attitude is rapidly growing. If you approach your veterinarian honestly with your desires and concerns, she will probably respect them and try to work with you. If you run into resistance or hostility, perhaps she can recommend a colleague who would be more comfortable working with you, or you can ask your friends for recommendations.

Remember that your veterinarian may be unfamiliar with homeopathy, and conventional medicine may be all she knows, so she will be most comfortable (and most effective) with the skills she possesses. Your companion relies upon you as his guardian, however, so you are in charge. Your veterinarian is a consultant, and you are the one who should make the decisions, but you must be responsible and use all advice wisely. Veterinarians have years of training and experience working with sick animals—don't ignore the contribution they can offer. And if you have success with holistic methods, any open-minded person will be appreciative and probably interested in your success.

Working with a conventional veterinarian can be tricky, though. It is easy to let his fears or opinions trigger your fears, and then to make a decision you may regret. Try to remain calm, and ask questions until you understand as best you can. You want to know what to expect, how serious the condition is, and how much time healing will take. You also want to know how much time you have to try treating a condition before you simply need to use conventional medicine. These are questions with which most veterinarians are not practiced, and with which many may be uncomfortable. So use tact, be respectful, and be honest.

If you can find a homeopathic veterinarian, so much the better. Even a veterinarian who leans toward or uses other holistic methods will usually understand your needs more readily than someone without holistic experience, though this certainly varies. Your notes and prescriptions up to the time of the consultation will help if the veterinarian is familiar with homeopathy.

Here are some situations where you should seek assistance:

- if your companion refuses to eat for more than a couple of days;
- if your companion has breathing difficulty;
- if your companion is vomiting more often than once or twice a day in chronic situations or more than once every few hours in acute conditions;
- if your companion has diarrhea that persists for more than a few days;
- if any condition persists beyond a reasonable time, or after you have tried three or four remedies;
- if your companion's condition is worsening;
- if your companion is weak or listless for more than a day or so;
- if you cannot figure out a good remedy to use or cannot understand your companion's condition;
- if your companion is unable to urinate or defecate.

Basically, any time you see that you cannot help or the condition is out of your grasp—if you have any concern—seek help. You don't want to learn at the expense of your animal friends. Always keep their best interest at heart.

Working with a Homeopathic Veterinarian

Many cases simply will require the expertise of an experienced homeopathic prescriber, and while it is not absolutely necessary that this person be a veterinarian, it can be beneficial. If you decide to work with a nonveterinary homeopath, you should also enlist the services of a veterinarian for assessment and monitoring as described above.

Your prescriber's success depends greatly upon communication between him and you, and upon your ability to convey the picture of your companion's illness to the homeopath. Since homeopathic prescribing depends so heavily upon the observations of the primary caregiver, you need to be attentive and complete in your presentation. Notes are imperative. Ask your homeopath what information he needs, and take notes regularly. Monitor all physical symptoms as well as how your companion feels and acts. Note any patterns such as times of day, association with moon phases, or periodic recurrences like every other day, once a week, and so on. Note any conditions that worsen or lessen the symptoms, such as cold rainy weather, heat of the sun, and food changes, and whether your companion wants attention or wishes to be left alone.

Next, if you can accurately summarize the notes into an overall report rather than a day-by-day presentation, it will streamline the conversation. The homeopath can then ask for details where he needs them. Try to be as objective as possible in the summary; it is easy to color the report either based upon your hope for improvement, your desire to please the homeopath, or your fear that treatment won't work. And do not hold back information out of embarrassment or the feeling that you will be judged for the care you give—this is not the case, and the information may be essential to the prescriber.

Read the chapters on disease and cure so you will have an idea of what to expect. This will aid your reporting as well as help you know when to wait and when to call if you aren't seeing improvement, or if you are seeing an aggravation. Generally, it is best to wait awhile—a day or so—before calling, as the aggravation will often subside on its own.

Finally, follow advice on diet, supplements, and other suggestions to help provide your dog with the ability to respond to the prescribed remedies. Poor nutrition and poor supportive care often become the major limiting factors in holistic treatment. Homeopathic medicines are very powerful, but they may work poorly if the patient does not have adequate nutrition to fuel the healing process.

Aids and Obstacles to Cure

Every intelligent physician, having a knowledge of rational etiology, will first remove by appropriate means, as far as possible, every exciting and maintaining cause of disease and obstacle to cure, and endeavor to establish a correct and orderly course of living for his patient, with due regard to mental and physical hygiene. Failing to do this, but little impression can be made by homeopathic remedies, and what slight impression is made will be of short duration.

—Stuart Close, MD[1]

Diet

Because we rely upon the body to heal itself, we must provide the best nutritional support possible. This is primarily a homeopathic book, so I am not giving detailed dietary guidelines, but it is so important that a few words are in order.

My nutrition training in veterinary school was minimal, to say the least, as it was for most of my contemporary colleagues. We were basically told to "feed a good brand of pet food and don't give anything else as it will upset the perfectly balanced formula." Table foods, we heard, were an absolute invitation to disaster. Dry food was considered the best choice for cats and dogs. Then we were given literature—something like today's infomercials—on a couple of brands of foods. Not surprisingly, these two companies command the major share of the marketplace, largely due to recommendations by veterinarians. I now believe much of this information to be incorrect. Furthermore, I see this misinformation as contributing to the deterioration in the health of our companion animals that we have witnessed in recent decades.

Diet and nutrition are sensitive topics in all of medicine. We have all seen (and probably bought) many of the numerous books available. There are hundreds of ideas out there; many have good bases, but often they are taken too far. Quite naturally I have my own beliefs, and I will summarize them here. But one key that almost all diet books (and surprisingly many homeopaths) overlook is individual nutritional needs. Each person is an individual, and thus nutritional guidelines must be tailored to the individual. The best parameter for evaluation of diet is the response by your companion. It takes a minimum of a month or two to see the response to diet changes. The change may not be discernible for three to six months in some animals. With very ill animals it sometimes takes a year or two to see the maximum impact of improved nutrition.

Generally, I support a home-prepared, fresh food diet whenever possible, as this comes as close as we can get to matching the diets that these animals have fine-tuned over eons of evolution. Raw meats, fresh-cooked grains and vegetables, and a few supplements to balance the diet make a great substitute for freshly killed animals. Use organic foods whenever possible, as it is not only healthier for your animals but also for you. Additionally, it is best for the planet because you'll avoid pesticides and drugs, and organic farmers usually use more humane methods for raising animals.

If you cannot afford organic meats and vegetables, at least buy organic liver and kidney, as these organs are great food, but they concentrate any drugs or chemicals to which the animal has been exposed. If you feed your companion nonorganic organ meats, you will expose her to high amounts of harmful substances like pesticides, antibiotics, and steroids. Liver, like all meats, should be fed raw. I am amused to occasionally hear my clients report that their conventional veterinarians react in horror about the raw meats. As a good friend says, I have never seen wild carnivores grilling their prey over a hibachi! And even though we domesticated these companion animals (or they domesticated themselves) millennia ago, their digestive systems have changed little. They evolved with raw foods, and these still work best in most cases.

Yet, some animals are too sick to make the transition; certainly it should be done gradually in all cases. This is where individualization is important. Some people recommend avoiding grains—this is good for some animals but not for others. We must in all cases use the response in our companions as the final guide. A few animals may do better on commercial foods. But I see the vast majority of cats and dogs on fresh, raw-food diets blossoming. Their coats are soft and shiny, and they fairly glow with life.

More and more reports arise about the horrible ingredients of commercial pet foods: rancid meats and oils, diseased animal parts, even cats and dogs killed at animal shelters.[2] Often these dead animals still wear their flea collars; these become part of the food, as do the drugs that killed them at the shelters. Some pet food companies, like many corporations, hold profit above all else. You simply cannot expect great health to arise from poor foods. And without good foods, sick people (this includes animals) generally cannot regain lost health, especially since it may be the foods that contributed to the disease in the first place.

The appendix lists resources for recipes for cats and dogs. See also Chapter Eight, "Digestive System," for more information. If you feel you just cannot feed your companion home-prepared foods, at least feed him a high-quality food that uses human food–grade ingredients and is without artificial flavors and preservatives. If you feed him commercial foods, use canned foods rather than dry foods *at least* 50 percent of the time for dogs and 75 percent for cats. Give your companion table foods frequently, as long as these are healthy (no fast foods). If the amount of added foods exceeds 10 to 15 percent of the total food intake, however, you'll need to use recipes or buy prepared frozen foods. Otherwise you may see some nutritional imbalances. Generally, though, anything you do toward fresh foods will help, even a couple of meals a week. It is not an all-or-nothing item, so don't give up if you cannot go 100 percent fresh. Do what you can, and keep moving.

Vaccination

Vaccination is the other major influence upon health in our companion animals. It is so important in my mind that I have included a chapter devoted entirely to the vaccine issue; read Chapter Sixteen for detailed information. Its place in this chapter is that vaccination often blocks any treatment efforts. The impact of prior vaccines is often reversible, but if you choose to continue to vaccinate, treatment may be unrewarding. I came to this point of view reluctantly and over many years. Having been trained conventionally, I initially supported vaccination, but my observations have gradually shown me that they create much more illness than they prevent.

I recognize that, since most state laws require rabies vaccines, this creates a difficult crossroad. I can only recommend here that you fight to change the laws in your state to reflect scientific knowledge, as current recommendations are not based in science. As a veterinarian, I am obligated to uphold rabies vaccination laws, thus I cannot recommend refusing rabies vaccination. If you contemplate avoiding rabies vaccination for your companion, you must realize that this is a legal decision as well as a medical decision. Rabies vaccines typically provide lifetime immunity, at least after two doses, so the need for further vaccination is legal, not medical (see Chapter Sixteen, "Vaccination"). With few exceptions (some communities may require other vaccines, though no state law requires them, to my knowledge), all other vaccines are optional. I recommend avoiding vaccination in almost all circumstances, as I believe it mainly creates illness rather than preventing illness.

Lifestyle

Alongside diet and vaccination, the lifestyle we can offer our companions greatly influences their health. We must respect these fellow creatures by always considering the impact that our choices have upon them. Before choosing to adopt a companion animal, ask yourself if you have the time, energy, means, and ability to care for him in the way you would wish to live. Don't make impulsive decisions, as you and they will bear the consequences for years. Do you have the room to keep and care for a dog, especially a large one? Can you let the dog or cat get outside for fresh air? Just because a cat or dog can live inside a small apartment does that mean she will thrive there.

We know that depression is a major cause of illness in humans; it is arrogant of us to assume dogs and cats to be unaffected by the same emotional states. I always ask guardians about the home stress when an illness arises. I am sometimes stunned at the responses, though the more I have asked this question the more I can anticipate the response. I see many animals with diabetes that arose after the death of another member of the household. I see many animals that react to stresses such as divorce. Do not assume animals to be immune to emotional damage. In fact, they are very susceptible. See Chapter Seventeen, "The Bigger Picture."

Toxins and Other Impacts

In today's world there are so many things that we encounter that damage health. We are all familiar with the problem with carcinogenic chemicals, but toxin damage extends way beyond this. Our drinking water is often contaminated with all sorts of drugs, from birth control pills to antibiotics and antidepressants. In the United Kingdom, men in record numbers have been undergoing breast reduction surgery because of estrogens in the drinking water that cause breast development. Many pesticides also have estrogenic effects; these enhance cancer development as well as creating many other problems. Air pollution also contributes greatly to disease, especially indoor air pollution. This is off-gassing of volatile organic solvents from paints, glues, plywood, particleboard, and other chemicals used in modern building techniques. And then there are electromagnetic fields (EMFs), which occur around wires and other electrical circuits, such as appliances, outlets, electric heaters, and so on. Compact fluorescent bulbs generate quite strong EMFs, as well as usually containing mercury, so while these consume less electricity, they can be quite health-damaging. And their production consumes much more energy than standard bulbs, so the gain is questionable. I was initially a fan of these bulbs, but I don't like being around them, and when I heard about the EMF issue with these, I understood why.

A huge issue today is the vast number of wireless devices we use, from radio stations to cell phones to wireless Internet routers. The invisible waves these produce actually cause a lot of damage. European studies have shown many problems, like increased cancers, with cell phones and cell phone towers. Even cordless phones in our houses generate very similar frequencies. Our bodies simply are not able to cope with these impacts. Not everyone notices the problems, but enough individuals suffer as a result of these electromagnetic pollutants that we know there are problems. I have a client who lives in rural California. She became quite ill two years ago with chronic fatigue–like symptoms. Doctors could not help, and no matter what immune- or energy-boosting herbs she took, she could not carry on her normal life. Her husband happened to speak with their neighbors, however, and found that they had installed a wireless router for their Internet service shortly before Laura became ill. The neighbors agreed to turn the router off when they were not using the Internet, and overnight all of Laura's symptoms disappeared. And these neighbors did not live too close, as they are in a rural, not an urban, setting.

What to do? I recommend not using wireless systems, including cell phones and cordless phones, as well as avoiding wireless Internet. Furthermore, resist strongly any attempts by cities or others to install wireless Internet services. A woman in Santa Fe, New Mexico, committed suicide a couple of years ago when she finally ran out of places to stay, as all the apartment complexes and even a campground where she had been saying installed wireless Internet. She could not live near these signals, and finally killed herself out of exasperation. Even microchips, regularly installed in animals, can cause problems. I have another client whose veterinarian convinced her to microchip her cat, but she subsequently found that she could no longer have the cat sleep on the bed with her. Fortunately she had the veterinarian remove the microchip. Imagine what the poor animals must feel if this woman could not be around the cat when he had the microchip in place. Granted, this is a woman with environmental sensitivity, but these things obviously affect everyone else; we just may not feel them.

If you are unwilling to dispense with cell phones and wireless routers, turn them off when not in use. As for air pollution, this is more difficult, though you can install air filters, but they must have carbon/charcoal filters to remove organic solvents. Install good water filters on your tap water. This is a better solution than buying water in bottles. First, there is the huge landfill issue with the millions of water bottles we now consume daily. And worse, in many ways, the bisphenol-A (BPA) and other plasticizers and petroleum products in plastics cause health problems on their own. BPA is an estrogen-mimicking chemical; it was developed in the 1930s as an estrogen replacement chemical but was deemed unsafe. It was replaced with diethylstilbestrol (DES), another terribly damaging chemical, but BPA was then found useful in the plastics industry. When drinking from plastic bottles, we get huge doses of estrogenic compounds. BPA is also in the white plastic material used for filling cavities; we also get bombarded there if we choose that material. Further, these fillings tend to begin leaking after only three to five years. Back to buying water in bottles, though: many bottled waters simply contain municipal water and are no different from tap water. Dasani is one of these, though they may have changed this.

Finally, avoid any drugs and chemicals where you can. Don't put pesticides on your animals (like Frontline and Advantage), and don't use pesticides in your home or on your lawn. See the sections on fleas and heartworm in Chapter Fifteen for further information. In short, our fascination with chemicals and technology must come to an end, or at least be hugely moderated, if we are to return to any semblance of health.

Promote Health, Don't Fight Disease

So, what is the formula for our companion's health? Good food, a loving family, opportunities for fun and growth—just like for us. We should not be surprised at that. And if we see our companion get sick, we should take the opportunity to examine our lives carefully—with care, for us all.

Safe health care is equally important; we don't want to create illness in our attempt to prevent illness. The vaccine issue is one that is sure to raise controversy and lots of resistance, but my experience reinforces daily that the damage from vaccines is vast. In my opinion (and the opinion of many colleagues) vaccine use must be curbed if we are ever to regain health. Additionally, drug use should be limited to situations where it is truly necessary. The common practice of administering drugs for any ailment, no matter the severity, is dangerous. So is the common use of antibiotics for viral infections. Use methods that promote health rather than fighting against a perceived outside threat. The only way to attain health is to strengthen the body. Methods that destroy, even if they are meant to destroy an invading enemy, are still destructive and only provide short-term gains. Antibiotics, for example, are the primary cause of one type of liver failure in humans.[3] Further, antibiotics generally wreak havoc on the beneficial organisms in the intestines, leading to digestive issues and sometimes candida overgrowth. Thus, while in some cases antibiotics save lives, in other cases they risk lives. It is important to weigh their necessity carefully in each case, as, like vaccines, these drugs are not as benign as we once thought.

Other Treatment Methods

Many animals I treat are quite ill and currently on conventional or other treatment. Whether or not this interferes with successful homeopathic treatment is controversial within the homeopathic community. One answer is that, as in all things, everyone is an individual. In some patients the drugs are a problem, while in others there seems to be no harm. The disease state probably creates sensitivity in some individuals. Furthermore, most interference comes when the homeopathic remedy is not really the best choice, thus it is more easily antidoted.

Generally, however, I prefer to treat without concomitant use of other modalities, as the picture is clearer even if there is no interference. This includes acupuncture. While acupuncture is a great method of treatment, it can occasionally interfere with homeopathic medicines (and vice versa).

Also, any therapy that changes the disease will change its appearance. As we depend upon symptoms to guide our evaluation of the response to treatment, this change can make evaluation more difficult. This, more than interference, may be the biggest impediment to using two modalities at a time. Once the situation is more stable, it is acceptable to add other treatment methods in some cases.

The clarity issue is twofold: first, the true disease picture is the unadulterated one with no suppressive treatment; this is the state we need to match with our remedy. Once a drug has altered the picture, it may be hard to see clearly enough to find the correct homeopathic medicine. Secondly, the suppressive drug will alter the response to the remedy, thus we are unclear if a change is due to the drug or the remedy, or if absence of a change means the wrong remedy or drug interference. *If changes must be made to the remedy and to supplements, drugs, or any other treatment, it is imperative that these be done at different times so that if there is a change in the patient's illness, we can determine which treatment was responsible.* This is important as we may need to change part of the treatment and we need to know what to keep and what to alter. In extremely ill animals, we sometimes must abandon this precept, as we need to use aggressive treatment, adding supplements and even other treatments if necessary to stabilize our patient in the short term. Even here this can be confusing and should be done with support from an experienced homeopath. Some homeopaths still resist using any other treatment even in these situations, so you must respect the person with whom you work. And in any case, these cases are not common.

In some cases, notably skin and ear affections, the biggest resistance to stopping drugs (usually steroids) is the perceived discomfort of the patient. This is very understandable, yet often these very drugs interfere not so much with the remedy as with the patient's ability to heal, as they impede the body's immune system—the very system responsible for healing. In like manner, antibiotics can also affect the immune system, so discontinuing them is beneficial whenever possible. You may need to taper these drugs slowly, especially with steroids, and once again this should be under the supervision of a veterinarian (or an experienced homeopath).

I remember once overhearing a conversation at a veterinary meeting about the paradoxical ability of antibiotics to impact upper respiratory infections in cats that were known to be viral rather than bacterial infections. (Antibiotics have no direct impact upon viruses. As with the common cold in humans, veterinarians often prescribe antibiotics for these viral infections because no other treatment is available.) My colleagues were understandably puzzled, as indeed they should be. The conventional model cannot explain this phenomenon. The homeopathic model, however, has an answer: the antibiotic merely creates a drug disease (an altered body state as a reaction to the drug) that is more powerful than the viral infection, thus the body must deal with the drug disease. When the drug is stopped, the viral infection often resumes. Antibiotics thus may interfere with the healing process by not allowing the immune system to fight the virus as long as the antibiotic is in the body (see Chapter Two, "The Nature of Disease").

Additionally, some antibiotics, notably the tetracyclines, have anti-inflammatory (immunosuppressive) properties, so they directly impede healing in the body. This is one reason why so many cases of Lyme disease are reported. Lyme disease is a rare but often-reported tick-borne infection in the joints that creates lameness, and tetracyclines are the drugs of choice for the infection. When tetracyclines are prescribed for noninfectious lameness, the anti-inflammatory effect reduces the pain, and the (incorrect) interpretation is that the condition must have been infectious (Lyme disease), since symptoms abate. This misinterpretation arises because the anti-inflammatory effect of the drug is poorly known; doctors then assume the improvement resulted from killing Lyme organisms. Similarly, most other drugs also alter the natural disease picture, as well as interfere with the immune system, often in ways we might not expect; this naturally also interferes with interpreting remedy choice and remedy response.

If a patient comes under my care and is not on medications, or I feel the medications can be stopped, that is my first choice. If the condition is too fragile to stop the drugs, then I start treatment and begin to taper the drugs as quickly as possible. Stopping conventional medicines abruptly is often too much of a shock to the system, so gradual decrease is the best route. This is due to the strong nature of conventional drugs and their resultant tendency to take over the body's internal systems. Slow withdrawal allows the body to begin to regain function. Homeopathic medicines can assist the return to function, but there can be interference from the strong conventional drugs, so I usually use lower potency remedies and repeat them. This allows the remedy to continue to stimulate the body in the face of repeated drug dosing. As the body improves, the drug can be withdrawn.

The bottom line is that while it is ideal to treat with remedies alone, this is often impractical and sometimes (though rarely) dangerous. Begin treatment alongside the conventional methods if there is any risk to stopping other treatment first. The remedy will still work if it is correct and will probably even help the body resist the damaging tendency of the conventional drugs. The drugs can usually be reduced over time, if not stopped altogether, and even if we cannot tell exactly which method did what, if our patient truly improves, it is academic or ego-driven to ask why.

If your companion is currently on medications that you wish to stop, it is imperative that you work with a veterinarian on eliminating the drugs. She will know which ones can be stopped quickly and which ones should be reduced more slowly. She can also help you determine if reducing the medication creates a problem, or if the medication itself was creating part of the illness.

Summary

It is important to recognize when your companion's illness is beyond your ability to treat him at home. See "When to Seek Veterinary Help" above as well as the specific treatment chapters to determine whether or not you should treat a particular problem. Always work with your veterinarian to obtain the best care. This does not mean that you cannot decide what treatment you want. You are the primary caregiver. But you should seek assistance from conventional and holistic veterinarians as needed.

Poor diet, vaccinations, drugs and toxins, stress, and other therapeutic methods may all interfere with healing. The first four conditions are especially critical. Without good support, many animals cannot respond to treatment. While it is clearest to use only one treatment method at a time, sometimes this is impractical or impossible. It is possible to use homeopathy in conjunction with other treatments, including drugs, though the response may be slower. It is also more difficult to evaluate the response. When you use more than one modality at the same time, it is especially important to have help with the evaluation.

Chapter Five
USING HOMEOPATHY AT HOME

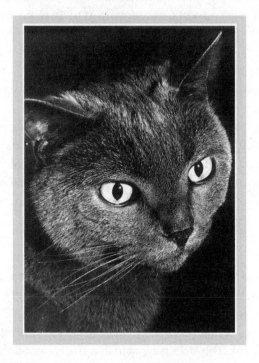

How to Take a Case and Choose a Remedy

Constitutional Prescribing versus Acute Prescribing

How to Use the Treatment Chapters

Dosage: How to Handle and Administer Remedies

Potency and Repetition

Monitoring Your Companion's Progress

Summary

THIS CHAPTER COVERS THE "NUTS AND BOLTS" OF HOMEOPATHY—how to actually use the remedies. I hope you have taken the time to read the previous chapters first, as they will have given you an understanding that will greatly aid your successful employment of the medicines. The focus here is upon the steps you will take when one of your companions is ill and needs treatment.

These steps include "taking the case" (observing and collecting the symptoms that guide you to the correct remedy), using the treatment chapters in this book, administering the remedy, and monitoring the progress in your sick animal.

How to Take a Case and Choose a Remedy

Perhaps the most difficult aspect of homeopathic medicine is case-taking and case analysis, since we approach illness from a different aspect than our conventional counterparts. We homeopaths consider illness as something that affects an individual *and becomes an integral part of that individual,* so we must find a remedy that fits the individual and not simply the disease. From our conventional training, we learned to consider the disease more than the individual, so this reversal of perspective takes time and a concerted effort.

Consider how we recognize a friend or acquaintance. We know them by an almost instinctual identification of their face. In fact, if asked to describe the face of a friend, we may find it quite difficult, yet we know them the instant we see them. All humans have essentially the same features, yet we can look very different. Sometimes, however, this difference is difficult to discern. People within racial groups, for example, share certain patterns that lend a commonality to their appearance, especially to those outside the group. When we first encounter a new racial group, we have difficulty in identifying individuals until we have learned the common characteristics of the group; only then can we separate out the individual.

Disease is much the same. While there are many common symptoms among diabetic dogs, for example, the differences are more telling. Our task is not to stereotype illnesses, rather to recognize the individuals with illness. We must have some understanding of which symptoms are common to a given illness and which are particular to the individual. Only then can we separate the common symptoms from the individual ones. We call the latter symptoms *characteristic symptoms,* in that they characterize the illness *in the individual.*

Diabetic animals, for example, generally have high levels of blood sugar (glucose), and as a result they urinate a lot and become very thirsty. Typically, their appetite is great also. These are the common symptoms. One diabetic dog may wish to be left alone when he feels unwell, however, while another may cling to his guardian. Or perhaps one cat eats ravenously and then regurgitates, while another cat merely picks at her food, but each time she eats, she runs to the litter box with diarrhea. All of these animals may have high blood glucose and be thirsty and urinate large volumes, thus they have diabetes mellitus. But they are individuals, as their other symptoms indicate. *It is in these other symptoms—the ones that are not of the disease but of the individual—that we will find the clue to the correct remedy.* This is especially true if the other symptoms arose at around the time the diabetes manifested.

Finally, as part of the characteristic symptoms, there are those we call the "strange, rare, and peculiar" symptoms. These symptoms are such that they stand out as so uncommon that they quickly identify the individuality. Often these are contrary to the expected finding, such as an animal that is cold to the touch but prefers to be in a cold environment, or one with nausea and vomiting that is improved by eating. Not every animal shows one of these unusual symptoms, but in those that do, the symptom may be very helpful.

I remember Sparky, a cat with an erosion of the tip of his nose. I thought the erosion was something like an ulcer and tried a couple of remedies to no avail, as I had no characteristic symptoms. Then one day his guardian said, "He just keeps rubbing his nose." That was odd, as the lesion looked sore—it was quite raw. But I realized Sparky's nose bothered him, and possibly he was creating the erosion by the furious rubbing. In the repertory, I found a rubric (a listed symptom with remedies that may be useful), "tingling in the tip of the nose, ameliorated by rubbing." Only one remedy was listed *(Belladonna)*, which cured the condition right away. The more peculiar the symptom, the more likely it is to point to a remedy—if the remedy is known and fairly represented in the homeopathic literature. Usually, we do not prescribe based only upon a peculiar symptom, however; the entire picture must still fit the case. In Sparky's case there was only one symptom, so this was all I had to go on. (We refer to these cases as "one-sided cases." They can be very difficult unless we get lucky with a strange symptom.)

A strange symptom may often be unrelated to the main complaint. Jesse was brought to me because of a severe disease that made her very unsteady in her hind legs, so she had a difficult time running with her dog buddies. After a couple of consultations, I discovered that she tended to drop food from her mouth when eating. I found this listed in the mouth section of the repertory; one remedy was listed. *Argentum nitricum* had this peculiar symptom and fit the hind leg partial paralysis quite well. I gave it to Jesse and she improved tremendously.

While these cases are exciting, they are not typical. More commonly, we work with a group of less striking symptoms and try to filter out the important symptoms. Once we have a grasp of the case through these characteristic symptoms, we begin our search for a remedy to match the symptoms. We typically go to the repertory (the listing of symptoms—rubrics—and possible remedies) at this time and see which remedies are listed and have the same symptoms as the patient. Next, we read the possible remedies in the *materia medica* to see which of these provides the best fit. If none really fit well, then we look at the symptoms again to be sure we did not overlook an important symptom or that we did not overvalue a common symptom (a symptom that is commonly present in animals with the same condition, such as increased thirst in a diabetic animal). The latter is the most common mistake.

Using the treatment section of this book is slightly different, as there is no true repertory. But the process is similar: find the characteristic symptoms, then go to the chapter and section that cover the primary symptom (the main complaint or problem). Read the overview to better understand the condition and to decide if home treatment is appropriate. Then go through the remedies in that section and write down the possible choices, remembering to look for the individuating symptoms. Finally, go to the *materia medica* (Part Four) to read the broad picture of each remedy under consideration to be certain the remedy fits your companion's disease picture. Each section basically groups remedies by the common symptoms they share, and then gives individual symptoms for the remedies so you can identify the correct remedy, or at least narrow your choice to two or three remedies. Then, hopefully, the *materia medica* section will further clarify your choice.

Let's look at a case to see how this works: Lily is an Old English sheepdog who developed kennel cough after a trip to the groomer. She was generally in good spirits, active, and normal except for a deep hacking cough. She coughed as if she had something stuck in her throat, and the throat was so sensitive that slight touch or barking would incite the cough. Also, she frequently coughed as soon as she lay down. Her temperature was normal, and she had been on antibiotics for a week without any change. In this case, almost all of the symptoms are common to kennel cough—the deep hacking cough, coughing as if something is stuck in the throat, and the sensitivity. Her sensitivity, however, was more pronounced than most, and most characteristic was the aggravation upon lying down (it's more common for coughing to worsen with standing or exertion). These characteristic symptoms show how Lily responded to kennel cough *as an individual.* They pointed to *Drosera,* which quickly cured her of the infection.

From a practical standpoint, here is how I recommend taking a case: first, gather all changes you have noted in your companion since she has been sick, starting with what caught your attention in the first place. It helps me to then ask about symptoms from head to tail and see if there are items I may have missed. Consider anything—stool, urine, appetite, thirst, tendency to seek warmth or cool, discharges, and so on. Don't forget the behavioral symptoms, but remember they may not have as much significance if they did not change when the illness arose. Make a list of the changes, and then try to separate them into common and characteristic symptoms. While you may not be an expert on animal illness, try to relate her sickness to one you may have experienced, or ask a friend. Consider which symptoms are common to most animals with the condition and which ones seem to represent your companion's individual expression. Then emphasize the characteristic symptoms, and add one or two of the most intense common symptoms—those that best describe the illness— so you ensure that the chosen remedy covers the symptoms of her illness *as she experiences the illness.*

From these symptoms you should have an understanding of the disease, and then you should be able to go to the chapter on the body system that is primarily affected and choose a remedy. If one remedy is not clear, pick two or three, then go to the *materia medica* at the back of the book and read the larger descriptions of each remedy to see if this helps. There may be another symptom or aspect listed there that one remedy covers better than the others. You can even look at other *materia medicas,* such as the ones listed in the appendix. These will give still broader descriptions that may clarify your choice, though these can be confusing for inexperienced homeopaths as they list so many symptoms, most of which will not be present. After awhile, all remedies can sound alike in these larger texts. They are very useful, but if you get confused, stick to my descriptions for now.

Furthermore, whenever you read remedy descriptions, you may read something that sounds like it is common in a remedy picture but which you do not see in your animal. Do not let the absence of a symptom or characteristic that is listed in a remedy description, but is not in your patient, deter you from a remedy if that remedy looks good otherwise. So do not ignore *Pulsatilla*, for example, if your patient is thirsty (*Pulsatilla* patients tend to not be thirsty, but nothing is absolute). Remember this general rule, however: *It is not essential that every symptom listed for a remedy exists in your patient.* (In fact, it will never happen.) *But it is important that the symptoms in your patient are represented in the remedy description;* at least the most important ones should be there.

Constitutional Prescribing versus Acute Prescribing

This term is somewhat unclear because different people use it differently, though it is a common term within the homeopathic community. I will define my usage, as it is an important concept.

You hopefully understand by now that the correct homeopathic prescription takes into account not only the primary complaint, such as vomiting, coughing, and so on, but also considers the entire state of the patient at the time of the illness. This includes emotional and behavioral aspects as well as physical conditions. Thus we might have two dogs with diarrhea, but one is very thirsty and prefers to stay to herself, while the other one has no thirst but wants to be close by her guardian. These dogs would receive different homeopathic medicines for essentially the same primary complaint.

This is essential in homeopathic prescribing, and it holds true for acute conditions as well as chronic conditions. For acute conditions, however, the disease is often rather superficially imposed upon the body. The changes we see in a sick animal may be minimal and focused around the primary complaint. Individual differences do occur, though they may be subtle in some cases and pronounced in others. Additionally, as acute conditions are short-term, we must base our prescription upon the state of the body during the time of the acute illness only. Thus the behavioral state may not be important *unless it changed during the acute illness.*

Acute prescribing, then, deals with conditions that visit the body, in a sense, rather than being a deep-seated, integral part of the individual. The individuality becomes visible as the individual responds to the acute illness. The more superficial the disease, the more the prescription matches the illness, whereas the deeper that the disease impacts the animal, the more the prescription must match the essence of the individual. There is thus a gray zone of transition between acute prescribing and constitutional prescribing.

Constitutional prescribing addresses the individual more deeply, since it is based upon the concept that disease is an individual response to external stress. Each individual (human or nonhuman) responds to stress differently, thus he will produce symptoms that reflect his inner self. His response comes out of his constitution, out of the essence of how he relates to the world. One person's anxiety, for example, may result in diarrhea, whereas another person would experience tightness in the chest. This difference would exist even if the trigger (flying, for instance) were the same in both cases. As a contrasting example, two people may suffer from occasional diarrhea, but one always gets diarrhea after eating a high-fat meal, whereas the second one develops diarrhea whenever she has an approaching deadline for a work project. These are completely different situations, even though the symptom (diarrhea) is the same. A prescription that only focuses upon physical common symptoms (again, the diarrhea in this case) will have little effect, as it addresses the disease (so to speak) and not the individual. Constitutional prescribing is thus necessary to address how the individual relates to the world. It is his relationship to the world that has caused him to develop illness, and only by harmonizing this relationship can we affect his illness. If we can assist him in developing a harmonious interaction with his world, he will have no need to react defensively, and he can then heal.

In reality, we need both acute and constitutional prescribing at different times and in different situations. Disease is often a blend of external stress and individual reaction. With food poisoning, for example, the stress is very similar for most individuals, so *Arsenicum album* is effective in most cases (in my experience). Emotional stress such as grief, however, expresses very differently in different individuals, thus we need many different remedies for the resultant illnesses among the different individuals.

In practice, the approach is similar in that we take the entire picture of the disease in the sick animal and find a remedy that covers this entire picture. What we sometimes find, though, is that the remedy that fits the current state will not cure the illness. In this case we need a remedy that matches the individual more intimately. We may need to go through her entire life history to find a common thread, to see who she is and how she relates to the world in all situations. Her constitution influences how she responds, even to an acute illness, and thus she needs a remedy that addresses her constitutional response rather than the acute illness. She needs a constitutional prescription because her way of responding to external stress is not maintaining her health. Instead, it is contributing to her disease.

Carrying this idea further, the constitutional remedy may be beneficial throughout the life of the individual. An occasional dose of the constitutional remedy can put someone back on course any time she begins to develop symptoms of illness. Thus we may speak of a *"Phosphorus* cat" or a *"Sulphur* dog." As individuality creeps into play, however, I find that this does not always hold true. While some practitioners hold steadfastly to the idea of finding the constitutional remedy and staying with it for the life of the individual, others believe that the needed remedy may change with time. In my experience, both situations occur. Sometimes one remedy does help a given animal time after time, but in other cases different remedies may be needed as healing occurs. This has inspired the concept of layers of illness. One disease state, or layer, is treated with a remedy, and then another layer emerges. In another scenario, sometimes an acute remedy is needed by an animal who generally responds to a different constitutional remedy.

It is part of the difficulty of homeopathy that many situations occur, thus hard-and-fast rules quickly create confusion. It is not necessary that you fully understand all of these variations, as you will be treating acute conditions only. I have endeavored to explain this so you can understand when your acute prescribing may be inadequate and constitutional prescribing may be needed. When this is the case, it generally means that your companion suffers from chronic illness, another way of saying that his constitutional response is not keeping him healthy. It will then be necessary to examine his life as an individual to see what remedy will assist him in all areas of his life. I recommend that you consult with an experienced veterinary homeopath for this.

How to Use the Treatment Chapters

This section describes the layout of the following ten chapters, which cover home care. Chapters Six through Fourteen cover one system at a time, explaining briefly how the system works and how it malfunctions. Treatment is then directed toward these malfunctions. As homeopathy is symptom-based treatment, this is an attempt to approximate the classical approach. Chapter Fifteen, "Therapeutic Indications by Condition," covers conditions that do not fit into other chapters for various reasons. These conditions are listed alphabetically, and each section is self-contained.

For a particular problem with your companion animal, one of the treatment chapters should provide information specific to his condition. You must first identify the main complaint and turn to the chapter that covers the affected system. Here you will find information that helps you determine the severity of the condition and gives treatment suggestions. If a condition is potentially serious, I list signs that indicate if you should seek veterinary care. For some conditions I have given different levels of severity and the relative urgency of seeking help. In any case, seek help if you are unsure. If your veterinarian assures you that the condition is not too serious, you have the right to choose home treatment. Inform the veterinarian what you wish to do and why. Keep her in the loop, and she will be more responsive to your needs if home treatment is unsuccessful. Make it a team effort.

If you determine that the disease is minor enough to treat at home, you need to evaluate the symptoms to help you see the character of the illness as it affects your companion. For most conditions I list things to look for to help you individualize the disease. This will help you choose the correct remedy.

Before getting to the remedy, though, I list supportive treatments. This may be therapies like hot compresses for abscesses, cleaning solutions for ear problems, or vitamin and herbal supplements to enhance healing. I have listed dosage and preparation instructions in each section to facilitate usage. For herbs and vitamins I give the dosage on a per-pound basis. Generally there is a range, and as long as you stay within the range you will be OK. This allows you to more easily match an available capsule or tablet strength to your animal's weight. Simply multiply the weight by the per-pound dosage to get the total dose. You may round up or down to get to a convenient total. As a general rule, smaller animals require a higher dose per pound than larger ones, so if you have a large dog, use the lower amount. For cats and small dogs, the higher amount is often appropriate. In some cases cats are very sensitive to supplements, and I may give a separate dose for cats.

I believe that most herbal use should be short-term. Medicinal herbs often contain potentially toxic substances, and these may accumulate in the body over a lengthy administration period. Use an herb for three to four weeks, and then stop for a week before restarting. Continue in this manner for a few cycles if necessary, but if you do not see a response, stop the herb. Some herbs, such as goldenseal, are even stronger, and a shorter usage is better, while some herbs, such as dandelion, are quite safe. Check with an herbalist or a reference book (Tilford's is good—see the appendix) if you are unsure and you wish to use an herb for a longer time.

Once you have read about your companion's condition and understand the general care, you will want to choose a homeopathic medicine to aid the healing. Keep in mind that the chosen remedy will work best if it matches not only the main complaint but also any other symptoms, including mental and emotional states. Anything that has changed in association with the main complaint is a part of the disease picture and needs to be taken into consideration when you select a remedy.

For each condition I list several remedies that may help. Each remedy has a slightly different picture, and hopefully you will find a remedy that will match your companion's disease state. When you find a remedy or two that seem possible, turn to the *materia medica* (Part Four) to read the broad description of each remedy under consideration. This should strengthen the case for one of the remedies.

I recommend that you always confirm your choice by reading about the remedy in the *materia medica* rather than making your selection from the treatment chapter only, as this will not only clarify your choice, but it will also teach you more about the remedy. The more you use homeopathic medicines, the more they become like good friends that you can rely upon in times of need. Purchase and refer to other *materia medicas* also; I list some good choices in the appendix. The better you know each remedy, the more easily you can decide which one to call upon in a given circumstance. With time, you will be able to prescribe for many situations from your own knowledge and experience, though it never hurts to confirm your idea by rereading the *materia medica*. Even those of us with a lot of experience do this daily.

If none of the remedies fit, make certain you have emphasized the appropriate symptoms. Reconsider the case from a different perspective if necessary to see if this helps. If you still come up empty, it is possible that the correct remedy is not listed, as this book is a general guide and is limited in scope (there are over two thousand homeopathic remedies available). If you cannot find an appropriate choice, or if you obtain poor response to your choices, you may need the help of a friend or practitioner with more experience. You may also need to read other homeopathic books for help. Check the appendix for other books on homeopathy. A repertory will give more remedy choices, and a book on the homeopathic *materia medica* may give you a different description that will help you see that one of the listed remedies is correct. While my book is very comprehensive, I fully recognize that no book can have an answer to every problem, and I encourage you to seek elsewhere if you don't find an answer here.

Dosage: How to Handle and Administer Remedies

Once you choose a remedy, you must give it to the patient. While not complicated, this is very important, as there are differences from conventional drugs. Remedies work at subtle energy levels, so they are sensitive to interference from other substances. We call this "antidoting," and it may occur before or after administration. For the best effect, homeopathic medicines must be given directly into the mouth. Mixing with food may neutralize the remedy, so avoid this method if possible. Even food particles remaining in the mouth can be a problem, so wait at least fifteen to thirty minutes after a meal to administer the remedy. It is not important whether the stomach is full or empty, just that the mouth is neutral. Additionally, some practitioners feel that exposure to sunlight, electromagnetic fields, and strong odors like camphor and mint can neutralize remedies in the vial. I don't know how commonly remedies are antidoted in the vial, but I recommend caution as the best course. Don't store remedies near spices, electric appliances, or windows.

Homeopathic remedies are available at many herbal and health food stores. Common remedies may easily be obtained locally, though you may have limited choice of potency. Further, the most commonly available remedies come in plastic vials. I do not like plastic, and at times I find these remedies less effective than those stored and sold in glass. I recommend ordering remedies in amber glass vials when you have the option. If you believe you have the correct remedy, but you do not get a response, it is possible that your remedy is not active. While this is uncommon, it does happen; try a different source in this case. Sometimes, even a different vial from the same company may work better, though it is best to change companies if you have the option. Additionally, if you can afford the initial expense, many companies offer kits that contain twenty-five to fifty of the most commonly needed acute remedies. The price per remedy is significantly less than purchasing them separately, and you will often have the remedy you need on hand instead of having to search for it when illness arises. And you can then have a supply of remedies in glass, which will keep better. See the appendix for a list of suppliers that sell homeopathic medicines by mail. Even though the Food and Drug Administration requires an expiration date on homeopathic remedies, they keep almost indefinitely in glass, as long as they are stored away from sunlight, electromagnetic fields, and strong odors.

Before you administer any medicine or supplement, make a connection with your companion to let her know what you intend. Just take a minute or two to calmly think about your desire to help. Speak this to your com-

panion. She may not understand the words, but she will understand the general intent. This is important any time you need to give her something, clean her ears, or do anything that she may not understand or that may induce discomfort. Homeopathic medicines are generally well accepted by animals, but it is still important to communicate prior to administration. See the accompanying photographs if you are uncertain about just how to administer homeopathic medicines.

Remedies may be dispensed as solids (pellets or tablets) or liquids.

Pellets are the most commonly available form, though tissue salts (a sub-group of homeopathic medications, also called cell salts) often come on tablets. To administer pellets or tablets (pills), simply drop a few of either into the mouth. Use the cap of the vial to hold them, as handling them may negate their effect in some cases. Most cats and dogs readily take pills since these have a pleasant taste, unlike conventional drugs. Another option is to use two spoons and grind a few pellets into a powder, and then pour this

into the mouth. This way the animal cannot spit the pills out, though I rarely find that to be a big problem. Pellets and tablets have a minimal, sweet taste, so animals tolerate these readily. Furthermore, when you mostly (or only) administer these acceptable-tasting remedies, your cat or dog won't resist being given medications as much as with conventional medicines. If your cat or dog does spit out the pills, usually they have already been exposed to the remedy, especially with pellets, as the remedy is on the surface of pellets. If the pellets were in the mouth even ten to fifteen seconds, the dose is probably sufficient. Wet dosing, however, obviates this concern altogether. We refer to pellets and tablets as dry doses, and liquid remedies as wet doses.

For one or a few doses, dry dosing is fine. Over the years, however, I've realized that wet dosing works better and more gently for most situations. As with dry dosing, for only a few doses you can simply dissolve a few pellets in a small amount of water. For example, I commonly put two to four pellets in one or two ounces of nonchlorinated water. Once these dissolve, I usually give a dropperful to a cat or small dog, and one-half to two teaspoonfuls to larger dogs. This solution keeps fine for a day or two, and stirring briskly before each successive dose improves the response. I recommend spring water or filtered water for homeopathic remedies because of the possibility of interference by the chemicals in most city tap water. Be cautious about bottled water labeled "drinking water" as the source may be questionable.

For longer periods, it is best to use a liquid remedy. You can purchase most remedies in liquid form from homeopathic pharmacies, though these are often more expensive than pelleted forms, and you won't find liquid remedies on the shelf in herbal or health food stores. It is simple, however, to make a liquid remedy from a pelleted form. There are a few reasons to do this. First, as I mentioned above, for some reason remedies in liquid form seem to work more powerfully yet at the same time more gently. Secondly, our bodies rather poorly tolerate repeating the exact same potency more than a few times. Following repeated "exact potency doses," the patient may aggravate for a time, or she may not respond well, if at all. Very low potencies, like 6X or 6C, do not seem as troublesome as higher potencies, but even with these it works better to alter the potency each time. How do we do this? We normally increase potency by dilution and succussion (See Chapter One). If we shake a liquid remedy, however, this succussion alone *slightly* increases its potency, even without further dilution, as it is the added energy that raises the strength. The remedy then works more powerfully, and the body does not react adversely to an exact potency repetition. Repeating the exact same potency sometimes also results in diminishing response or no response. Often poor response comes first, and further repetition gives aggravation. This is similar to a palliative response, but can also occur with exact potency repetition. Third, with liquid dosing, as soon as the remedy touches the mucous membranes of the mouth, the remedy begins to work, and we need not worry about spitting out pellets or some of the dose. And the liquid quickly spreads out, hitting many more nerve endings than pellets, improving the exposure to the remedy. Finally, with liquid remedies we can readily alter the dose (the amount of remedy), fine-tuning the dose for optimal effect without aggravation.

I was taught that the dose does not matter, and that we only need concern ourselves with potency when administering remedies. In the decade or so since I wrote the first edition, however, I have found that dose matters in many cases. I learned this from some clients, who said such things as, "I tried four pellets, as you suggested, but it did not help, so I gave him ten pellets, and he's much better." After hearing this a couple of times, I began to experiment with different doses in my patients, and I soon verified these reports. Further work with liquid remedies has broadened my understanding and improved my results.

Here is how it works: we have four steps, including (as step one, if necessary) making the stock liquid remedy. Step two is succussing (shaking) the bottle to increase the potency. Step three is putting some of the liquid remedy into a second container for dosing, and step four is giving the dose.

The first step, if necessary, is to make your liquid remedy. This only need be done once with each remedy at a given potency. To make a liquid remedy from dry pellets (I don't believe tablets work as well for this), take a one-ounce dropper bottle and fill it with one-third brandy or vodka and two-thirds nonchlorinated water. (A one-ounce bottle is a common size, used for most herbal tinctures. You can reuse one of these; simply wash it well, being sure to separate the dropper from the bulb so you can wash out the bulb. Use a bottle with a glass dropper.) Place four pellets of your remedy into the bottle, and allow them to dissolve. Shake the bottle three or four times. This becomes your stock remedy.

Dosing is then a three-step process, which you will do for each dose, or at least each day. First, succuss (shake) the bottle by holding it in one

MAKING A LIQUID STOCK REMEDY FROM PELLETS

←——— One-ounce dropper bottle

←——— One-third brandy or vodka

←——— Two-thirds non-chlorinated water

←——— Add four pellets of your remedy

fist and hitting the heel of the other hand with that fist. This increases the strength. I typically use five shakes, though you can vary from one to ten successions, depending upon your patient's sensitivity. (See below for variations in any of these three dosing steps.) Next, put one to ten drops into one-fourth to one cup of water. As with successions, I usually use five drops as a middle ground, again depending upon sensitivity. And I almost always use one-quarter cup. Finally, take your dose from that water dilution. Use a clean dropper, spoon, or syringe for the dose—not the dropper from the bottle. The dose can be from one drop to one teaspoonful. I usually give one dropperful to cats and small dogs, up to one teaspoonful to larger dogs (forty-five pounds and over). Give about one-half teaspoonful to mid-size dogs. One teaspoon is about five cc (milliliters); one dropper is about half a cc.

The wide range of shakes, drops into the water, and doses from the water provides great flexibility, especially for sensitive animals. Sensitive animals may easily aggravate, so using minimum shakes, drops, and doses helps them tolerate the remedy better. If you give a dose and your patient worsens, especially if this occurs rapidly, he may be sensitive. Try one shake, one drop, and a smaller dose. You may also place the one drop into a larger water volume, for example one-half cup, or even one cup. This further softens the dose. At the other end of the spectrum, less sensitive animals may need more shakes and drops, and a larger dose, to respond. If you feel your

LIQUID REMEDY DOSING

Shake stock bottle five times
Put five drops into ¼ cup water
Stir, and then give:
    One dropperful to cats and small dogs*
    One-half teaspoonful to medium dogs
    One teaspoonful to large dogs
    *use a different dropper

Vary amounts as needed (see text)

remedy choice is correct but you don't see a response, try increasing these amounts before changing remedies. I realize this is probably confusing, but with time you will better understand these subtleties. These situations will probably be very uncommon, so generally you can follow the instructions for average animals, as follows.

As a starting point, here is how I would use this for average animals— the vast majority: I usually use five succussions and put five drops into one-quarter cup of water. Then I give one dropperful (with a clean dropper) to cats and small dogs, up to one teaspoonful for large dogs (over forty to fifty pounds). Then I watch to see how my patient responds. If she overreacts, I'll reduce the amounts; if there is a poor response, I'll increase the amounts, assuming I still believe I have the best remedy. To increase or decrease the strength, I usually increase or decrease the number of succussions and drops, usually together. So I might use three succussions and three drops, but the same dose from the one-quarter cup of water. If my patient is very sensitive, I may use one cup for the dilution, and then only give one drop out of that cup to the patient. It is even possible to take a few drops from the first cup and put these into a second cup, and dose from there for extremely sensitive patients. You will rarely or never need to do this, though. I do it rarely myself, usually with chronically ill patients who are quite debilitated, wherein I would not recommend home treatments. If you are working with an experienced homeopath, however, you might use this.

To recap, then, make your stock bottle with one-fourth brandy or vodka and three-fourths nonchlorinated water in a one-ounce dropper bottle. Into this, put four pellets of your remedy. For each dosing, shake the bottle five times, put five drops into one-fourth cup of water, and give one dropperful to one teaspoonful to your animal, depending upon size, and using a clean dropper. Throw out the balance of the water mix, making a new dilution for each dose (but not a new stock bottle; this you keep). Adjust your dose if needed. If you need to give several doses in one day, you can keep the water dilution, stirring briskly before each successive dose, and then make a new dilution each day, though there may be a slight advantage to mixing the water dilution freshly each time. (You may wonder why I said above that when simply dissolving pellets into an ounce or two of water, you could keep the solution for one or two days, whereas here I suggest keeping the solution no longer than a day. In this latter situation, we wish to change the potency with more certainty, and shaking the stock bottle and then diluting in a fresh solution does this. In the first case, by contrast, where we merely dissolved pellets into water, we are only administering the remedy for a short time, wherein potency change is not as critical.)

For dry dosing, here are some guidelines for amounts: whereas tablet size is standard, pellets come in three primary sizes. The number thirty-five is most common and is about the size of a BB; the number ten is tiny, about the size of a poppy seed, and the number twenty is about the size of a sesame seed—about one-half the diameter of the number thirty-five and twice the diameter of the number ten. Put another way, the number thirty-five is about one-eighth of an inch in diameter, the number twenty is slightly larger than one-sixteenth of an inch, and the number ten is slightly larger than one-thirty-second of an inch in diameter. I therefore consider that one number thirty-five pellet equals about two number twenty pellets or five number ten pellets. Here are average dose quantities for number thirty-five pellets: for cats and small dogs I usually give two to three pellets; for medium-sized dogs I use four to six pellets; and for large dogs I give six to ten pellets. I consider tablets as basically equivalent to number thirty-five pellets, so use the same dosage (they are slightly larger, so use the minimum number).

Table 5-1

PELLET SIZE	CATS AND SMALL DOGS (up to 15 pounds)	MEDIUM DOGS (16–45 pounds)	LARGE DOGS (over 45 pounds)
Number 35 (BB-sized)	2–3 pellets	4–6 pellets	6–10 pellets
Number 20 (sesame seed–sized)	4–6 pellets	8–12 pellets	12–20 pellets
Number 10 (poppy seed–sized)	10–15 pellets	20–30 pellets	30–50 pellets
Fine granules (celery seed–sized)	15–30 granules	30–40 granules	40–75 granules
Tablets (primarily cell salts)	2 tablets	4 tablets	6 tablets

Adjust accordingly for smaller pellets—multiply by two for number twenty pellets, and by five for number ten pellets. Some British pharmacies offer "fine granules," which are about the size of celery seeds. For these, use the number ten amounts, or a little more. With the smallest sizes, your count can be approximate, and after a time or two you can "eyeball" the amount.

Potency and Repetition

Choosing the Right Potency

Another area of confusion is the different potency scales. Remember that remedies that are diluted tenfold at each step are referred to as "X" potencies (Roman numeral X = ten), and those that are diluted one hundredfold are "C" potencies (Roman numeral C = one hundred). Thus a 3X remedy has been diluted one part in ten, three times. A 6C remedy has been diluted one part in one hundred, six times. See "Potentization: Dilution and Succussion" in Chapter One if this is unclear. Centesimal (C) potencies are stronger than their numerical decimal (X) counterpart because of the greater dilution. So a 6C has greater impact than a 6X. Just why this is the case is unclear, but succussion probably imparts the strength, and one theory is that the greater dilution provides more "room" for the strength to accumulate. One chemical explanation involves tension because of hydrogen bonds between molecules, and the tension increases with greater dilution. The reason is unimportant; experience validates the empirical observation of the greater power of C potencies. Similarly, a 6C potency is separate from a 12C potency. *Whether you give one or ten pellets of a 6C remedy to your companion, you have still given a 6C remedy. Two 6C pellets do not equal a 12C pellet.*

○ 6C + ○ 6C does not = ○12C

We cannot directly correlate the two scales, but experience lends comparative value. The most commonly used decimal potencies are the 6X, 12X, 30X, and (less commonly) 200X. These are *approximately* equivalent to 3C, 6C, 12C, and 60C in my experience. Among the three lower strengths, the corresponding X is probably slightly stronger (12X slightly greater than 6C, for example). The highest potency sold without a prescription is 30C; among the decimal potencies, 30X is the highest available without a prescription. There is no 30C equivalent, as the X potencies jump from 30X to 200X.

Table 5-2

APPROXIMATE POTENCY EQUIVALENTS BETWEEN C AND X POTENCIES			
6X	12X	30X	200X
3C	6C	12C	60C

If we require stronger potencies, we use the centesimal remedies. Although 60C and 100C potencies are available, as are others in this range, we typically step up from a 6C to a 12C to a 30C, and then to a 200C. Higher C potencies are usually designated with the letter *M* (Roman numeral M = 1,000). This usage means the number of dilution steps, i.e. 1,000C = 1M, 10,000C = 10M, 50,000C= 50M. A potency of 100,000C is designated as CM, and a potency of 1,000,000C is called MM. The latter would be a substance diluted 1:100—one million times! These high potencies (above 30C) should only be used under the guidance of an experienced homeopath.

Potency choice is a complex area with few hard and fast rules, so it is difficult to describe accurately. Every case is a little different; it is part of the individualization of homeopathic treatment. I do have some guidelines to help, and with time you will get a feel for choosing the correct potency. The main variables to consider are the intensity of the illness, the overall strength (vital force) of the animal, the certainty of your remedy choice, and the strength of the remedy.

- **First:** Match the intensity of the disease process with the intensity (potency) of the remedy. An acute, aggressive disease, such as a high fever in a young animal, will respond more quickly to high potencies. Experienced homeopathic veterinarians often use 200C, 1M, or 10M potencies here. I do not recommend using greater than 30C or possibly 200C, however, without assistance from someone who is experienced. It is possible to cause serious problems with higher potencies if they are repeated too often or too many times. A longer-lasting disease process with a slow, steady onset cannot heal rapidly—it must be reversed slowly in turn. Thus, we usually start with lower potencies such as 6C, 9C, or 12C. These may be repeated daily to every few days depending upon the case and the response to the remedy.
- **Second:** Match the strength of the vital force with the potency. This is very important. A weak individual simply cannot tolerate a big

jolt that may be the result of a high potency. In this case, it could cause serious worsening of the condition, or even death. With older or frail animals we use 6C, sometimes 6X, given very infrequently. Here also, liquid dosing works much better; see the previous section. Strong symptoms generally indicate a strong vital force, as a weak vital force cannot muster the strength to produce symptoms. Extremely aggressive conditions like canine parvovirus disease or food poisoning can rapidly deplete the body, however, so if the condition does not improve rapidly in the early stages, lower potencies must be used as the disease progresses and the body weakens. A strong vital force will tend to localize the disease to one area of the body, and to the periphery (skin) or to less important organs such as the ears.

- **Third:** Match the strength of the potency with the accuracy of the prescription. The wrong remedy usually has little impact, but occasionally it may cause problems by simply aggravating the disease without providing a curative response. If there is any question about the correctness of the remedy, it is best to start with a low potency. You can always raise the potency with successive prescriptions. Some practitioners always start with a 6C, for example, particularly in chronic cases. While I do not generally like rote prescribing practices, this is a safe one. If the potency is too low, however, even the correct remedy may not have an effect in a strong disease state, so successive potency increases may be needed to determine the accuracy of the prescription.

- **Fourth:** Match the potency with the strength of the remedy. Some remedies are simply more powerful than others, and some remedies are more likely to produce aggravations. This is particularly true when starting a case. *Sulphur* and *Lycopodium* are two remedies that are very deep and powerful. Accuracy is a must when starting a chronic case with one of these. Most of the polychrests (broad, deep-acting, major remedies) are in this category, while more specific or more superficial remedies are less troublesome when inaccurately prescribed. The nosodes, like *Tuberculinum, Medorrhinum, Syphilinum,* and *Psorinum,* as well as vaccine remedies, fit into this category as well. For this reason, these should only be used under the supervision of an experienced homeopath. This concern primarily applies to chronic disease treatment and involves *materia medica* study to know which remedies are in each category. Most people will not be concerned with this aspect, as these cases should be treated by an experienced prescriber, but use caution with these remedies and don't repeat them too often.

Repeating the Dose

How often should you repeat a dose of the chosen remedy? Waiting is almost always preferable to repeating or changing the remedy. This is because it is the body's response that does the work once the remedy acts as a stimulus. It may take time for the body to respond, so we must allow adequate time. Furthermore, with lower potencies we may need a few doses before beginning to see a response. The response will depend upon the same basic factors that aided our choice of potency: More intense and rapidly changing illnesses demand quicker action, while slower states require waiting. Waiting is perhaps the most important and the most difficult part of homeopathy. We must know what to expect in our response (see Chapter Three, "The Nature of Cure") so we can tell if the response is good. We must also have a sense of the illness at hand (see Chapter Two, "The Nature of Disease"). And sometimes we just have to be patient and allow the body to do the work.

Remember that the best indicator is behavior, and that we like to see evidence that the patient feels better early in the treatment. In severe cases this may be as subtle as improved brightness of the eyes, or the fact that your companion follows your movement around the house rather than remaining withdrawn. Or perhaps she sniffs at food without eating, whereas before she turned away from food altogether.

There are some general principles. Higher potencies require and tolerate less repetition. Lower potencies may be repeated as needed or on a schedule. Beyond that statement, there is much difference in individual styles of prescription. Classically, the midpoint between high and low potencies is 30C.

As I have stated, I recommend using 30C and under unless you are experienced, so I will emphasize these potencies. I can only give ranges of time since each case is different, but this will give you a good idea of where to start, and your patient will guide you further. You will need to repeat the dose more often or use a higher potency for more intense states, but if you start with a low potency and give the remedy less often, you can always go higher or dose more frequently. The following chart gives a general guideline for potency and repetition according to the intensity of the condition.

Table 5-3

POTENCY	REPETITION			
	Intense	Moderate	Slow	Chronic
6X	every 5–30 minutes	every 1–4 hours	3–4 times per day	1–4 times day day
6C, 12X	every 5–30 minutes	every 3–6 hours	2–4 times per day	every 3 days to 4 times per day
12C, 30X	every 5–60 minutes	every 8–12 hours	1–2 times per day	every 1–7 days day
30C	every 5–90 minutes	every 12–24 hours	every 1–4 days	weekly to monthly or less

"Intense," "moderate," and "slow" refer to the severity or intensity of the illness, and "chronic" is for treatment of chronic conditions. An intense condition would be shock, collapse, or other life-threatening situations (these conditions should only be treated as you seek veterinary help). Moderate conditions might include gastrointestinal illness like parvovirus infections or severe respiratory distress—these conditions should also have veterinary supervision. Slow conditions would be feline upper respiratory infections, milder cases of diarrhea and vomiting, and so on. Intense, moderate, and slow conditions correspond somewhat to the medical categories peracute, acute, and subacute, respectively. Chronic conditions include asthma, seizures, skin disease, thyroid disease, ear infections, and autoimmune diseases. Chronic cases comprise the majority of my practice. They are very slow-moving and should be handled by a competent homeopathic veterinarian if possible. Of course, these divisions are somewhat arbitrary, and there is quite a gray zone between them, so use them as guideposts but not immoveable barriers.

The classic method of timing the dose is to give a remedy, wait for a response, and as long as there is improvement, do not repeat the dose. This method works best with higher potencies, so we tend to repeat low-potency remedies as often as we deem necessary, trying to approximate the duration of effect. If the remedy is not administered often enough there may·be a roller coaster effect, though the patient will still improve overall if the remedy is correct. If the repetition is too frequent, we may get an intensification of the symptoms over time; this intensification tells us to stop the remedy until the symptoms settle and then to use it less often. Evaluating the response is critical here, as the wrong remedy can do the same things if palliation is occurring (see Chapter Three, "The Nature of Cure"). You may also need to alter the dose—see the section on dosage above. This assessment can be tricky, but the main factor is that your patient should be improving in all aspects, especially her behavior. She should feel better as time elapses, but this will shift in relation to the intensity and the duration of her illness. As I mentioned above, liquid dosing can aid you in these cases, as you can repeat more frequently without aggravation, and adjust the dose for better effect without excessive reactions.

As she improves, reduce the frequency of administration until you can stop the remedy. She should continue to improve without the remedy when the cure has gotten some momentum. At this point you can use 30C, 30X, or 12C strengths on an as-needed basis, repeating only when she slips.

Occasionally an animal will worsen shortly after a remedy is given. This may be an indication that the remedy has resonated with the patient, and improvement may follow the worsening. These "curative aggravations" are generally short-lived, and the animal's attitude may indicate that improvement is coming. If you see a worsening, watch cautiously to see if improvement follows. Don't be in a hurry to change remedies or to repeat the dose. You should know within a reasonable time if your companion is going to improve.

Curative aggravations generally last only a few minutes in an intense illness, perhaps thirty minutes or an hour in a moderate illness, and a few hours to a day in a slow illness. Improvement will follow closely on the heels of the aggravation if the response is curative. If the remedy is incorrect, the animal will either continue to worsen or simply return to the state that existed prior to administering the remedy. Although the homeopathic aggravation is well-known and some people feel it is a necessary precursor to healing, it is not always present. In fact, if the potency is correct, there will not be an aggravation. The patient simply improves until she is cured.

Monitoring Your Companion's Progress

I was talking with a neighbor and expert gardener today, during a break between writing, asking her advice on gardening in the harsh New Mexico climate, and she emphatically said, "Keep good notes on everything you try. You think you'll remember, but you won't." I thought that to be apt advice here as well. Use your notes from taking the case as a starting point, and periodically check everything on the list. Often my clients tell me they see no change, but when I ask about different symptoms, these may have improved a lot. Once things change it is easy to forget the original condition. By the same token, sometimes I hear a good report, but the details do not support the initial assessment. We sometimes wish to see things so much that we color our vision. I have found this to be true with my household companions—it is very easy to be inaccurate without good notes. And if you have to seek outside homeopathic help, your notes will be valuable for the prescriber.

Use a notebook to track the progress, making new entries as necessary. The frequency will depend upon the illness itself; allow time for the body to heal. In slower cases, a calendar might work well. This is another area where you must use judgment. Err on the side of too often until you see what interval works best. If you must take a temperature, try to keep this at a minimum, since the invasiveness may add to your companion's discomfort. (It is possible to take the temperature under the "armpit" as with children; the reading will be about one degree Fahrenheit below the rectal temperature.) You must balance your need for information with his need for comfort, as comfort and a good state of mind encourage healing.

Always keep in mind that the emotional state is of primary importance when evaluating progress; these symptoms often improve before the local physical symptoms. Hering's Rule of Cure provides help here as well, particularly the observation that symptoms often improve in the reverse order of their original appearance. If you see this pattern of improvement, you can generally relax and watch the improvement continue.

If you do not see improvement in a timely manner, however, you must make a change. See a veterinarian if necessary, or change your remedy choice if your patient is not too sick but not improving. For an intense condition, you should seek immediate advice in any case, but even while you are on the way to the veterinary hospital, change the remedy if you don't see improvement quickly. If the interval between doses is correct, you will usually know within two or three doses if your companion is responding. Switch remedies if he is not responding, and continue to treat even during the conventional care if allowed.

For less urgent conditions the same two-to-three-dose rule of thumb applies as well—dose according to the chart above for repetition times, and two to three doses should give enough time for an evaluation. Improvement may be subtle, so if you are not sure of the response, you should wait a bit longer. This is especially true for slow-moving conditions. Changing remedies too soon is one of the biggest mistakes of novices, and understanding how long to wait is something you learn with time—even as an individual case progresses.

Summary

Once you have determined that your companion's illness is safe to treat at home, the following steps are the basis of treatment.

Taking the Case

Look at the entire picture of your companion's state *since she became ill.* Consider not only the main complaint, but also any other changes that accompanied the main problem. If there are behavior changes, these are especially important. Try to create an image of her illness as it affects her, especially how it differs from a similar illness in another animal. Try to see the individuality of her illness.

Choosing a Remedy and a Treatment Plan

Once you have the image of your companion's illness in your mind, read the appropriate section in the treatment chapters for conditions that may warrant taking her to a veterinarian for supportive care and for remedy suggestions. Once you find possible remedies, read about each one in the *materia medica* to determine which one is best for your companion. Remember that homeopathic medicines are very specific and must be individually matched to your companion's condition. Don't simply give a remedy that covers the primary complaint, but find one that matches the overall picture.

Dose, Potency, Repetition

Use the chart in this chapter to determine the appropriate repetition time for your remedy, depending upon the potency you choose (or the available potency). Any potency under 30C is acceptable for home treatment, but the time between redosing will vary according to potency. Don't repeat the remedy more than a few times if you are not seeing a good response. Liquid dosing generally works better than dry dosing, though the latter is acceptable if few doses are needed.

Monitoring

Keep good notes and check all symptoms for improvement. It is especially important that your companion's attitude and behavior improve as the physical symptoms improve. If you do not see improvement in a timely manner, reevaluate the case and change the remedy as needed. Don't change too soon, however. Give the body time to heal. Remember that occasionally you may see a slight worsening after giving the remedy, though this should not last very long. Improvement should then follow. It is not necessary that this worsening (aggravation) occurs, however.

Seek Help If Needed

Finally, if you do not see improvement right away, seek help. This may be from a homeopathic veterinarian or a conventional veterinarian, depending upon the urgency of the illness and the availability of homeopathic care.

Chapter Six
SKIN AND EARS

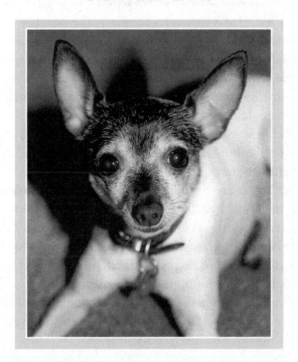

Overview

Function

Skin Infections and Eruptions

Overview

I have included ear problems with skin symptoms, since the external ears (including the ear canals) are essentially part of the skin. Both organs originate from the same type of tissue in the embryo, and they generally respond similarly when illness occurs. As superficial parts of the body, these organs tend to be affected early in the course of chronic illness. They also seem to have a large capacity for disease in the sense that the body can limit disease symptoms to the skin and ears for a long time, even though the illness is worsening. Remember that homeopathic disease theory groups all symptoms as part of one illness rather than separate diseases, and that the skin is typically affected first since it is exterior. I recommend that you read Chapter Two, "The Nature of Disease," before reading this chapter. This will assist you in understanding that skin disease is an outwardly visible manifestation of serious internal chronic disease.

The body attempts to keep the disease centered in organs that are not essential for life or that can take a lot of insult before becoming life-threatening. The skin and ears fulfill this requirement nicely. Because they are affected early and can be severely damaged without major limitations to health, these organs are sort of a "dumping ground" for chronic illness—very unsightly but not necessarily dangerous.

The importance of this is that almost all skin and ear ailments are external manifestations of internal, chronic disease and must be treated as such—not as local, isolated conditions. These diseases are usually of great substance (the animal is much more ill than he appears), though this is often misunderstood because it is "only" the skin that is perceived to be affected. Although they may appear suddenly, they often have been developing over a long period of time, thus the great substance or mass they carry; the skin symptoms are like the tip of an iceberg. This "mass of illness" has great inertia, thus skin and ear ailments are extremely difficult to treat and slow to cure. Veterinarians (other than those brave or foolish enough to become dermatologists) generally consider skin disease to be the bane of our practice. It certainly was a great motivator for me in my search for better methods of treatment.

Skin and ear diseases are very frustrating for veterinarian and guardian alike because the symptoms are very visible and the patient may be quite uncomfortable. Recovery takes a long time and requires a lot of patience and trust—this can be difficult in the presence of an itchy, constantly scratching dog—especially if he keeps you up at night. Full recovery from chronic skin affections may take two to three years, though improvement begins within a month or so on the correct remedy and diet. Diet is important in all situations, but with skin and ear symptoms it is crucial; I believe that healing of these ailments is almost impossible without an excellent diet that includes fresh food and raw meats. Many other factors may interfere, such as allergens (the substances to which the animal is allergic), toxins, and emotional stress. As discussed elsewhere, topical pesticides, often used on animals with skin ailments, cause damage to the liver and kidneys, and sometimes directly induce itching, so these are not good choices for skin ailments. See the section on fleas in Chapter Fifteen.

Allergies are not caused by the allergen—they are an internal problem first. The immune system becomes overreactive and then develops an allergy to whatever potential allergens are around. A flea allergy is not caused by fleas; rather the dog is already potentially allergic and fleas are common, so he develops an allergy to the flea saliva. The immune system must be compromised first, and this is often caused by other stressors like vaccines, toxins, and poor foods. Once the allergy is present, however, the continued allergic reaction may keep the dog from responding to treatment, so the allergens must be avoided as much as possible until the sensitivity can be diminished. If fleas are the problem, holistic flea control is essential; if food allergies are present, those foods must be avoided until the allergy lessens through treatment.

In my experience and according to research,[1] vaccination is a major factor in initiating skin problems. Immune system sensitization and stimulation creates fertile ground for allergic and autoimmune skin reactivity, and in practice we see that skin diseases often arise in four- to eight-month-old animals—during the time of intensive vaccination. Additionally, many skin allergies worsen within a one- to three-month period following a booster immunization (see Chapter Sixteen, "Vaccination," for more information).

The role of toxins and poor indoor air quality has been overlooked in both human and veterinary fields for years. Although gaining attention these days, the impact of environmental illness is continually dismissed by many medical experts despite a growing base of well-documented evidence. Toxins can readily damage the body and disrupt the immune system, leading to allergies and many other problems. I believe poor indoor air quality may be as large a deterrent to recovery from skin disease and other ailments as diet and vaccination.

Finally, emotional stress is a well-recognized cause of skin problems, from psychosomatic itching to self-mutilation from boredom or intense emotional discomfort. This has been recognized in cats for years, often because of the notion that cats can live comfortably in a small apartment without going outside. In reality, many cats become quite stressed when kept inside, especially when they are alone a lot or when there are too many cats in a house and not enough room for each cat to have its own space. Dogs can also suffer from these stresses, usually from similar circumstances—being left alone a lot, kept in a pen, not getting enough exercise—in short, from poor emotional care. Some veterinarians today use drugs like Prozac in these cases, but in my opinion drugs are a poor substitute for proper care.

Since skin and ear ailments are not usually externally caused, topical treatment is almost always risky, though mild substances that can relieve but not suppress the symptoms are safe. Strong treatments that stop symptoms can force the body to move the symptoms of illness to other organs, usually with serious consequences. Products like tar and sulfur shampoos and "cortisone" or antibiotic ointments can easily suppress symptoms, leading to deeper disease symptoms. Oral or injected drugs are even riskier. Homeopaths consider suppression of the skin symptoms to be a major factor in worsening of chronic disease; suppression occurs most commonly following conventional drug therapy, but any method has the potential to suppress if it is incorrectly applied.

For these reasons, I can give little advice regarding treatment of most skin and ear problems. Treating these problems from a guidebook such as this one is generally unsuccessful because the response to treatment is very hard to interpret and the indications for the correct remedy are too complicated. Prescriptions thus tend to be superficial and not too effective. Typically, you may get relief from symptoms for a time, but they tend to recur despite repetition of the remedy. Excessive repetition of homeopathic medicines has the potential to suppress symptoms, though this is not likely with lower potencies. As in all cases, if you do not obtain relief according to the principles of cure (see Chapter Three, "The Nature of Cure"), seek help from an experienced homeopathic practitioner. *Do not just keep giving remedies in an attempt to mask symptoms; this is little better than conventional drug therapy.*

I do not mean to imply that these conditions cannot be treated with homeopathy, or even that you will not have success. But many cases prove very difficult even for experienced homeopathic veterinarians. In this chapter, I will give suggestions to relieve minor problems and will list some major remedies, but I recommend you seek help for most conditions.

Function

The skin primarily serves as a barrier to the outside world, and in a sense it defines the individual—it creates our appearance and demarcates where our physical bodies end and the outside world begins. Hair provides insulation and a protective layer against injury and abrasion. Glands in the skin secrete oils that both condition the hair and coat the skin, providing further protection from water and other chemicals that may irritate the skin. These same glands act as an organ of elimination, so the skin belongs with the liver, kidneys, lungs, and intestines in this capacity. In fact, skin illness may stress these other organs by increasing the demands put upon them; conversely, keeping the skin clean can reduce the load required of the kidneys or the liver when these organs begin to weaken.

Not only does the skin provide an outline for the body, but the coloration and conformation identify the individual visually, while the oil odors identify the individual by smell, so the connection between skin and self-image is great. Some speculate that skin illness in people represents a poor self-image; it may also be said that skin disease represents a failure at maintaining boundaries. Perhaps this is a philosophical reason for skin eruptions following vaccination: the body never has the chance to maintain its boundary because the organisms are injected directly through the skin. Whether or not animals develop psychosomatic illness in this manner is certainly controversial, but the evidence in humans seems strong to me, and I believe nonhuman animals have the capacity to react similarly, if not to the same degree. To assume otherwise seems arrogant to me. I certainly see animals who appear embarrassed following having their fur clipped off, and cats and dogs recognize others who look similar or differently than they do. In fact, after having a couple of clients point out to me that cats more readily accept other cats when the newcomers look like them, I began to observe this myself. As hard as it may be to accept, I have seen that our orange tabbies accepted other orange tabbies much more readily than a black and white cat. And one very observant client, who primarily introduced this idea to me, sticks to black and white cats, as when she attempted to introduce a differently marked cat, things did not go as well. And purebred dogs also accept other dogs of the same breed better than different breeds in many instances. If they are so aware of their appearance, could they develop skin issues like we do, from poor boundaries and poor self-image?

Skin Infections and Eruptions

Skin infections and eruptions, like all symptoms, represent the body's attempt to rid itself of disease. Though we commonly speak of infected skin and ears, the bacteria we culture from these areas are almost always common species that are normally found in these regions. The most common skin infection, known as a "staph" infection, occurs when *Staphylococcus aureus*, a bacterial species that is on virtually everyone's skin, grows in large numbers in sores on the skin. The obvious question is, Why does this occur in one animal and not another if the bacteria are the cause of the problem? The answer lies in Louis Pasteur's opinion from his later years: "The microbe is nothing, the terrain everything." The bacteria have merely seized an opportunity to grow because the body provided the opportunity. It is the same when we clear-cut an area of forest. Blackberry bushes and brambles quickly invade the area, but they did not cause the clear-cut.

Even in "infections" the body is responsible—thus it is extremely difficult to treat an infection of the skin or the ears with antibiotic therapy. Without changing the terrain, the infection will return again and again. Antibiotics may help alleviate the symptoms and slow down an aggressive bacterial growth that has taken a strong hold, but *regaining immune health is the only hope for cure.*

Itching

Itching is probably far and away the greatest reason for calls and trips to the veterinarian, and a source of anguish for all people concerned. Watching a beloved companion scratch and scratch will try the patience of even the most dedicated homeopathy aficionado. Homeopathy can work here, but it may be frustratingly slow. Deep constitutional and antivaccinosis treatment is usually the only way to give permanent relief, and *if your cat or dog is under constitutional treatment, you should not give other remedies.*

General Care for Itching

Obtain a veterinary examination to rule out serious problems if the itching persists for long. This is especially important in puppies, as mange is a possibility. Also in cats with itchy ears, there may be ear mites, but be sure these are confirmed with an otoscope or magnifying glass and not diagnosed simply on the appearance of the discharge. Check for fleas and ticks as well anytime there is itching. Mange does occur on cats, as do lice, but these are uncommon.

Have your companion checked right away:
- if you notice an unusual or foul odor;
- if there is appetite loss or lethargy;
- if *you* develop itchiness and you have a puppy (possibly mange).

Have an examination soon:
- if itching persists more than a week or two;
- if open sores or crusts develop;
- if the condition spreads to other parts of the body.

Mild topical solutions may alleviate the itch enough while homeopathic treatment begins its work. Oatmeal baths or soaks help some animals, as does topical application of a tea or infusion of yellow dock. This herb is available at most health food or herbal stores. Use about one tablespoonful of dry herb to one or two cups of water; prepare by pouring boiling water over the herb and let this sit until cool. Strain off the herb and use the liquid topically as a spray or rinse. Other topical products that may help include aloe, calendula, and green tea.

Fasting can provide temporary but significant relief from itchiness. This is partly because it helps keep the intestines clean; this in turn relieves some of the stress on the skin by reducing the need for elimination through the skin. A two- to three-day fast with a broth and honey or broth and blackstrap molasses (for calories) works well if the animal is strong. A one-day-per-week fast is a good maintenance plan.

Oral supplements that may help include vitamin E (5–10 mg/pound of mixed tocopherols daily), vitamin C (5–10 mg/pound two to three times a day; use a natural form if you can, and use a low dose), pycnogenol (1 mg/pound one to two times a day), and flax seed oil (¼–½ teaspoonful/10 pounds, one to two times a day). Flax seed oil provides omega-3 fatty acids;

other sources (fish, pumpkin seeds, greens, and commercial omega-3 supplements) are fine also. When using these oils, be sure your cat or dog is getting adequate calcium, as these oils promote calcium entry into the skin, and this reduces itching; without the calcium the benefit is minimal. A low dose of slippery elm bark may help some animals, as often food allergies or toxin absorption from the intestine aggravate the skin. This occurs with leaky gut syndrome, wherein intestinal inflammation allows toxins or large proteins to pass through the gut wall, allowing the body to react. The slippery elm bark can heal the gut. Marshmallow root can help here as well. Use about ⅛ teaspoonful for small dogs and cats, up to ½ teaspoonful for large dogs. Give this once or twice a day for two to three months.

Cucumbers or cucumber juice internally can help animals whose skin condition seems especially hot, as cucumbers are cooling. Additionally, cucumbers are mildly bitter, which helps settle the liver, and with skin conditions the liver is often inflamed or congested. See also the section on liver conditions in Chapter Sixteen. Nettle tea may also help internally, or topically on irritated skin.

Bathing helps some animals and aggravates others, and the water temperature will also have an effect. Experiment with different methods, and this information may help determine a useful homeopathic medicine. Use very mild shampoos with minimal ingredients and no conditioners. Try it on your own hair first. It should leave your hair soft and clean with no residue, stiffness, or itchy sensation. Surprisingly, baby shampoos are not very mild. Be sure to rinse very thoroughly, as soap residue can greatly aggravate itchiness and dry skin. Chamomile tea works also as a rinse; this will remove some toxins and calm the skin.

If you find you simply cannot tolerate the itchiness and decide to use drugs, use antihistamines like Benadryl rather than "cortisones" (steroids) like prednisone and prednisolone. Especially avoid the long-acting injections of steroids (like Depo-Medrol), as these are particularly hard on the adrenal glands. Ovaban (also known as megestrol acetate) is occasionally recommended for cats with chronic skin problems, but this should *never* be used as it is highly dangerous, causing diabetes and breast cancer in cats, among other problems.

Homeopathic Medicines to Relieve Itching

Don't give one of these remedies to an animal who is already on another homeo-

pathic medicine. Use these remedies for a short time only, or use them intermittently. Constant repetition of homeopathic medicines can worsen the overall condition just like strong medicines can. If you find you are using remedies daily for more than a few weeks, seek help.

Apis mellifica

Apis is the venom of the honeybee, so its use is indicated for intense burning and itching that is usually accompanied by hot red swollen sores, reminiscent of bee stings. Generalized white puffy swelling may also occur, as may a general redness with intense itching. The face is often swollen and the eyelids shut. The itching tends to be worst at night. Heat worsens while cool air and bathing helps the itching and swelling.

Arsenicum album

Burning is a part of the *Arsenicum* picture here as everywhere. These animals often start with dry, scaly, itching skin, but they may quickly develop infected sores if the condition persists. They may also itch intensely without any eruptions. Restlessness is quite common, especially just after midnight. These animals are usually chilly and, almost paradoxically, warmth relieves the itching.

Astacus fluviatilis

This is crawfish, and can relieve itching on the entire body, especially if associated with liver disease. The *Astacus* picture also includes terrible mouth and gum inflammation (scorbutic gums), so if you see itching with gum inflammation, consider *Astacus*. It will not be needed frequently.

Formica rufa

This remedy is made from red ants, so you can likely imagine the itching that might call for its use. Redness with itching and burning is common; it looks like a nettle rash. Ants have formic acid in their saliva, which stings the skin. There is even an old medical term, *formication*, which means a sensation as if numbers of ants were crawling over a part of the body.

Gout and arthritis are part of the chronic picture of this remedy, especially on the right side, so if your dog has this along with itching, this remedy is a possibility. The itching may be better with warmth like *Arsenicum,* but is also better after midnight—the opposite of *Arsenicum.*

Galphimia glauca

This is a "small remedy," but it has indications in skin allergies: urticaria, herpetic dermatitis, allergic eczema, and mycotic (fungal) eczema. It sometimes provides temporary relief. It is also indicated for recurring herpes of the lips or genitalia, so it could provide help with feline eosinophilic granuloma of the lips.

Histaminum

This remedy is made from histamine, which is a normally occurring bodily chemical that causes the redness and itching in allergic reactions. Histamine is a messenger that comes to an area and induces itching; it does not cause the allergic reaction in the first place. Sometimes the remedy can temporarily alleviate allergic itching, though constitutional treatment will still be required to eliminate the allergies. Best used short-term.

Ledum palustre

Ledum has its greatest use in puncture wounds and thus has been reported to be helpful with itching due to flea bites. The itching is worse with warmth, especially after warming up in bed. Cold air and cold bathing often relieve the itching.

The plant produces a rash similar to that from poison oak/ivy, thus it may alleviate a similar rash on the body. Dogs and cats are not typically affected by these plants, though they will commonly bring the oils to their guardians as an unwanted gift. A bumpy red-and-white rash similar to that of poison ivy may respond to Ledum.

Curiously, Ledum also has use in rheumatic affections like arthritis, and honeybee venom is used conventionally in some cases of arthritis, so there may be some connection between skin and joint problems. Rheumatoid arthritis is an autoimmune disease, as are most skin ailments, so skin disease may serve as a warning of possible later development of arthritis.

Mezereum

I have seen some good responses to this remedy with constantly itchy animals who have no other symptoms. Like those needing Arsenicum, these poor animals often itch furiously, but the skin appears normal—itching without eruptions. Itching is worse at night in bed, and touch often incites intense itching. Warm bathing usually worsens the itching as well. Vaccination may initiate the *Mezereum* state.

Rhus toxicodendron

This is poison ivy—no explanation needed for those who have experienced the joy of a reaction to this plant! In mild cases, the resultant rash is bumpy and very, very itchy; in serious cases, large blisters form, and the itching is so intense that it never stops. Heat and warm bathing intensify the itching initially, though it may relieve the itch after a time. Motion may alleviate the itch, so these animals may move constantly.

Rhus tox is yet another arthritis and skin-itching remedy. The joint pains are better with continued motion and with warmth.

Silicea (Silica)

This remedy is a great one in skin affections, particularly when they began after a vaccination. The skin eruptions often get infected, and these animals may suffer from recurrent abscesses. Itching may not be as intense as with the above remedies, but it is persistent. These animals are usually chilly and may be rather listless.

This is a very deep-acting remedy, so don't use it too long or too often without assistance from an experienced prescriber. It is commonly needed in animals because of the numerous vaccinations.

Urtica urens

This is another plant remedy—this time the stinging nettle. Nettles have formic acid on them, so the itching will be similar to that of *Formica rufa*—burning and stinging. Itching is violent, though rubbing or scratching the area relieves the itch. Exercise worsens the *Urtica* itch, and rest ameliorates the itch. There may be red blotches that are quite itchy.

Urtica is also a good remedy for bladder inflammation with constant straining to urinate, and here again is another remedy for gout and arthritis alternating with skin rashes.

Hotspots

A hotspot is an area of intense skin inflammation that usually occurs in warm months when dogs (rarely cats) begin to exhibit allergies to fleas, pollens, or whatever. One or more spots will apparently itch intensely, and the dog then scratches the spot violently, removing the hair and creating a bright red, weeping sore that may become infected. When infected, these sores usually turn greenish and develop a foul odor. Even though they are very sore, the underlying itchiness drives the dog to continue scratching, sometimes until it bleeds.

General Care for Hotspots

Though not dangerous, hotspots can spread or can be difficult to heal, though most respond well to appropriate treatment. Veterinarians tend to use antibiotics for these cases, but the infection is usually superficial and will heal without antibiotics in almost all cases.

Have an examination soon:

- if the hotspot does not begin to heal within a couple of days— sooner if the hotspot is very painful or spreading.

The first step is to clip the hair away from the hotspot. Though most hair will be gone, some will remain, particularly at the edges. Additionally, some hair will stick to the sore because of the oozing of serum from the raw skin. An electric clipper works best, but you will need to clean the blade frequently to keep the serum from accumulating. The blades tend to get hot also, and you can easily burn the sensitive skin; some hotspots even begin with a clipper burn. Scissors will work also, but extreme caution is necessary. Be especially careful if you pull up a tuft of hair because it is very easy to cut the skin, as it lifts with the hair. I have seen many experienced groomers, veterinary technicians, and veterinarians make this mistake. I have even done it myself. Don't think it can't happen to you. Hotspots can be very sore, so clipping and cleaning them can be difficult. If so, make a solution of bee propolis and spray this on the wound; this should numb the skin somewhat and make the job easier.

Once you have the hair clipped away, you need to clean the wound. I find witch hazel a great cleanser and astringent. Even though there is some alcohol in witch hazel, it generally does not sting much, and the astringent property helps dry up the serum, which is essential to facilitate healing. Thayers Original Witch Hazel has aloe vera in it, and this is a great combination for hotspots and other uses. The aloe soothes the wound and is antibacterial. If your pharmacy doesn't have this brand, check a health food store, or ask the pharmacist to order the product. You can also add aloe juice to witch hazel; use one-third to one-half aloe juice. Soap and water can work for cleaning also, but use a mild soap and rinse well. This method requires more manipulation and may be more painful, and you don't get the astringent effect. Iodine solutions can be used also, though these are rather harsh. Yellow dock tea can also help, as it is somewhat astringent; use one to three times daily.

After cleaning, apply a mild disinfectant herb such as *Calendula*, aloe vera, or *Hypericum* (St. John's wort). Use an infusion (tea) rather than an alcohol-based tincture as the alcohol is irritating. Apply these three to four times a day, and clean as necessary. I usually refrain from using the witch hazel more than once a day, as too much repetition sometimes irritates the skin. Grated cucumber, applied topically, can reduce the heat and inflammation as well.

Fasting can help here as well by reducing any heat in the body and reducing toxin production, as hotspots may represent a sudden need to detox. Cucumber juice can even help orally here by cooling the body and assisting the liver, as explained above in "General Care for Itching." Nettle tea may also help, orally as well as topically.

Homeopathic Medicines for Hotspots

Apis mellifica
See above under "Itching." The *Apis* hotspot will usually be swollen, red to white, and quite sensitive to touch, like a bee sting.

Belladonna
Belladonna conditions tend to occur suddenly and violently, so think of this remedy if an intense hotspot arises "overnight" (most hotspots do arise quickly, though the itching may have been present longer and given a hint of trouble). The sore will be bright red, even glistening—the heat will be quite obvious, and even the pulse may be accelerated. The dog will likely be irritable and restless, maybe even violent, with dilated pupils—though only in the most severe cases. These dogs are generally very hot and cannot tolerate external heat, and they are usually thirsty, differentiating this remedy from the thirstless *Apis* state—although some patients needing *Belladonna* are thirstless as well.

Graphites
These hotspots characteristically ooze a sticky, yellowish, or honey-colored substance. They are often located in bends of limbs or in skin folds. There

may be cracks along the margins of the sore. Although the animals are usually chilly, warmth worsens the itching and the eruption. Obesity is common.

Hepar sulphuris calcareum

The *Hepar sulph* hotspots are very similar to those needing *Graphites*—moist eruptions in skin folds, with discharge. The discharge here tends to be foul, though—the odor precedes the dog into the room. And the sores are intensely painful, so the patient is fearful and very aggressive if anyone tries to touch the sore. These dogs are also chilly, and warmth soothes the condition.

Mercurius (vivus or solubilis)

When this remedy is needed, the hotspot will often be ulcerated, with a moist discharge that easily becomes infected and turns greenish, or it may develop a yellow crust. Pimples may occur in the area of the sore, and the lymph nodes ("glands") in the region may enlarge. These dogs may be irritable, especially upon examination—they distrust others, believing them to be enemies. Diarrhea or salivation may accompany the skin ailment. In any *Mercurius* state, *Mercurius corrosivus* may be needed if the patient is a male.

Nitric acid

These hotspots will usually become very ulcerated, looking like raw flesh. They bleed easily, and they are intensely painful—very similar to the *Hepar* sores. The pains are described by people as splinter-like. Irritability is common here as with many of the other hotspot remedies—the painful sores drive the dog to violence. Cold aggravates and warm applications alleviate the *Nitric acid* hotspots.

Rhus toxicodendron

Here the hotspot tends more toward itchiness rather than pain and may have a bumpy appearance. The skin is often thickened and stiff—even dry and scaly, sometimes infected. Hot water lessens and cold water worsens the itching. Motion also relieves the itch, so these dogs may move about a lot. Stiff joints that loosen up with walking may accompany the hotspot.

Acne

We primarily recognize acne in cats, usually localized on the chin. Orange-yellow tabbies seem to suffer more than others, and the condition is almost always evidence of deeper chronic illness, though it is not serious at this stage. I recommend treatment by a qualified homeopath. Affected cats may have acute stages that resemble hotspots, however, so the above remedies may be helpful. The suggestions for cleaning hotspots will often work well to alleviate acute acne also. Treat the acute episodes if necessary, then see a veterinary homeopath for treatment of the underlying chronic disease. *Gunpowder* (the homeopathic remedy) may help nasty-looking acne when it is reddened and pustular, but you still should consult with an experienced homeopath for chronic treatment.

A good diet is important here as in all conditions. Additionally, be sure you are not using plastic dishes for food or water as these can off-gas chemicals that irritate the chin, and I have occasionally seen acne disappear upon changing to glass, ceramic, or stainless steel dishes. Cheap stainless steel bowls may be of poor quality and may contain toxic heavy metals, so buy good bowls—usually you are safe with American-made or European-made dishes. Furthermore, stainless steel contains nickel, which can be toxic for many animals, so glass and ceramics are the best choice.

Mange

Although this term is often erroneously applied to any scruffy dog in poor health, mange refers to an infestation by one of two skin parasites (mites). The first type of mange is called sarcoptic mange and is also known as scabies. This mange mite commonly infests young stray puppies, though it may affect adults also. It is very contagious, so caution is necessary. Affected animals scratch constantly and violently, as the mites burrow under the skin and this creates great itchiness. The itchiness is similar to chigger bites, so if you have experienced these, you know how your dog feels. The ears and abdomen are the most common sites of infestation, as these areas are slightly cooler than the rest of the body. The ear tips are usually crusty, and scratching them causes the puppy to immediately move the back leg on that side in a scratching motion. The mites will even transiently invade people, but they do not spread or multiply; you may get a few bites that look like chiggers. The bumps are quite red and itchy. No treatment is usually necessary for people once the dog's problem is controlled.

Conventional treatment is dipping the animal with strong petrochemicals. I recommend avoiding this if possible. Lavender oil diluted 1:10 in almond oil is recommended as an alternative[2] along with a fresh food diet. Yellow dock tea is an alternative to the lavender. Use these daily for one to three weeks until you see improvement, then once a week for two or three more applications. If you must use an insecticide, try pyrethrin shampoos before using stronger dips. See below for homeopathic medicines. Mange can be slow to respond to treatment, so you must have patience.

The second type of mange is demodectic mange, also called follicular mange and red mange. This is an immune system problem in that these mites are basically on all dogs, but only those with poor immune systems have problems. I have seen a lot of chow chow dogs with this type of mange. I have also seen a mild case deteriorate dramatically after a booster vaccination because of the immune-compromising effect. The first area typically affected is around the eyes. There will be hair loss and mild reddening, but this mange is only mildly itchy. If it worsens, it may spread to the head and then to other parts of the body. In most dogs, this mange clears as the dog ages and his immune system reaches its full strength. This usually happens around nine to eighteen months of age.

In a small percentage of dogs, the mange spreads to the entire body and overwhelms their system. These dogs cannot rid themselves of the mites without help. This is called generalized demodectic mange, and it can be serious. Many people have given up and opted for euthanasia in these cases.

Conventional treatment calls for even stronger chemicals than those used for sarcoptic mange. These chemicals deplete the immune system even more. I believe this is part of the reason for the failure of the treatment. The answer is in building up the immune system. Fresh raw foods are essential. Vitamins can help also—see above under "General Care for Itching." Echinacea, cat's claw, and astragalus are good immune-system-building herbs. For up to twenty-five-pound dogs, give one-fourth the human recommendation; for twenty-five- to fifty-pound dogs, give one-half the human dose; and give a full dose for larger dogs. Use the herbs in alternation, two to three weeks at a time for maximum effect. Use yellow dock, calendula, or echinacea tea as a topical rinse as needed. Sage tea may also work here.

These cases take time—weeks to months. As long as the patient doesn't worsen and his energy and attitude are good, just keep up the foods, supplements, and herbs. Try one of the following homeopathic remedies as well. You may need to try them all (one at a time) to see which one works best. This is local treatment, so the general symptoms are not as important. If you cannot decide, start with *Silicea*, then try either *Sulphur* or *Psorinum*. If you have no success, call a homeopathic veterinarian.

Psorinum

This remedy is made from the human scabies mite. I have found it success-ful in several cases of mange of both types. These dogs usually smell very strong and may be oily. They can be chilly. Use a 30C potency once a week. It may be hard to find, so contact a homeopathic pharmacy rather than a health food store. You may need a prescription.

Silicea (Silica)

This remedy is often needed during part of the treatment, probably due to the vaccine impact upon the immune system. You may need to use it in alternation with either *Psorinum* or *Sulphur.* By alternation, I mean use one remedy as long as it is working, and switch to the other when the first stops working. *Silicea* is a good place to start; then try one of the others.

Sulphur

This remedy is also good for skin parasites. These dogs are dirty, but not as dirty and smelly as those needing *Psorinum,* and they are more often warm than chilly. They may be very thirsty.

Insect Bites and Stings

Cats and dogs occasionally get stung by bees and wasps or bitten by spi-ders. Usually these resolve on their own, but sometimes assistance is needed. Sometimes the face will swell after a sting—if this occurs, keep a close eye on the animal for an hour or two to see if the swelling worsens. See also the section on allergic reactions in Chapter Fifteen, "Therapeutic Indications by Condition."

General Care for Insect Bites and Stings

Obtain veterinary help immediately if your dog or cat swells intensely or develops breathing difficulty after a bee or wasp sting, as the lungs can fill with fluid and cause death. Though this is rare, it is not worth taking the chance. You can try one of the remedies listed below while on the way to the clinic. Benadryl (1–2 mg/pound) or another antihistamine may help also, but don't use either method in lieu of obtaining veterinary care; rather use them in the interim.

An old folk remedy is tobacco juice applied topically—this will reduce the sting and may reduce swelling. Crush the tobacco in some water and apply it to the sting. Dandelion tea given orally is a diuretic and may help reduce swelling also. Arnica tincture also provides fast relief; this is my bee-keeping wife's first choice.

Homeopathic Medicines for Insect Bites and Stings

Apis mellifica

This remedy, made from honeybee venom, sometimes helps since the symptoms are essentially those of a bee sting. This is often recommended first for bee stings, but I find that it doesn't always work. Consider it, however, for the typical bee sting, with a bright-red smooth swelling, sometimes white at the edges due to swelling. *Apis* may work best when facial swelling occurs or with inordinate swelling around the wound.

Arnica montana

Margaret Tyler, MD, reports that "A drop of the strong tincture applied to a wasp sting cures it an once."[3] This definitely works for bee stings, although I have not tried it for wasp stings.

Cantharis

Consider *Cantharis* when the sting or bite becomes intensely inflamed and looks somewhat like a burn. It may even form blisters.

Carbolic acid

These patients have severe reactions to bee stings, including weakness, collapse, swelling of the face, and respiratory difficulty. There may also be an intensely itching eruption all over the body as an accompaniment.

Histaminum

As with general itching, this remedy can interrupt the histamine reaction and so can reduce inflammation following bites and stings.

Lachesis

When *Lachesis* is indicated, the area around the sting will often turn a dark purplish red and will be very painful. This remedy may be useful for older stings that worsen rather than improve; they may even become infected or bleed a dark red-bluish blood. I find *Lachesis* and *Ledum* the two best remedies for bee stings. Both are also good choices for spider bites.

Ledum palustre

This remedy is well known for its effects in any puncture wound, and bites and stings are well within its realm. The wound may be cold to touch, yet it feels better with cold applications. *I generally recommend* Ledum *first for bites and stings unless there are indications for another remedy.* Scorpion stings may respond well to *Ledum* also.

Rhus toxicodendron

Rhus has swelling of the eyelids and conjunctivitis, often itchy. If the eyes swell up and become red and produce a discharge, *Rhus* may help.

Tarentula cubensis

This medicine is made from the venom of the Cuban spider. It is good for spider bites or insect stings that become deep red and infected. They are violently painful to touch. This state is similar to the *Lachesis* condition, but the pain may be greater when *Tarentula cubensis* is indicated. This remedy is not to be confused with the remedy *Tarentula hispanica*.

Vespa crabro

This is the European hornet, and can be indicated as with *Apis,* above. Symptoms include redness, intense itching, burning, boils, stinging and soreness. Pains are stinging and burning, as if pierced with red hot needles. Animals needing this remedy will be in some distress. Bathing with vinegar may relieve the intense discomfort.

Burns and Scalds

General Care for Burns

Seek veterinary help immediately if the burn is anything other than a minor one. Burns are classified into three categories: a first-degree burn results in redness only; second-degree burns progress to blister formation, and with third-degree burns the blisters rupture and the flesh is opened and raw. First-degree and minor second-degree burns (minimal blistering) that do not cover much area may be amenable to home treatment, but seek help for anything more than this. Use one of the following remedies, but obtain treatment also.

A burn is a sudden acute inflammation following exposure to heat. Chemicals released into the tissues carry out the inflammatory process.

These chemicals increase blood flow to the area, bringing nutrients and other immune system chemicals and cells along to speed healing. When we put cold water on a burn, it does reduce pain by limiting the effect of the inflammatory chemicals, but the burn may worsen dramatically because the body cannot do its job. Hahnemann postulated that, following the homeopathic principle of "like cures like," we should put warm rather than cold water on a burn. This often does work much better. The pain is worsened at first, so we tend to shy away from the warm water and toward cold water, but the warm water accelerates the healing process by improving circulation, and the burn heals more quickly. Try it next time you get sunburn or another minor burn.

Nettle or arnica tea may help topically for minor burns.

Homeopathic Medicines for Burns

Apis mellifica

Apis, with its burning, stinging pains and swelling (edema), could be indicated for a burn. If Apis is needed, there will likely be a white area as well as redness, with puffy swelling; this could be useful if burns approach second degree. Sometimes severe burns can cause kidney shutdown, and while this would obviously warrant hospitalization, Apis could prevent further damage.

Arsenicum album

More noted for burning sensations than for actual burns, Arsenicum is nevertheless a good remedy for a burn if the symptoms fit the general picture of chilliness, restlessness, and thirst. The restlessness worsens just after midnight. The wound will probably be swollen and even infected or ulcerated and quite painful. The patient may be extremely listless—out of proportion to the apparent injury. Most Arsenicum skin conditions are better with warm applications.

Cantharis

This is generally the first remedy to consider for burns and scalds, especially right when they happen. Cantharis is best given before any blisters form, but it may still be useful once the blisters erupt. Sunburn is especially amenable to Cantharis, so it may help white cats who tend to get burns on their ear tips (although these cats should receive constitutional treatment for the underlying sensitivity). If a deeper Cantharis state occurs following a burn, you may see excessive straining during urination as well as sexual behavior. Cold water lessens the pain in a *Cantharis* state (but see general care for burns, above).

Causticum

This remedy is generally needed for worn out, broken-down states, but it has application for some cases of burns as well. Generally, *Causticum* is suited for older burns that will not heal well—the wounds keep reopening and don't ever completely scar over. These patients will often be sluggish and chilly, possibly just since the burn.

Urtica urens

A tea of *Urtica* (stinging nettle) applied topically can quickly reduce the pain and inflammation of a first-degree burn. The homeopathic medicine may be used internally as well. When *Urtica* is indicated, the burn often itches as well as being painful.

Ringworm

This is actually a fungus infection and is not caused by a worm. Ringworm lesions are typically circular, dry, and crusty; they usually itch mildly. The hair falls out over the affected area. Ringworm is contagious to humans, so use some caution, though cleanliness is usually sufficient to prevent contagion. On people, the lesions are usually raised, slightly red, crusty, and itchy. Due to the possibility of contagion, I recommend having a veterinarian confirm a diagnosis of ringworm.

Ringworm may be either a local infection or evidence of systemic weakness. Local infections tend to be small areas and readily respond to topical treatment, whereas systemic ringworm occurs in multiple areas on the skin and requires constitutional treatment to eliminate the disease. Cats in catteries often develop systemic ringworm infections, possibly due to stress, genetic weakness from inbreeding, diet, vaccinations, or all of the above. Treatment is best done under the care of a homeopathic practitioner when the disease is systemic, but I have seen many responses to *Thuja*, so you could try a 30C potency once a week for three weeks. I have tried many remedies reputed to treat ringworm with little success, but then I started using *Thuja* and have had several good responses. This is interesting to me, as *Thuja* is so well known as an antivaccinosis remedy—which suggests that at least some of these systemic ringworm cases must result from vaccine stress.

If the ringworm is limited to small areas, you can try topical treatment. Be sure to wash your hands after handling the affected animal (cats are more often affected than dogs). Tea tree oil is a very good antifungal medicine. It can be irritating, so dilute it before application. A mixture of one-half ounce olive oil, 200 IU vitamin E, and one-half teaspoon tea tree oil is a good solution for topical ringworm treatment. The better-quality tea tree oils are less irritating. I have found the Desert Essence brand to be mild. I'm sure there are other good ones also, but this one has worked well for me. Apply the oil daily for three to six weeks. It is quite safe for people as well, should you develop a spot. I have heard reports that tea tree oil can be toxic to cats, but I have never seen any problems. A tea with calendula and sage is a pretty effective antifungal rinse as well. Calendula ointment sometimes works also. It is very soothing and may be used alone or in alternation with the tea tree oil mixture. Clipping the hair around the perimeter of the lesion helps, as this is the most active area of infection.

If topical treatment (with or without *Thuja*) is unsuccessful, and especially if the ringworm spreads, you'll need to seek professional help. Other remedies to consider are *Bacillinum, Sepia, Sulphur, Tellurium, Graphites,* and *Dulcamara,* under professional guidance.

Ear Problems

As with skin disease, most ear troubles are an external manifestation of internal chronic disease. Local treatment is not generally of much help in the long term. Although conventional veterinarians tend to consider ear discharges and wax buildup to be infectious, this is rarely the case. There may be bacteria or yeast present, but these are usually opportunists. The "infection" occurs in only a few animals who have an underlying weakness that allows the organisms to proliferate. If the animal were healthy, the bacteria would not reproduce in large numbers. If the bacteria (or yeast) were the cause, then almost all animals would have ear infections, skin infections, intestinal infections, lung infections, and so on.

While topical treatment can help alleviate symptoms, it cannot typically cure an ear infection. Only those that occur secondary to an injury or from an insult such as a foxtail (grass seed head) are truly local and may respond to local treatment. The vast majority of ear problems do not respond to topical treatment. This results in a similar frustration with ear "infections" as with skin ailments. Additionally, there is an observed connection between the ears and the brain. Suppressed ear disease can lead to brain problems—and curative treatment of brain disease may be followed by an ear discharge. Suppressive treatment of the discharge may reawaken the brain illness (See Dolly's case in the "Palliation" section of Chapter Three). Topical drug therapy may be dangerous as well as frustrating.

Other than for minor problems, I recommend that you seek the help of a homeopathic prescriber for ear diseases. Even though they may appear simple, they are not. If you skipped the first part of this chapter, please read it for an explanation, as skin and ear problems are in many ways the same.

General Care for Ear Problems

Mild cleaning solutions and soothing herbs will help the body do what it is attempting to do—cleanse the ear to remove overgrowing organisms and possibly toxins. If wax is especially heavy and thick, an oil-based cleaner will help dissolve the wax. I use a mix of one-half ounce olive oil with 200 IU vitamin E and one-fourth teaspoon tea tree oil; this is a good cleaner and mild disinfectant. The tea tree oil is optional. Occasionally, an animal is sensitive to this, and it irritates the ears. Mullein and garlic can be substituted for their soothing properties. You can also use the oil mix (or straight olive oil) before a bath or swimming to keep water out of the ears. Vinegar and water is a good cleaner when the wax is not too thick. Use one part vinegar in five to twenty parts water, less if the solution irritates the ear. This solution can also be used to dry the ears after swimming or bathing, and it kills yeast. A tea of St. John's wort *(Hypericum)* is another good topical herb as it is anti-infective and will soothe irritated, painful ears. Aloe juice mixed with witch hazel (two parts aloe to one part witch hazel) can help also, though it could sting if ears are raw and inflamed. Nutribiotic Ear Drops, with grapefruit seed extract and tea tree oil, can be helpful in some animals. This preparation is available at many health food stores.

Avoid chemical rinses and antibiotic solutions. These are not necessary, and they are generally too strong. Also avoid "cortisone" solutions or ointments, as these can suppress the symptoms.

Ear Mites

These are primarily a problem in cats, although dogs can be affected. Kittens and cats scratch the ears violently, often creating a sore behind the ear. Lightly touching the ear will incite the scratching, as will any attempt at topical treatment—though this is necessary. The mites are at the limit of our visual range, so we usually won't see them without magnification. The body produces a dark brown, crumbly wax as a response, and this along with the itchiness may indicate mites, though I recommend getting a veterinarian to inspect the ears for mites or mite eggs, as other ear conditions can produce a similar discharge. Be sure the veterinarian examines the ears with an otoscope or looks at the debris under magnification to verify mite presence.

Oregano oil (put one-half teaspoon of dry oregano into one-half to one ounce of olive oil, and let it sit for twenty-four to forty-eight hours) will help with ear mites. Alternately, you can use commercially available oregano oil *if it is prepared for use in the ears,* or use the essential oil and put about fifteen drops into one ounce of olive oil. Put five to twenty drops into each ear daily, depending upon the patient's size. *Do not use the essential oil directly in the ears.* Another good treatment for ear mites is an infusion (tea) of yellow dock. Pour one-half cup of boiling water over a teaspoonful of dry herb. Allow it to cool, and then pour the liquid into a bottle. Place one-half dropperful into the ears once or twice daily. This is very effective and relieves the itching as well.[4] You may alternate the oregano oil with the yellow dock infusion. The ears are usually irritated, so don't use the tea tree oil mix. It is also possible to make an oil infusion of yellow dock, using one teaspoonful of dry herb in one ounce of olive oil. Use five to twenty drops in each ear, once a day.

If the mites persist, either the cat is too unhealthy to eliminate the mites, or there may be other animals that continue to reinfect each other. In the latter case, all animals will need treatment. If reinfection from an outside source is not likely, the cat needs homeopathic treatment. You can try a few doses of homeopathic *Sulphur,* but if the problem does not resolve within a couple of weeks, consult a homeopathic veterinarian for treatment. Some veterinarians recommend using pesticide shampoos or dips when animals have ear mites, but I do not find these necessary. You could use the yellow dock tea on the head around the ears if mites do not readily disappear.

Foxtails and Foreign Bodies

A foxtail is a grass seed head that has spines on it that attach to hair (these are primarily found in the western United States). This unique feature facilitates spreading the grass seed, but it can be a problem for dogs and cats. Occasionally, foxtails will work into the ear canals, where they cause an intensely painful irritation and secondary infection and can even penetrate the ear drum. They can also invade the nose and eyes or into the tissue between the toes. Check your companion after any walks through grassy areas, and remove foxtails before they can cause problems. If you notice a persistent discharge from the ear, and if you see evidence of pain, have the ears checked. If a foxtail is present, it will likely require removal by a veterinarian, probably under anesthesia. *You can try the following homeopathic remedies, but not in place of veterinary care.* Go ahead and give the remedy, but take the animal in for an examination.

Myristica sebifera

Myristica is a great remedy for inciting the body to expel foreign bodies, and it may push out a foxtail in a few cases. It is so good at pushing out splinters and such that the old homeopathic masters said that *Myristica* "often does away with use of the knife."

Silicea (Silica)

This is the other main remedy for expelling splinters and other foreign bodies. Try *Myristica* first if available, but *Silicea* is more common and thus easier to obtain, and it has great power in its own right at pushing out foreign bodies.

Aural Hematomas

Occasionally the pinna, or ear flap, will suddenly fill with blood for no apparent reason. This problem occurs primarily in dogs, though I have seen it a couple of times in cats. We used to believe this to be the result of an ear infection and the resultant violent ear shaking. It was thought that the shaking ruptured a blood vessel in the ear. We now understand that this is primarily an autoimmune disease, the bane of twentieth-century health. The body's immune system attacks the circulatory system in this case, leading to an inability to clot and to increased permeability of the ear veins. Thus, the weakness and tendency to hemorrhage are the primary cause of the hematoma. In some cases, shaking the ears may initiate bleeding due to the preexisting weakness, but normally shaking does not lead to bleeding.

As with "infections," it is helpful to ask, Why this dog and not all dogs? to understand whether a suspected cause is indeed the culprit (see "Skin Infections and Eruptions" above, and Chapter Two, "The Nature of Disease").

Once again, we see that what appears to be a local problem is instead evidence of deeper illness. I thus recommend constitutional prescribing for aural hematomas. The conventional treatment for this condition is surgical draining followed by suturing the outer and inner skin of the pinna together like a mattress. Many cases actually do not need this if the hematoma is small, but some cases will require surgery. Your homeopathic veterinarian may be able to help decide which is right for your dog. Typically, surgery for aural hematomas involves anesthesia, then lancing the hematoma, removing accumulated blood and fibrous clots, and then suturing the outer and inner surfaces of the pinna back together. I have found over the years, however, that often this is unnecessary. In many cases, quickly lancing the hematoma, then bandaging the pinna over a thick roll of cotton gauze allows the ear to heal, often with less scarring than with the suture method. This can be done without anesthesia, and while this may seem harsh, I think it is less stressful than undergoing anesthesia. Bandaging the ear is tricky, so you'll need a veterinarian's help. Many times, following surgery and suturing, the pinna scars badly. *Thiosinaminum* 6X, given twice daily starting a week after surgery for two to three weeks, can minimize the scarring. I'll give a few other homeopathic medicines below for treating the hematomas, but as with other skin diseases, seek professional help if the condition does not resolve promptly.

Belladonna
Belladonna conditions arise suddenly and with much heat, so when this remedy is needed, the ear will rapidly fill up with fluid and will generally be red and hot. Additionally, the dog may be very restless and irritable, even violent, and the pupils may dilate when he is aggressive. *Belladonna* states tend to affect the right side more than the left.

Crotalus horridus
This remedy is made from the venom of the timber rattlesnake. As with most snake remedies, this one has a tendency to hemorrhage. *Crotalus* affects the right side predominantly. Those needing *Crotalus* are often generally

weak and sluggish with tendencies to serious illness, so it is not likely needed in a young, vital dog—more often this remedy is used for older dogs.

Lachesis

Another snake remedy, this time from the venom of the bushmaster snake from South America, *Lachesis* also has bleeding tendencies but tends to be left-sided. The ear may be dark, even bluish in appearance. The *Lachesis* state tends to worsen with sleep, so these cases may occur during the night—the dog may wake up with the hematoma.

Millefolium

This remedy is a small remedy that has hemorrhage as its primary indication. I have used it successfully when there was a hematoma in an otherwise healthy dog without indications for a constitutional remedy.

Phosphorus

As one of the major remedies for hemorrhage of any type, *Phosphorus* should be considered for aural hematomas. These dogs tend to be thin, outgoing, vocal, thirsty, and hungry. The left side is more predominantly affected when this remedy is indicated. Hemorrhaged blood tends to be bright red, unlike *Crotalus horridus* and *Lachesis* with their dark blood. You may not see the blood with hematomas, but if surgical lancing is required, you can inquire about the blood color.

Fly Strike

Fly strike occurs mainly in humid climates where flies are plentiful and the humidity keeps many wounds moist and irritated. Certain types of flies bite the tips of the ears (primarily of dogs) repeatedly. The ear tips become raw and painful, and they itch and burn. Treatment is primarily limited to using repellents and healing salves. Try *Calendula* ointment, aloe vera, or a diluted tea tree oil (see "General Care for Ear Problems" above) to heal the wound. Lavender or eucalyptus may help repel the flies.

The homeopathic medicine *Caladium seguinum* is especially effective in some cases of fly and mosquito bites with this type of reaction and thus may assist in the healing of and resistance to fly bites.

Chapter Seven
MOUTH, GUMS, AND TEETH

Function

Food intake is the primary function of the mouth. This involves not only acquisition but also initial processing of foods. Procuring foods begins with the incisors and canine teeth. Incisors, the small teeth at the front of the mouth, are more important for herbivores (along with the tongue) than for carnivores. As grazers, herbivores chop off grasses and other plants with the bladelike surface of their incisors. Carnivores, on the other hand, primarily utilize their canine teeth for obtaining foods, since the foods must be caught. The length and sharpness of these "fangs" securely grasps prey animals, as well as contributing to the kill by puncturing deeply into body tissues. Evidence suggests that the spread of the canines in cats corresponds to the space between the neck vertebrae of their larger prey animals, allowing the teeth to slide between the vertebrae and sever the spinal cord. This efficiency greatly aids these solitary hunters in killing prey animals their own size or even larger.

Dogs and cats also use their teeth for grooming. Fleas, ticks, lice, burs, porcupine quills, and many other objects can be grasped and removed with a good set of incisors. Last but certainly not least, teeth are a formidable means of defense against those who might prey upon these carnivores.

Once a carnivore has successfully caught and killed an animal, he uses his premolars and molars to slice and chop it into pieces small enough to be swallowed. For dogs, this does not need to be very small, as they will swallow very large bites (thus the adage of "wolfing" one's food). Cats chew their foods a bit more than dogs, but neither species follows the dictum about "one chew for each tooth." In carnivores, this might be amended to one chew for each fang. The only real chewing involves bones, and cats as well as dogs consume large quantities of bones to obtain their calcium needs. They simply crush the bones into small pieces and swallow them, allowing the digestive juices to complete the breakdown. Why, you may wonder, do the bones not cause problems? Very rarely they may, but the problems we associate with splintered shards of bone result from feeding cooked bones. Raw bones do not tend to splinter. Additionally, in the wild the bones are consumed last, on top of a large feast, and the foods in the stomach lend some protection against any sharp edges until the strong digestive fluids begin the breakdown process.

Obviously, strong gums and healthy teeth provide an essential foundation to a successful predator. The best program for maintaining these healthy teeth and gums is the one the predator developed over eons of evolution. Fresh foods and chewing on bones are the major components of the carnivore dental-health preventive-care program. Chewing dog biscuits is no substitute; in fact, dry foods and biscuits have little impact upon dental health or tartar accumulation. Some dogs, with relatively weak enamel, may wear down their teeth or crack teeth with hard bones, but this is not common, and for most dogs the emotional and health benefits of bones outweighs the risks. (Chewing bones is a great stress reliever for dogs.) The key to good gum health is a healthy immune system, and this comes from a healthy diet, as well as avoiding stressors that compromise the immune system, such as vaccination, drugs, and other toxins. With raw food diets, at least some meat in the diet should be in chunks, so the animal must chew her food; this also helps strengthen gums and clean teeth.

The mouth, and especially the space between the teeth and gums, is a point of contact with the world of microorganisms. Bacteria normally live in the mouth (as well as the entire digestive tract) and bring no harm to healthy individuals. A functioning immune system maintains the margin and keeps the bacteria outside the body tissues. (Technically, the mouth and digestive tract are outside the body in the sense that they are cavities that connect to the outside.) Saliva contains two types of components that inhibit bacterial growth. The first type is thiocyanate ions, which can kill bacteria, especially once the ions get inside the bacteria. The second component, lysozyme, is an enzyme with three main properties: it digests food particles, thus removing nutrients for bacteria. It can directly attack bacteria, either killing them or limiting their growth. Finally, lysozyme aids thiocyanate ions in entering bacteria.[1] The adage about saliva's healing properties is indeed correct.

When immunity weakens, however, microorganisms begin to invade the body, starting at the gum line. Red gums, or a red line at the gum margin, indicate the depth of this invasion, as the body initiates inflammation in an attempt to push the bacteria out. With continued weakening, the invasion and redness intensifies, and ultimately we recognize the "infection" and call it gingivitis (which simply means "inflammation of the gums").

While antibiotic therapy may help reduce this inflammation for a time by helping the body push out the invading bacteria, permanent cure is not possible with this method. If the body is not strengthened, microorganisms will continue to invade, and they rapidly become immune to antibiotics. Additionally, antibiotics weaken the immune system, thereby contributing to the gingivitis in the long run. Clinical experience supports this observation, as the benefit derived from antibiotic treatment of many conditions is short-lived, necessitating frequent changes of dose or medicine. Ultimately, antibiotics stop working altogether when the body has weakened to the point that it cannot provide any fight on its own. The body's resistance is a necessary (though often overlooked) part of antibiotic therapy. Only by boosting immune function can these conditions come to successful conclusions.

Tartar accumulation begins with deposition of plaque on tooth surfaces. This film of food residues adheres to teeth after eating, and the rougher the surface, the more easily the plaque sticks. Bacterial secretions may worsen this deposition. If not removed within twenty-four hours, the plaque hardens into tartar. Gradually, the tartar accumulates. Chewing on bones cleans the plaque off the teeth before hardening can occur. Dry foods and dog biscuits simply do not provide enough friction or time to accomplish this task, and there are usually sugars in the foods that contribute to plaque formation. Salivation aids tartar control by rinsing teeth and digesting the plaque, as well as by limiting bacterial growth.

Poor foods contribute to gum and tooth disease by several means. First, and most obvious, high levels of sugars and simple carbohydrates provide rapidly available nutrition for oral bacteria. Secondly, poor nutrient quality simply does not support the immune system. Third, and probably most important, though commonly overlooked, rancid foods contribute greatly to degeneration of all body tissues. The gums are either particularly sensitive or are just easily visible, but I commonly see inflamed gums in an otherwise apparently healthy animal. In either case, this provides an early warning signal for the beginning of chronic disease.

Cats are particularly prone to develop inflamed gums. I believe rancid foods play a large part in this tendency.[2] The severe problems with inflamed, ulcerated gums we see so commonly in cats is a pathetic sight and is reminiscent of historical descriptions of scurvy among sailors. We understand scurvy to be a deficiency of vitamin C in humans, since these early sailors responded dramatically to foods containing vitamin C. I believe this may be only partially correct. Scurvy developed on long voyages, and fresh foods were often nonexistent for long periods of time. Refrigeration was not available, and undoubtedly the meats and grains these ships carried became quite rancid over time. We know now that rancid foods create large numbers of oxygen free radicals, which in turn cause severe tissue destruction. Vitamin C is an antioxidant, meaning it neutralizes these free radicals. This may be why it was so effective against scurvy.

Cats evolved eating only freshly killed animals. During the evolutionary process, they abandoned the liver's ability to detoxify certain types of chemicals. As one consequence, cats are very sensitive to rancidity. Terrible gum inflammation is probably one result, and I think it appropriate to consider this a form of scurvy. Unfortunately, these cats do not respond to antioxidants as well as the sailors did. This may be due to the more effective detoxifying systems of humans as well as to the overall cleaner environment of the time. Additionally, the extra stress of vaccination further weakens the feline immune system. Homeopathy can help, but this condition in cats can be quite difficult to cure. As with skin conditions, gingivitis may heal very slowly. Prevention is always easier, so start puppies and kittens out with fresh foods, and spare the vaccinations—help them keep those healthy, strong teeth.

Gingivitis and Mouth Inflammation

General Care for Gingivitis and Mouth Inflammation

Gum inflammation develops over a long period of time—months to years—so improvement will be slow as well. As you know from reading the prior section, food quality is the most important limiting factor in gum health. By providing the freshest, best food you can, you improve the possibility for healing. Antioxidants will help, but these do not supplant the need for good food. Give vitamin C *with bioflavonoids* (10 mg/pound, two to three times a day; use natural vitamin C if available) and vitamin E (5–10 mg/pound, once a day; use mixed tocopherols). Pycnogenol, a powerful bioflavonoid, sometimes benefits greatly (0.5–1 mg/pound). Grape seed extract (not grapefruit seed extract) contains a similar compound and can be used interchangeably with pycnogenol. Coenzyme Q_{10} (1–3 mg/pound, once a day) may help also. The oil-based formulation of coenzyme Q_{10} is much more effective than dry forms and can be given at the lower end of the dose range. Folic acid is also important for gum health, so you can give this separately or in a B complex supplement. Use 25–75 mcg daily for cats, up to 400 mcg in a large dog. *Cordyceps* (a medicinal mushroom) helps circulation to the gums and is available from Eclectic Institute in a capsule (as well as from other companies). Here, use one-half capsule once or twice a day for cats and small dogs, and one capsule per twenty to twenty-five pounds for larger dogs, up to three capsules twice daily in large dogs.

For a topical rinse, you can mix a solution in a dropper bottle or small cup, though this solution needs to be mixed fresh daily. Use a small pinch of vitamin C, acidophilus, and digestive enzyme powders. Rinse the mouth with this solution three to four times a day. The enzymes clean the teeth somewhat; the vitamin C is healthy for the gums, and the acidophilus puts "good" bacteria in the mouth to compete with the ones that have overgrown.

You can also brush the teeth with a soft pediatric toothbrush, using baking soda or dentie tooth powder. Dentie is available in health food stores and is made from charred eggplant and salt; it is a Japanese formula that is healing and not too strong tasting. You can also mix equal parts hydrogen peroxide and water and add a small amount to the baking soda to make a paste. The peroxide drives the baking soda into the gums, and it is also a good antiseptic for the anaerobic bacteria that live in the gum spaces and tend to overgrow and cause problems. Of course, there are also toothpastes and brushes for cats and dogs, though some toothpastes have artificial preservatives and flavors in them, which are not healthy. If you cannot use a toothbrush, you can use a cotton terry cloth or a finger brush. The latter are often available at pet supply stores. It can be difficult to brush a dog's teeth, and even more difficult with cats, but if you can manage to do this, it will help. At least use the rinse, though, if your dog or cat suffers from gingivitis.

If you find that your cat or dog has tartar that you cannot remove, she may need dental scraping to remove the tartar and have her teeth thoroughly examined. This generally requires anesthesia, which has some inherent risks (albeit small) but which may cause minimal but accumulative brain damage with successive anesthesia events. Furthermore, the possibility exists for enamel damage from overzealous cleaning with ultrasonic scalers. One study from years ago demonstrated enamel damage with these scalers if more than one gram of pressure is applied. This is akin to the pressure of the needle on an old turntable for LP albums ("vinyl"). It is very light. I have seen many cases wherein tartar builds up more easily and faster following teeth cleaning, so this is a real possibility. Thus, anesthesia and dental cleaning have their disadvantages. It is possible in many cases to hand-scale teeth without anesthesia. Of course, this is not as thorough as cleaning with anesthesia, but often is more than sufficient, especially with home care and improved health with diet changes. Obviously this depends upon the ease of working with individual patients. But it is worth pursuing; many areas of the country now have technicians who come to the home and do hand-scaling. If your animal's mouth is not too bad, I suggest giving this a try, at least some of the time. And you can ask your veterinarian for hand-scaling in any case, even if she is unwilling to attempt scaling without anesthesia, although it does not hurt to ask for this. Even if the no-anesthesia scaling does not get under the gums, it still helps many animals. With cats, sometimes it is possible to flick the big tartar pieces off the teeth, and even this is helpful. Cats primarily get tartar on their upper teeth, and mostly on the last two large cutting teeth on either side. If you can get your thumbnail above the tartar, but below the gum, you may be able to flick the tartar off. You can then see if her gums improve over the ensuing month or two; if not, you may want to get an examination to see if more intervention is needed, keeping in mind your options and the potential drawbacks and advantages of anesthesia.

As I noted above, gingivitis has been very difficult to cure, even with homeopathy. This is especially true in cats, who suffer so frequently with this complaint. Conventional treatment is no better, however, as previously discussed. Many practitioners now recommend extraction of all the cat's teeth as a treatment for severe gingivitis; this seems barbaric to me, although I can understand the frustration that leads to such a decision. The theory is that without the opening between the teeth and gum, the bacteria cannot invade and incite inflammation. Apparently, many cases are successful—if one accepts the loss of teeth as a satisfactory compromise. Not all cases accomplish the desired result, however, and either way this is a drastic, last-ditch procedure.

The best approach is, of course, prevention. At the first sign of red gums, even a small red line, I recommend working with a homeopathic practitioner to provide constitutional treatment. Treatment at this stage may be difficult, as often the red line is the only symptom. But it is worth taking preventive measures, as the prognosis worsens considerably as the severity increases. And I cannot emphasize enough the importance of diet. If the condition has progressed to the point that a lot of tartar has accumulated, then a dental cleaning is warranted. This can often be accomplished without anesthesia if the buildup is minimal. Many clinics recommend anesthesia and cleaning far too frequently and for animals whose teeth are not too bad. Be sure the anesthesia and comprehensive cleaning are really necessary before opting for this procedure. While anesthesia is very safe today, repeated use can weaken the body, and it should not be taken too lightly. It may even contribute to senile dementia, in humans as well as cats.

If your dog or cat has gingivitis, I recommend working with an experienced practitioner for the above reasons. There are, however, some remedies that may provide relief, especially in acute flare-ups. To decide which remedy may be helpful, try to determine patterns or circumstances:

- Are the gums painful?
- Does the condition interfere with eating?
- Do the gums bleed? Profusely or easily?
- Is ulceration present, and is the tongue or the roof of the mouth affected?
- Is there a foul odor?
- Is there pus?

Note: The presence of ulceration may indicate kidney failure and toxin accumulation, so be sure to obtain a thorough veterinary examination if this symptom is present.

Homeopathic Medicines for Gingivitis and Mouth Inflammation

Arsenicum album

Arsenicum may be indicated for gingivitis, especially in an animal with kidney disease. The gums will be quite painful and the mouth odor quite strong. Bleeding may accompany the inflammation, which often includes ulceration. These animals are often thirsty and will drink often, usually in small sips. If inflammation is severe, cold water (which they desire) can be painful to teeth or gums, so they may try to drink but quickly stop. Other common *Arsenicum* symptoms will usually be present, such as worsening after midnight, restlessness, chilliness, and fear of strangers. The right side may be more severely affected.

Arum triphyllum

This remedy, made from the root of the jack in the pulpit, is very effective in relieving some cases of severe gingivitis. The root is very irritating to mucous membranes, thus the affinity to gum disease. A keynote of *Arum triphyllum* is cracks at the corners of the mouth. The mouth is intensely painful, and eating and drinking are often very difficult. Ulcers are usually present and may affect any surface in the mouth. The tongue tends to be red, even beet red. Salivation is common due to the painful mouth, and the mouth usually has a foul odor. There is a tendency for the condition to be worse on the left side.

Astacus fluviatilis

This remedy, from the crawfish, has a marked affinity to the mouth and gums, and it can be helpful in severe gingivitis. There may be general skin itchiness along with the gum disease. The lips may be chapped or cracked as well. The breath may smell fishy.

Borax

This remedy has quite a reputation for relieving ulceration in the mouth, though I have not had much luck with its use. The main keynote of *Borax* is fear of downward motion, whether going down stairs, jumping off of furniture, or being placed on the floor or ground after being held. Even rocking or riding in a car may be intolerable, as is air travel. These animals may also be extremely sensitive to sudden noise, especially that of a gunshot, even at great distance. They may be very irritable and fidgety, with amelioration after eleven at night.

The mouth symptoms primarily involve ulceration on the tongue and on the inside of the cheeks. There may be a white coating or growth, as with thrush (incidentally, Clarke reports that a simple yet effective treatment for thrush is eating large quantities of strawberries).[3] Urination and defecation may be very painful, causing crying out during the action.

Carbo vegetabilis

Carbo veg obtains its usefulness in gingivitis in that it is well suited to conditions of poor vitality and degeneration. The gums would naturally be one of the first and most visibly affected regions. Hemorrhage is common, and blood will usually be dark rather than bright red. The mouth, as well as the extremities, are often cool to cold. Gums will be swollen and receded from the teeth, often with a purulent discharge. Bluish discoloration is common and should bring *Carbo veg* to mind, along with *Lachesis*. Salivation may be pronounced, and the mouth has a bad odor.

These patients tend to be quite sluggish, fat, and flatulent. They may readily weaken into a state of collapse. Though they are often cold, they need fresh air and may sit in front of a fan or open door. They are very ill, and healing will take a long time.

Kali chloricum

Like *Arsenicum*, *Kali chlor* is often indicated when the disease center is in the kidneys. These animals will have swelling in most surfaces in the mouth, with grayish ulcers. The tongue may be cold and swollen. Inflammation tends toward gangrene—circulation is poor, and tissues begin to die and rot, giving off a foul odor. This is obviously a severe state. Mucous membranes are often bluish.

Diarrhea or dysentery is a common accompanying symptom, as is incessant vomiting of greenish-black mucus. The patient may have a right-sided nosebleed. These animals may alternate between feeling low-spirited and feeling perky. *Kali muriaticum*, a closely related remedy, is one of Schüssler's tissue salts and is commonly available in health food stores and herb shops. While it is not exactly the same remedy, some authors consider its action similar enough to consider it the same, and if you cannot readily obtain *Kali chlor*, you might try *Kali mur*.

Kali phosphoricum

All of the *Kalis* have affinity to the mouth and nose, and *Kali phos* finds usefulness when the gums are spongy, bleed easily (all *Phosphorus* remedy states have bleeding tendencies), and recede from the teeth. The tongue may have a mustard-colored coating and may be partially paralyzed—the animal may struggle to eat or drink. As with most remedies for gingivitis, the breath may be foul; in this case it smells like a dead animal. The mouth may be dry in the morning, with the tongue stuck to the roof of the mouth.

Weakness and despondency are often profound, and young animals tend to need this remedy more than older ones. It is particularly useful when they are teething.

Kreosotum

This homeopathic medicine finds its main indications in conditions with burning, irritating discharges. Like *Borax*, *Kreosotum* has a great reputation in mouth inflammations, though I have not been so rewarded with its use. Dentition is a major time of *Kreosotum's* action and may be so painful as to interfere with sleep. The teeth decay rapidly, becoming dark and brittle, even developing black spots as soon as they appear. The gums are spongy, bleed easily, and may be bluish. The left side may be primarily affected. The mouth odor will usually be putrid.

These animals will be very restless at around three in the morning and may even cry out. They may also cry out while passing their stool. Vomiting several hours after eating is a keynote for *Kreosotum*.

Mercurius (*vivus* or *solubilis*)

Mercury, primarily as the compound calomel, was a standard of conventional medicine for many years. It was commonly administered until the patient began to salivate profusely. This was due to the affinity to the mouth and the impact upon the gums. Frequently, the patient lost part or all of her teeth as a consequence. George Washington's famous false teeth (they were probably not wooden) were a reward for his syphilis, which was treated with mercury by his doctors, among them Benjamin Rush, one of the signers of the Declaration of Independence and one of this country's foremost allopathic physicians.

As a homeopathic medicine, *Mercurius* retains this affinity to the mouth. Gum disease with profuse salivation is a hallmark of the *Mercurius* state; salivation occurs even during sleep. The gums are usually spongy, red, and painful, and they bleed easily. The teeth become quite loose due to bone loss, and they fall out easily. Yellow discharges are common from any orifice; the tongue may be coated yellow, with indentations from the teeth. Nasal discharge and inflammation often accompany the mouth symptoms. Yellow or yellow-green foul-smelling pus is usually present.

The animal needing *Mercurius* is often like a thermometer in that she is sensitive to both hot and cold temperatures. There is often a foul odor, not only to the mouth but to the entire body. Diarrhea with straining is common. This state is usually serious, with many body systems affected. Typically, all symptoms become worse at sundown, only lessening as morning approaches, and they may be quite restless at night. These animals may be angry and quick to bite, especially if disciplined.

Mercurius corrosivus

As with *Merc v,* this remedy has great affinity to the gums, and I have seen good result in some cats with calicivirus infections with *Merc corr,* wherein there was great salivation, foul odor, and ulceration. This is not the only remedy for calicivirus, though; as with all conditions, individualization is critical. *Merc corr* may also be more useful in males, though this is by no means universal.

Muriaticum acidum

All "acid remedy" states share the symptoms of weakness and irritating discharges, with inflammation of mucous membranes. When these remedies are needed, the animal's curative powers are often poor. *Muriatic acid* is no exception, and one of the focal points for this remedy is the entire digestive tract, but particularly the mouth. Deep ulceration and inflammation suggest this remedy. The tongue, however, tends to be dry, even leathery, and may be difficult to use. It may be dark red and covered with a grayish-white membrane.

These animals may have an aversion to eating meat (very strange for a carnivore) and will often have watery diarrhea, which irritates the anus, creating great pain and sensitivity. Urination is usually accompanied by diarrhea, often because urination is difficult and requires much straining. Listlessness is pronounced, though the animal may be irritable. They feel worse in open air, so they prefer to be indoors.

Natrum muriaticum

This polychrest remedy (from common table salt) is a sodium salt of muriatic acid, so it has similar symptoms, especially relating to the mucous membrane irritation and ulceration. The gums are spongy, sore, and bleed easily, and frothy saliva collects at the edge of the tongue. Salivation is greatest in the morning. The tongue feels heavy and is difficult to use, as with *Muriatic acid*. Vesicles (small blisters) may be present on the tongue; they are quite painful when eating.

These animals are almost always very thirsty and cannot tolerate much heat, especially the heat of the sun. They often do not like petting and prefer to keep to themselves. Illness frequently follows grief, as when a household companion dies or leaves. They may be hungry, yet not eat very much—either due to the grief or to the mouth inflammation (if present). There is often a desire for salty foods and fish.

Nitric acid

Nitric acid has the acid remedy's affinity for mucous membranes, causing irritation and ulceration in the mouth, urethra, eyes, nose, and anus. These ulcers are usually quite painful, as though from a splinter or hot wire. Ulceration commonly erupts on the soft palate and the inside of the cheeks. The tongue may have a furrow down the center and pimple-like eruptions on the sides.

These animals crave fats and salty foods and are very irritable, even vicious; they will bite or strike with little provocation, and they go for blood. They are often chilly, and while not as weak as some others that require acid remedies, they still become tired and weary easily, especially emotionally.

Phosphorus

The gum inflammation seen when this remedy is indicated is often behind and around the incisors; these animals may lose their incisors at a young age. Bleeding from the gums occurs readily, even from light touch. There may also be eroded and bleeding areas inside the cheeks.

Thirsty, friendly, vocal, chilly, demanding, and easily startled encapsulates the *Phosphorus* personality. He is usually lean and tall and vomits easily.

Sycotic co

This remedy, one of the bowel nosodes, has great affinity for the mouth and nose, with mucus and ulceration. It is good for feline calicivirus and herpesvirus (rhinotracheitis) infections. The tongue may appear scalded, and there may be ulcers on the tongue or gums, with salivation and foul odor, similar to the *Mercurius* family. There also may be cracks in the corners of the mouth or in the nose. A great remedy if available; it is generally a prescription remedy.

Syphilinum

I list this remedy primarily for practitioners; it is deep-acting and can be quite useful in ulcerative inflammations. As a nosode, this medicine is available by prescription only to licensed practitioners. I recommend that its use be under the direction of an experienced homeopath.

These animals may be very similar to those needing *Mercurius,* with the irritability and the aggravation at sundown. The mucous membranes are affected, as are teeth and bones. The teeth decay quickly, and easily loosen. There may be paralysis of the tongue. Salivation can be profuse and occurs while asleep.

Ranula

A ranula is a translucent, cystic (fluid-filled) swelling under the tongue. It results from an obstruction of the duct of one of the sublingual salivary glands, although the cause is unknown. In my experience, it is more common in dogs than cats. An affected dog may have difficulty drinking or eating due to the swelling. Frequently, he will constantly move the tongue and mouth until it becomes obvious that there is a problem. It is not serious and often will recede on its own, though many need to be surgically lanced.

Homeopathic Medicines for Ranula

There is not much differentiation in the local symptoms of ranulas, and most of the remedies are covered in this chapter for other conditions, so please refer to those descriptions as well as to the *materia medica* section. Your choice of remedy will need to be based upon other, accompanying symptoms as well as mental and general states.

Calcarea carbonica, Fluoric acid, Mezereum
See below, under "Abscessed or Decaying Teeth."

Mercurius, Natrum muriaticum, Nitric acid, Syphilinum
See above, under "Gingivitis and Mouth Inflammation."

Thuja occidentalis
The ranula might be bluish-red, and the veins under the tongue may be prominent. See also below, under "Abscessed or Decaying Teeth."

Abscessed or Decaying Teeth

These conditions result from an inability to mount an effective immune response, as with gingivitis. The difference, however, is that gingivitis and ulceration are conditions of immune system overactivity; abscesses and decay often result from underactivity, though the underactivity is a degeneration, when the body is wearing out (even if young), not a psoric (congenitally weak) condition. It is as if, in the initial stage, the body throws everything at the illness, thus the intense inflammation of an acute gingivitis. If the body is weak, this intense response is impossible, so a slow insidious response occurs. Pus forms from the constant death of white blood cells, bacteria, and local tissue cells. The body gathers the white blood cells to the area to fight bacteria that are multiplying in the weakened area, but the body cannot move the debris out fast enough, and it accumulates as pus. Put another way, the body tries to rid itself of infection by mounting an intense short-lived response; if this is impossible, then the slower response must suffice. If enough immune strength remains, the abscess will eventually heal, though it may require several days. In many cases, however, particularly with tooth abscesses, the infection and the low-grade inflammation persist.

Tooth decay can be from several causes. Persistent inflammation and infection will result in decay due to chemicals released by bacteria as well as from body tissues. Animals that are born with weak vitality often produce poorly formed teeth, and particularly a poor enamel coating, leaving them susceptible to early decay. Some viruses, such as the canine distemper virus, cause poor enamel formation in infected puppies. Those that survive the illness carry these malformed teeth into adulthood as evidence of the puppyhood infection.

Treatment with homeopathic medications will not reverse decay, but it may help slow or stop the process. This treatment, however, usually requires deep constitutional prescribing and is beyond the scope of this book. My focus will be upon decay associated with infections, though I will mention a few of the main remedies for decay due to poor development.

General Care for Abscessed or Decaying Teeth

In most cases, dental abscesses create a persistent, slowly developing condition that warrants slow immune-building treatment. Antibiotics, though commonly prescribed, often will not effectively stop the abscessing. Persistent chronic infections can lead to secondary inflammation of the heart valves and kidneys, so seek veterinary care to help assess the condition, and do not let an infection go on too long. Sometimes, however, the abscess is more acute and needs immediate attention. In either case, a dental cleaning may be necessary to allow healing, especially if there is a lot of tartar accumulation. (See above, under "General Care for Gingivitis and Mouth Inflammation," for more information about dental cleaning.) In especially severe cases, the affected tooth may require extraction.

Modern veterinary medicine now includes many dental procedures formerly available only for humans. Some of these are good, like better equipment for cleaning, X-rays, and so on, but veterinary dentists now offer root canals and cavity treatment. I do not recommend root canals in any circumstance (for human or nonhuman animals), as these use toxic substances as well as leave foci of bacterial infection, and have been associated with cancer, heart disease, kidney disease, and other chronic illness in humans. It is best to pull the tooth. Filling cavities is less black and white; plastic fillings contain estrogenic compounds and do not last long, and mercury amalgams are dangerous as well. Gold inlay is best, but I don't know anyone using this in animals. For minor cavities, filling them may be acceptable, but if they are large, I'd probably just have the tooth extracted.

To enhance the immune system, herbs like astragalus, echinacea, and goldenseal can help with infections. Use goldenseal only in severe conditions and for no longer than one to two weeks in dogs and one week in cats. Echinacea is safe for two to four weeks, and cat's claw for one to two months, although I prefer to stop all herbs periodically to rest the body. As with gingivitis, vitamin C, vitamin E, coenzyme Q_{10}, and pycnogenol may be helpful as well. See the "Gingivitis and Mouth Inflammation" section above for dosage.

To strengthen tooth enamel and teeth, dandelion, oats, cleavers, and nettles can help. Osteoherb, a prepared supplement for humans, is available from Herbalist & Alchemist (800-611-8235 or www.herbalist-alchemist.com) and is a great dental support supplement; use one-half capsule for cats and small dogs, up to two capsules for large dogs, given once to twice daily. You can mix this in food.

Have your companion checked right away:
- if she is weak and listless;
- if there is a swelling under the eye or elsewhere;
- if there is pain or intense inflammation—especially with lethargy;
- if there is a fever above 103.

Have an examination soon:
- to determine the overall health and to assess the impact of the infection/inflammation;
- if an abscess does not improve within one to three weeks (sooner if vitality wanes).

Next, try to determine patterns and circumstances:
- Is the abscess or tooth painful?

- Is the pus especially foul-smelling? (Perhaps an unfair question, as it all stinks—but some is worse than others.)
- Is the animal irritable? Weak? Easily startled?

Acute Tooth Abscesses

If your companion's energy is good, it is appropriate to treat the abscess with homeopathic medicines and immune-strengthening methods rather than antibiotics. The correct remedy will open the abscess and encourage healing at least as quickly as antibiotics and with greater therapeutic benefit to the animal. It is almost always better to allow the healing to come from the individual rather than drugs—long-term health will be better. Valerian root may help relieve tooth pain when there is an abscess.

Homeopathic Medicines for Tooth Abscesses

Calcarea carbonica

One of our main remedies for poor development (as are all the *Calcarea* family), *Calc carb* is classically suited to overweight, sluggish, lazy, big-boned individuals. They may be awkward in their movements. Teeth and bones are often poorly formed, slow to erupt, and easily broken. These animals generally have slow, minimally reactive abscesses, usually associated with enlarged glands under the jaw.

Calc carb animals are very sensitive to cold and damp weather. Sometimes they emit a sour odor or discharges from the body, mouth, and/or ears. They can be quite fearful of change, and they like a consistent schedule. We usually find them friendly, easygoing individuals.

Calcarea fluorica

As with *Calc carb*, this can be useful for abscesses, but animals needing this remedy often look like they are decaying, with poor coat, teeth, and generally poor condition.

Gunpowder

Gunpowder is useful for abscesses anywhere, and tooth abscesses are no exception. It is especially useful if there is septicemia—a systemic infection in addition to the local one. You would see an animal that is usually running a fever and listless. There may be bone infection as well, though you would not know this unless you either have a dental X-ray or the bone is visibly enlarged. Recurring abscesses may respond here as well.

Hecla lava

This remedy is made from volcanic ash found near Mount Hecla in Iceland. Sheep in the area develop exostoses (bony growths) on the jaws at much higher rates than elsewhere—this substance has great affinity to the jaw. Cancerous and noncancerous growths on the jaw often respond to *Hecla*. Tooth abscesses may also respond, and often there will be damage to the bone as well, either growths or deterioration. The glands will typically be enlarged also, and the glands and bony growths are painful to touch. The right side may be more prominently affected.

Hepar sulphuris calcareum

Hepar sulph provides relief in perhaps one-third of simple abscesses in cats and dogs. Only *Silicea* proves to be of greater importance in this realm. When *Hepar sulph* is indicated, the animal is usually irritable and chilly, and the abscess is very painful to the touch. The combination of irritability and pain may result in injuries to caregivers, as light touch can provoke a bite or scratch. The pus is especially foul-smelling.

Hypericum perforatum

This remedy is more for tooth pain than abscesses, but can be of great service in reducing discomfort, whether before or after an extraction, since it has such an affinity to nerves.

Mercurius (vivus or solubilis)

In addition to its usefulness for inflammatory diseases of the mouth, *Mercurius* may be indicated in abscesses if the other mouth symptoms fit. See above, under "Gingivitis and Mouth Inflammation," for a description of these symptoms. The pus tends to be acrid, causing irritation to any skin that it touches.

Caution: *Mercurius* and *Silicea* are very similar in some ways, but they should never be used after one another. If you have given one without effect, do not give the other right after. Use another remedy in between—*Sulphur* and *Hepar sulph* are good choices. The disease may intensify otherwise.

Phosphorus

Although not a major abscess remedy, *Phosphorus* does have an affinity to the lower jaw. Abscesses of teeth in the lower jawbone may call for *Phosphorus*, especially if accompanied by hemorrhage. When I have used this remedy for abscesses, the affected animal was easily startled and jumpy—a classic *Phosphorus* reaction.

Pyrogenium

When abscesses continue to recur, think of *Pyrogenium* (or *Gunpowder*). The abscess will usually be very painful, and tissues around the abscess are heavily damaged. The infection often spreads into the blood stream, so these animals may be quite ill. They are often in great pain, especially in the back, and they move constantly, as if they are unable to remain in one position long due to the pain. They are very chilly.

Silicea (Silica)

Silicea is far and away the main remedy for abscesses. Indications for *Silicea* include weakness, poor reaction, chilliness, and sensitivity to noise. The pus is typically rather bland and not so foul as that of the *Hepar sulph* or *Mercurius* states. Teeth may be brittle and malformed, as when *Calcarea* is needed, but the animal needing *Silicea* is more likely to be fine-boned rather than heavy.

Staphysagria

This is a good remedy for dental abscesses, especially with an animal who can be sweet alternating with reactive. The abscess is usually painful and especially sensitive to touch.

Homeopathic Medicines for Decaying Teeth

Note: As I mentioned above, homeopathy will not reverse decay, but it may stop or slow its progress.

Calcarea carbonica

See above, under "Homeopathic Medicines for Tooth Abscesses."

Calcarea fluorica

All remedies with fluorine as a component may be indicated for bone and tooth decay, because of fluorine's tendency to replace calcium, weakening these structures. When *Calc fluor* is indicated, the teeth have very minimal enamel and crumble easily. Glands may be enlarged and are often rock hard. Malnutrition occurs due to poor assimilation of foods as much as a poor diet. These are weak, scrawny individuals. They may have rickets.

Fluoric acid
The teeth come in late and then decay rapidly, especially at the gum line. The upper jaw is primarily affected. Although weak and sickly, these animals are intolerant of heat. These animals are very ill, with much degeneration, and even young animals may look quite old.

Mezereum
Mezereum may be needed for animals whose teeth decay rapidly at the roots. This may be accompanied by extremely itchy skin with no other evidence of skin disease.

Thuja occidentalis
The *Thuja* state includes the propensity to get decay at the gum line, and the teeth may be quite sensitive. Warts are common as well, even in the mouth. These animals may also develop urinary tract disease. The "neck lesions" (decay at the gum line) so common in cats resemble the description of the *Thuja* type of decay. *Thuja* is known to be a major remedy for vaccine-induced illness, as is *Mezereum*. Could vaccination play a part, along with poor foods, in the recent "outbreak" of these cavities in cats?

Homeopathic Remedies for Dental Care and Extractions
Teeth have extensive and sensitive nerve roots and can become quite painful as a result. Whether following extractions, or even just dental cleaning, the pain can be severe. Pain-minimizing medications can be helpful, but often, homeopathic remedies can also minimize pain quite well. From personal experience, I find that different remedies work at different times. Furthermore, even following one procedure, sometimes one remedy works for a time, then stops working. I then move on to another remedy, trying a few until I find one that works. Sometimes a remedy that did not work initially will work later, after taking another remedy for a time. The following are remedies that can help.

Arnica montana
The great trauma remedy; I tend to use this before and immediately following any surgical procedure.

Bellis perennis

The daisy; closely related to *Arnica*. *Bellis* is indicated for deeper trauma, such as abdominal, breast, testicle, and dental trauma. It can be effective when *Arnica* is not.

Calendula officinalis

This is a great post–dental extraction remedy; it helps heal as well as often helps with pain.

Hepar sulphuris calcareum

Mostly indicated in infections and abscesses, *Hepar sulph* can be helpful following extractions where there was infection, and can also help with dental pain in some cases.

Hypericum perforatum

"The *Arnica* of the nerves." *Hypericum* is helpful anytime there is great nerve involvement and nerve pain.

Nux vomica

Nux can help with the postanesthesia "drugging" effect as well as in some (but not many) cases of dental pain. The animal may be irritable following recovery, usually from the "hangover" resulting from the drugs.

Phosphorus

This remedy is great for postsurgical hemorrhage, as well as to help animals recover from surgery. Use this if bleeding or slow recovery is an issue.

Staphysagria

This remedy is good for incisional pain and more superficial pain of wounds, but it can be a very good analgesic for dental pain.

Chapter Eight
DIGESTIVE SYSTEM

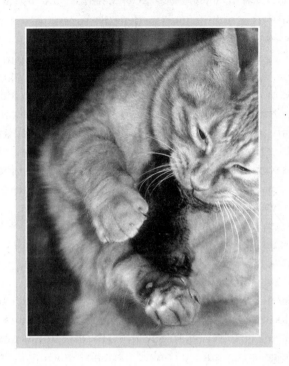

Foods

I have always liked the adage, "We are what we eat," and this applies as well to dogs and cats as to humans. The digestive system will usually bear the brunt of poor food intake. Other organs affected secondarily include the liver, pancreas, kidneys, and skin: the liver and pancreas as part of the digestive process, and the liver, kidneys, and skin as organs of elimination. Ultimately, of course, the entire body will suffer without adequate nutrition. Further, as the bowel goes, so goes the organism. In other words, if the digestion proceeds well and smoothly, and the foods move through the digestive tract from mouth to anus steadily and regularly, health tends to be good. As with humans, fresh foods provide the healthiest source of nutrition. This is partly because many nutrients such as vitamins and enzymes are extremely sensitive and easily destroyed by processing.

Another explanation relates to an absence of the life force, known as Qi in traditional Chinese medicine (pronounced "chee"—see Chapter Two, "The Nature of Disease"). Without Qi, foods may provide physical nutrients but no nourishment of the life force of the body. Dr. Francis Pottenger demonstrated this in his studies of cats in the 1930s. Pottenger separated the cats into three main groups. All groups received the same basic diet of meat, milk, and cod liver oil. In one group the cats ate raw meat and milk. The second group consumed cooked meat and raw milk, while the third group had raw meat and pasteurized milk. Dr. Pottenger observed that the cats feasting upon all-raw ingredients flourished, while those offered part of the diet cooked became weak and obviously malnourished. Even more fascinating, however, he noticed that the plants growing in the pens with each group reflected the diet as well: manure from the all-raw-food cats produced lush growth while that from the cats on part-cooked food produced poor, spindly growth.[1] Chemical analysis would show the same ingredients in all three diets, yet something was depleted by cooking the foods. That something is Qi. No Qi from food to cats, so no Qi from cats to plants.

Carnivores derive their primary nutrition (in cats, their entire nutrition) from the consumption of other animals. This is critical for health, and attempts to feed vegetarian diets to carnivores ultimately lead to malnutrition. Evolution ushered these animals into a predatory niche, and while dogs may tolerate a large quantity of nonmeat items in their food, inadequate meat quantities will not sustain them. Cats are obligate carnivores, that is, they must consume an almost all-animal diet to maintain health.

As a longtime vegetarian myself, I fully understand the desire to limit consumption of animals as food. Yet, I believe feeding carnivores a vegetarian diet to be tantamount to abuse. I have seen cases of severe malnutrition due to (well-intentioned) limitation of animal products in the diets of companion animals. Imagine the situation if we were the pets of our animals. Our canine and feline companions would joyfully provide us with freshly killed animals for our consumption (raw, of course)—as indeed cats often do when they present a fresh mouse at our doorstep each morning. Having evolved as primarily herbivores, we do not always appreciate the gesture; I do not believe carnivores much appreciate our offers of cereal-based meals either. The only fair choice, if buying and feeding animal products seems impossible to you, is choosing an herbivore rather than a carnivore as a companion. Another option is simply reducing the numbers of companion animals; see Chapter Seventeen, "The Bigger Picture," for more on this topic.

Function

The gastrointestinal (GI) system is a common site of problems in dogs and cats. As the first line of defense against toxins or organisms taken into the body via the mouth, this element is second only to the skin in importance as a barrier to outside forces. In many ways, the GI tract is an interior extension of the skin, as it constitutes a tunnel through the body. In essence, the body is like a long, hollow cylinder with the skin providing the outside surface and the GI tract the inside surface.

Just as the skin has a normal population of microorganisms within the pores and hair follicles of its exterior, the intestine hosts a variety of life forms within the nooks and crannies of its interior. These organisms live in harmony in a healthy body, and they aid in digestion as well as provide a source of vitamins for the host, particularly the B group. Even the notorious E. coli is a normal inhabitant of virtually every intestine on the planet. Generally, these organisms cause no problems unless the host organism is unhealthy prior to the overgrowth of the bacteria.

The basic function of the GI system is digestion of foods into usable and "waste" portions. Initial breakdown of foods begins with chewing and the concomitant addition of saliva, although minimal chewing occurs when dogs and cats eat foods. As carnivores, they simply tear food into pieces small enough to be swallowed. The only exceptions are with bones and dry foods. Chewing bones is actually quite healthy for carnivores, and they rarely encounter problems. Dry foods, however, are generally very unhealthy, particularly for cats, and *do not mimic bone chewing* as a method of keeping teeth clean and gums healthy.

Digestion begins in the mouth. Chewing begins to break down the foods, with the assistance of saliva, which contains mucin (a lubricant) and ptyalin (a form of amylase, an enzyme that digests starches). The stomach continues the breakdown of foods into a sort of mush. Hydrochloric acid plus enzymes provide the major chemical force, along with mechanical contraction of the stomach walls, changing the food into a consistency that is ready for further digestion in the small intestine. In contrast to humans, dogs and cats produce stomach acids only when they eat. Having evolved as predators, carnivores gorge themselves when they have the opportunity and rest between kills. Due to their high-meat diets, fasting between meals provides the important benefit of allowing the system to empty somewhat and clean itself. As seen in humans, residue from meats can be carcinogenic (this is a factor in colon cancer), thus periods of cleansing are essential. Additionally, carnivore systems are not used to the constant presence of stomach acids that occurs with continuous feeding. Intermittent feeding is essential to maintain health in carnivores. One or two meals daily are sufficient for most animals. An observation study on feral cats found that these cats ate, on average, about once every twenty-eight hours. Essentially, they ate when they caught something, and if it was large, they slept and lounged until they were hungry again. This is normal and healthy. Based upon this, once-daily feeding is probably preferable for cats and dogs, but twice daily is an acceptable substitute. It is important to pick up food between these meals, though, even if you still choose to use dry food (which I do not recommend). Feeding more often proves detrimental, and it encourages them to "hound" us for food all the time.

From the stomach, the food passes into the small intestine, where further breakdown occurs. Secretion of bile acids from the liver and gall bladder into the intestine aids in fat digestion, as does pancreatic secretion of the enzyme lipase. Amylase, another pancreatic enzyme, assists in starch digestion. Trypsin and other enzymes begin protein digestion. Bacteria living in the intestine aid in digestion and conversion of food products into substances that are utilizable by the host animal. The process of assimilation, or uptake of nutrients, also begins in the upper small intestine and is basically completed by the time the food residue passes into the large intestine, or colon.

The colon functions primarily as a storage and evacuation organ, sort of the body's solid waste disposal department. An important aspect of this is recovery (by reabsorption) of water and electrolytes from the waste before excretion. This greatly improves the efficiency of water metabolism.

In healthy animals, food and water consumption occurs in appropriate quantities at an appropriate rate. By the same token, solids and liquids exit the body at proper rates and in proper quantities and consistency. Most of the liquid excretion occurs via the urinary system. A certain amount does exit with fecal matter and keeps feces soft.

When illness occurs, symptoms of GI disturbance represent an inability of the body to carry out these normal functions. Food may not go down or stay down, thus regurgitation occurs, which is ejection of swallowed undigested foods shortly after eating. If foods have been in the stomach or even the small intestine longer and digestion is well underway, expulsion of these is called vomiting. Evacuation problems may be too rapid or too slow. Too-rapid passage leads to poor assimilation of foods and poor reabsorption of water, resulting in diarrhea. If movement is slow, excessive water resorption occurs and stools become dry and hard, resulting in constipation. With diarrhea or constipation there may be mucus or blood, straining (tenesmus), improper color or odor, undigested foods, or gas. Poor digestion or poor foods may also lead to irritating discharges, causing inflammation around the anus.

Regurgitation and Vomiting

To some degree, these are normal for cats and dogs. Both species have some voluntary control of the muscles involved in expelling foods through vomiting or regurgitation, as these functions provide a means of ridding the body of spoiled foods previously eaten. Dogs, as scavengers as well as hunters, more often consume potentially rancid foods than cats, so regurgitation and vomiting may occur frequently in dogs that "eat out." This may be normal in some cases. Cats also depend upon these functions for survival, but for a different reason. Unlike most species, felines have limited ability to break down many toxic chemicals found in rancid foods. As a result, poisoning is an ever-present risk, and without the ability to eliminate these toxins via the mouth, cats would die. (For this same reason, cats handle many drugs poorly. As an example, acetaminophen—Tylenol is the most common brand name—is highly poisonous and should never be administered to a cat). Cats have developed acute senses of taste and smell rather than detoxification mechanisms to protect against rancid foods, as they evolved eating freshly killed animals only. This creates the "finicky cat" stereotype: their senses tell them not to eat rancid foods. Unfortunately, most commercial foods contain large quantities of rancid animal products.

Rancid foods thus often lead to gastrointestinal illness in dogs as well as cats on commercial foods. A significant number of cases will respond well to a simple change in the diet to fresh food. Fresh raw meats, as mentioned above, retain enzymes to aid digestion and thus often assist problems of digestion and malassimilation of foods, a common cause of vomiting as well as diarrhea.

Essentially, then, vomiting is a means of ridding the body of toxins or unhealthy food by-products. If there is no obvious source for these toxins, they may be generated by poorly functioning internal organs, such as the liver, pancreas, or the kidneys. If vomiting occurs (especially if it persists) and there is no obvious cause, such as eating garbage or spoiled foods, it is a good idea to get an exam to see if there is a serious problem underlying the vomiting.

General Care for Regurgitation and Vomiting

If your companion experiences vomiting or regurgitation, you must first assess the severity the problem.

- Is this an isolated incident, or does this happen regularly?
- What is coming up? Digested food, undigested food, mucus, blood, bile?
- Is the vomitus foul-smelling (putrid, rotten)?
- How frequently is it occurring?
- Is she weak and listless?
- Is she dehydrated? (To check for dehydration, pick up some skin over the back and let it drop. It should return to its original position immediately. Any slowness of return indicates dehydration. Compare the response with a healthy animal if possible.)

Have your companion checked right away:

- if you notice weakness or dehydration;

- if vomiting occurs more than two to four times a day, especially if it lasts for more than three days;
- if you see blood (bright red to black), or if the contents are foul-smelling;
- if vomiting persists even with fasting (see below).

Have an examination soon:

- if vomiting/regurgitation occurs more than once a week;
- if the condition persists after correcting diet and after home treatment;
- if you see bile (yellow fluid) more than one or two times.

Next, try to determine patterns or circumstances. Are there triggering conditions such as:

- eating, or eating a large quantity of food (how soon after);
- spoiled foods, garbage;
- drinking (how soon after);
- times of day (morning, before breakfast, night, etc.);
- stress or anxiety?

Acute Vomiting

If the condition seems mild and the energy is good, fast her for twenty-four hours to allow the stomach to calm down. You may offer broth after four to eight hours in small quantities (one tablespoon for cats and small dogs, one to four ounces for medium dogs, and eight ounces for large dogs) at fifteen- to thirty-minute intervals. It is best to prepare fresh broth rather than using canned broth. If broth is not retained, wait another three to four hours and try again, or wait overnight if she seems OK otherwise. After twenty-four hours, begin offering food in small quantities, about the same as for broth, above. Use the well-cooked meat from preparing broth, and combine with well-cooked grains (white rice, millet, or oatmeal) in equal volume or two parts grain to one part meat. If vomiting recurs, go back to broth for twelve to twenty-four hours and try again.

After twenty-four hours on small meals, you may transition back onto a normal diet. This should be home-prepared if possible, but if you have not been using homemade foods, use 50 to 75 percent of the previous diet and 25 to 50 percent fresh homemade food. Increase 25 percent homemade per week until the transition is complete. Diets should not be switched abruptly, because in some animals this provides a shock to the system. With sick or older animals the introduction of fresh diets must be very gradual (start with no more than 25 percent), as these individuals are more likely to suffer reactions to quick changes.

If your dog develops pancreatitis, vitamin C (10 mg/pound) and selenium (0.5 mcg/pound) can offset acute episodes. You may need a few doses. The Pet Pancreatitis Tonic by Sharon Hubbs-Kreft works well for cats and dogs with chronic pancreatitis. See www.localharvest.org to order this product.

Chronic Vomiting

Have a thorough examination to assess the reason for the vomiting. These animals should be under the care of an experienced homeopathic veterinarian unless the vomiting is infrequent. Change the diet to a fresh one, as this will improve most cases and eliminate the problem in some. If you suspect stomach or upper small intestine ulceration, DGL (deglycyrrhizinated licorice) wafers are excellent for this. Give one chewable wafer per fifty pounds to dogs. It is safe for cats, but difficult to administer. Broccoli sprouts also help heal stomach ulcers.

For cats with hair balls, *Nux vomica* sometimes helps. Also, giving butter or adding butter to the food often works as well as the hair ball remedies and is much safer. Use real butter (preferably organic), and give about one-half teaspoonful daily (about one-half pat). You can also give flax or olive oil by dropperfuls in acute hair ball episodes, or mix it in food at the same dose as for butter.

As with acute vomiting, changing the food to a healthy, fresh food–based diet may alleviate chronic vomiting in some cases.

Homeopathic Medicines for Regurgitation and Vomiting

Arsenicum album

A major remedy for vomiting as well as diarrhea, *Arsenicum* is well suited for conditions ranging from mild to life-threatening. Hallmarks of the *Arsenicum* state include the triad of restlessness, chilliness, and thirst. Typically, the thirst is for small amounts at a time, though it may be for large quantities. Often, after drinking there is a tendency for regurgitation within a short period of time. In animals needing *Arsenicum*, diarrhea and vomiting may occur at the same time. In severe cases, extreme weakness or even collapse may occur, with coldness. Nausea may be so profound that animals cannot stand the sight or smell of food. There may also be thirst without desire to drink. This will show as the animal that hangs his head over the water bowl. The vomitus is often foul-smelling, even hard to distinguish from feces (fecal vomiting). Vomiting may be quite painful, as seen in cats who cry out before vomiting.

Arsenicum has served well in parvovirus disease in dogs, and it is a major remedy for food poisoning, garbage eating, and other toxic conditions.

Bismuth

This element is situated just below arsenic on the periodic table, thus its properties are similar to *Arsenicum*, though more intense. The keynote is the stomach pain, which is pronounced. *Bismuth* animals may be clingy with their guardians, and they crave cold water but vomit immediately. This remedy is not commonly indicated, but it can be useful with stomach pain, even with cancer.

Cocculus

Cocculus is my first choice for motion sickness, including nausea and vomiting from riding in a car. These animals may also become nauseated from looking at or smelling food, as can those needing *Colocynthis* and other remedies. *Cocculus* patients may also be drowsy and have issues with inco-ordination.

Ferrum metallicum

These animals will regurgitate immediately after eating, often without nausea, and food may be brought up by the mouthful. There is an aversion to meat, which would be very unusual in a carnivore. The appetite tends to alternate between increased and diminished. Anemia and pale gums may accompany the *Ferrum* state, as well as a throbbing headache. Mentally, these individuals may be hard (like iron) and intolerant of contradiction, as one might expect with a severe headache. The headache may also make them shy about petting or being touched on the head.

Ipecac

Ipecac finds its best use in vomiting. The keynote here is nausea and vomiting with respiratory conditions. Nausea is profound and not relieved by vomiting. Overeating and rich foods may bring about the *Ipecac* state. Vomiting of infants while nursing also can indicate *Ipecac*. The vomitus often contains blood.

Iris versicolor

With this remedy, there is burning throughout the digestive tract, colic, and recurrent episodes of vomiting. Pancreatitis can sometimes respond well to *Iris*. Vomitus tends to contain bile and recurs every four to six weeks, often lasting two or three days. *Iris* can be a good remedy for animals with recurrent vomiting. These animals may be irritable, like *Nux* animals. The liver may be affected as well.

Nux vomica

Nux is another remedy for garbage poisoning and toxic conditions, especially drug reactions (vomiting, diarrhea, or constipation as a side effect of drug therapy). It is not quite as broadly indicated for vomiting as its name might imply, though. *Nux* patients tend to be chilly and irritable. The irritability may come in part because they have cramping pains and forcible, painful vomiting as well as diarrhea. Animals needing *Nux* often feel better after vomiting and worse from eating, especially overeating.

Phosphorus

The *Phosphorus* state is generally one of regurgitation rather than vomiting. Animals needing *Phosphorus* bring up food and drink as soon as it is warmed by the stomach. Cats eating dry food will often bring it up rather quickly, and the food has generally been swallowed whole. This is because *Phosphorus* animals are usually ravenous. The thirst matches the hunger and is for cold water. *Phosphorus* animals tend to be thin, tall, friendly, and vocal.

Pulsatilla

Two characteristic *Pulsatilla* symptoms are thirstlessness and vomiting of undigested food several hours after eating. These animals typically crave attention, so they stay by people and can be quite persistent about petting. Although generally chilly, *Pulsatilla* animals cannot tolerate warm closed rooms, so they crave fresh air. Additionally, they are usually very sweet animals, so they capture our hearts.

Spongia tosta

I include *Spongia* in this section because it can be useful for pancreatitis. Vomiting is not such a major concern here, though these patients may vomit. These are the animals who may hunch after eating, due to abdominal pain. They tend to have rumbling in the abdomen, often before stool. This has been described as a snarling noise (now, that's descriptive!). Eating may help the *Spongia* cough, especially with warm food and drink, but it worsens the stomach distress. Thus these animals may be very hungry but stop eating before satisfying the hunger, due to the discomfort.

Veratrum album

This remedy is similar in many ways to *Arsenicum*. The *Veratrum* state is one of intense nausea, violent vomiting, collapse, and coldness. Like *Phosphorus* patients, these animals crave food and cold water. Water is immediately regurgitated, and this typically induces intense retching. Vomiting may be painful in these animals and is often accompanied by diarrhea. The onset is generally sudden, with rapid deterioration to a collapsed, cold state. The gums and other mucous membranes turn blue due to rapid dehydration and poor blood circulation. These animals need immediate veterinary care, but the remedy can be administered on the way to the hospital as well as in conjunction with critical care. *Veratrum* animals may be very irritable if they have the strength. *Veratrum* is also useful for food poisoning.

Diarrhea

As with vomiting, diarrhea is a way for the body to remove toxins and waste materials quickly. With acute diarrhea, this is virtually always the case, and these situations will often resolve themselves once the purging has finished. Causes include ingestion of toxins or bacteria as in food poisoning, virus infections (canine parvovirus, feline panleukopenia), and parasites (worms, *Giardia*). Acute diarrhea is common with many drugs also, as the body tries to rid itself of the toxin.

As with other chronic diseases, chronic diarrhea is a systemic problem, a symptom of a poorly functioning immune system. Many causes are possible, including poor diet. Repeated vaccination for viruses that cause acute diarrhea may lead to chronic diarrhea through establishment of a chronic form of the disease (see Chapter Sixteen, "Vaccination").

General Care for Diarrhea

If your companion is having diarrhea, try to ascertain the severity of the situation:

- Is this an isolated incident, or does it happen regularly?
- How frequently is the diarrhea occurring?
- What does the diarrhea look like? Is there mucus, blood (bright red or black), undigested food? What color is the diarrhea?
- Is she dehydrated? (See the "Vomiting" section.)
- Is she weak and listless?
- Is there a lot of straining?

Have your companion checked right away:
- if he is weak or dehydrated;
- if you see blood (black or red);
- if diarrhea occurs more than six to eight times in a day.

Have an examination soon:
- if diarrhea lasts more than three to four days;
- if diarrhea persists after home treatment and correcting diet;
- if diarrhea episodes occur more than once a month;
- if there is weight loss or poor appearance of coat and skin.

Next, try to determine patterns and circumstances. Are there triggering conditions such as:
- eating, or eating certain foods;
- spoiled foods or garbage;
- stress or anxiety;
- times of day or night?

Acute Diarrhea

If your companion's energy is good and the condition seems mild, simply modifying the diet to a simpler one may resolve the diarrhea. Try one-half to two-thirds white rice or millet and the balance boiled meat. Fasting for the first twenty-four hours will often speed resolution of the problem. Prepare fresh broth by boiling meat, and offer this for the first day. Follow this with the grain-meat mix (above) until the stool is firm, and then transition back to a balanced diet. Cats can be quite resistant to a high-grain diet, so use the twenty-four-hour fast and then reverse the above ratio of meat to grain (i.e.

one-half to two-thirds meat). Baby food works well also, but be sure to use one without onion powder, as onion powder may cause anemia. Slippery elm bark is a good herbal remedy for diarrhea and is available in most health food stores. Give one capsule per twenty to twenty-five pounds, three times daily. For cats and small dogs, you can make a syrup: add one teaspoonful of slippery elm bark to a cup of cold water, bring to a boil, and then simmer for a couple of minutes until it thickens. Add one to three teaspoonfuls honey to sweeten. Give about one-half to one teaspoonful per ten pounds. You may also use Floressence, a version of Essiac tea, in acute or chronic diarrhea. Give about one teaspoonful of prepared tea per ten to twenty pounds, two or three times daily. You can double this if necessary. Charcoal capsules can help also for dogs, especially if you suspect food poisoning. Use one capsule per twenty pounds, and give one or two doses.

If signs of weakness or dehydration develop, have a veterinarian examine the animal right away, as supportive treatment may be necessary.

Chronic Diarrhea

First, have a veterinarian perform a complete evaluation to determine the cause of the diarrhea, if possible. Don't accept a prescription for antibiotics, however, as these are rarely indicated for gastrointestinal disease (although they are frequently prescribed). If worms are discovered, you may opt for conventional deworming medications for expediency and efficacy, or use an herbal regimen (see Dr. Pitcairn's book for herbal deworming, listed in the Appendix). If *Giardia* is diagnosed, be sure it is confirmed by microscopic examination. Grapefruit seed extract (available at health food stores) will often eliminate this pathogen; use it for ten to fourteen days. Basil is helpful as well, and for dogs can be mixed in food—one-half to one teaspoonful daily for two weeks. Neem is also an antiparasitic herb that is safe for dogs. Use capsules and give one-fourth the human dose per twenty-five pounds. Give one dose daily for ten days. Homeopathic treatment can also succeed by improving immunity. If you find drug treatment necessary, penicillin G is often quite effective and much safer than Flagyl (metronidazole), which is most commonly prescribed but is much more toxic. (The dose for pen-G is 40,000 units per kilogram, every six hours, should you need to use this. The sodium and potassium forms are equally effective.) Panacur (fenbendazole), given daily for five days, is much more effective than metronidazole (90 percent versus 70 percent effective) and much safer as well. Most veterinarians are more familiar with Panacur for giardiasis than penicillin G. It can be helpful to bathe your cat or dog on the last day of treatment to get any organisms off the coat.

As with cases of chronic vomiting, diet improvement will correct many cases of chronic diarrhea. I suggest using food enzymes for the first month or more, as often the animal is not adequately digesting food. Most health food stores and some pet stores have food enzymes. You need not use ones designed only for animals, as the ones sold for humans are fine. If you can obtain a powdered form that is made from pancreas enzymes (amylase, lipase, trypsin), those are best, but plant-based enzymes (papain, bromelain, etc.) will work also. Be sure the product has no artificial ingredients.

Gradually change to as much home-prepared foods as you can (see the Appendix for resources) and be patient, as diet-related improvement may take from one to six months. If inflammatory bowel disease (IBD) is present, expect a longer response time. It is best to work with an experienced homeopathic prescriber with IBD. At the least, you should work with a cooperative veterinarian to monitor the progress.

Supplements that can help with chronic diarrhea include slippery elm bark, at half the doses listed for acute diarrhea. Floressence is also useful; see above under "Acute Diarrhea." A good probiotic is helpful in most cases; Primal Defense is excellent, though expensive. Give one scoop or one tablet per twenty-five to forty pounds, once a day. Give one-quarter scoop to cats and one-quarter to one-half scoop to small dogs. You can also use acidophilus, like Jarrowdophilus PB-8, and Megadophilus. Marshmallow root is helpful as well; like slippery elm, this herb heals damaged mucous membranes.

Homeopathic Medicines for Diarrhea

Aloe

Animals needing *Aloe* as a homeopathic remedy have such loose and flatulent diarrhea that urging is sudden, so they may not make it outside or to the litter box. Additionally, urine and feces will usually be passed together. The anus is often very sore, with burning pain. Diarrhea occurs in the early morning, often forcing the animal up from sleeping. Mentally, these patients are sad in the morning and cheerful in the evening. They are easily fatigued.

Arsenicum album

The diarrhea in an *Arsenicum* patient is often very foul-smelling, like rotting meat. It may be black and/or quite watery and often is irritating, so the anus may be red and inflamed. Typically there is much straining, and the anus may protrude. Vomiting and diarrhea may occur at the same time. Generally the triad of restlessness, thirst, and chilliness predominates unless weakness has developed. The animal will shift position frequently, as no position remains comfortable. Weakness may be profound, as with parvovirus infections.

Baptisia

The *Baptisia* state is one of rapid debilitation and severe prostration. This remedy is well suited to canine parvovirus and other infections of the blood and intestines if the symptoms match. If your dog or cat develops a disease condition corresponding to *Baptisia,* you will need to seek veterinary care, but give the homeopathic medicine as well. These animals have offensive, watery, dark, bloody diarrhea. Animals rapidly become very weak and listless. Vomiting generally occurs in these individuals as well. They may be thirsty but not hungry. The gum color is usually dark, a pointer to this remedy.

Chamomilla

Diarrhea during teething is a keynote indicating *Chamomilla,* and stools may be grassy green and slimy with a foul odor. The diarrhea is irritating, so the anus may be sensitive. Mentally, the *Chamomilla* patient is sensitive as well as irritable and restless. Whining often accompanies the restlessness. The only relief comes when being carried about and petted constantly. These animals are generally hot and thirsty.

China (Cinchona) officinalis

Individuals needing *China* (pronounced "keena") tend to become excessively weak with diarrhea or any fluid loss. The diarrhea may be undigested food, bloody, and yellow; it is often accompanied by flatulence. Colic may occur with sensitivity to touch. Curiously, light touch is more painful than hard pressure. Diarrhea may be more likely in summer. Puppies and kittens that develop diarrhea after weaning may need *China.* In adult animals, the diarrhea often accompanies kidney disease. Debility and apathy are often prominent in these animals.

Colocynthis

The diarrhea often contains jellylike mucus in these animals, and the least food or drink will initiate an evacuation of stool. Flatulence is generally present also, and the stool may contain shreds of white material. Extreme abdominal pain accompanies any intestinal condition. Animals may lie on their stomachs or curled up, as bending double or lying on the abdomen relieves the pain. Even the slightest touch creates intense pain, leading to crying and moaning.

Croton tiglium

Yellow, squirting stools often guide us to this remedy. Like the *Aloe* state, urging is sudden in these animals, but the diarrhea of *Croton tiglium* is more explosive and projectile. Coccidia infections often produce this type of stool and thus are relieved by this remedy. The diarrhea may alternate with a skin rash that resembles poison ivy *(Croton tiglium* is often indicated for the poison ivy rash).

Lycopodium clavatum

A *Lycopodium* keynote is intestinal and urinary symptoms in the same individual, although not necessarily at the same time. Another characteristic symptom is excessive flatulence. These animals have been known to clear a room because of their gas. While this remedy is frequently needed for chronic diarrhea, it is not so often indicated in acute episodes. The diarrhea will commonly be associated with liver disease. These animals generally do not want a lot of attention, but they like to be in the same room with their caregiver.

Mercurius (solubilis or vivus)

Straining and tenesmus are almost always present in animals needing *Mercurius*. The straining is especially evident after passing a stool, as the feeling persists that there are more feces to be passed. Stools may contain mucus and blood. There may be a straining to urinate along with the straining at stool.

Mercurius corrosivus

Merc corr presents a more intense version of the *Mercurius* state. The main differences are that the straining and tenesmus are constant, and there are shredded particles in the feces. Males may need *Merc corr* more frequently than females.

Natrum sulphuricum

Two characteristics guide us to *Nat sulph:* the diarrhea occurs suddenly in the early morning (five to six or upon rising), and cold and dampness aggravate the diarrhea. Thus, wet weather, cold food and drink, and vegetables may incite an outbreak of early-morning diarrhea (as well as inciting other *Nat sulph* symptoms, such as asthma). These animals tend to be sad, and they may have liver disease as part of the picture.

Nux vomica

Animals needing *Nux* have often (though not necessarily) had a lot of medications in the past. Constipation may alternate with diarrhea, and much urging accompanies either condition. Absence of desire for defecation virtually rules out *Nux* in intestinal disorders. Overeating or eating poor foods, including garbage, often initiates diarrhea. These animals may be quite irritable, and they may be sensitive to noise.

Phosphoric acid

Copious diarrhea, which may be watery and may have undigested food in it, is a hallmark of this remedy. The diarrhea may be persistent, but it has little odor and does not normally weaken the animal. This is unusual, as weakness is common in animals needing *Phosphoric acid* for other conditions. Another keynote for *Phosphoric acid* is that diarrhea often arises from fright or anxiety.

Phosphorus

In contrast to *Phosphoric acid, Phosphorus* diarrhea can be quite foul and normally weakens the patient significantly. In this way, *Phosphorus* is similar to *Arsenicum,* with which it is closely related. Keynotes for *Phosphorus* include bleeding and a protrusion of the anus, with the anus often partially open. The anus may be painful. These animals tend to be nervous and skittish. They can be quite vocal and demanding—for food as well as attention.

Podophyllum

Podophyllum is a good remedy in many cases of diarrhea, as it will often provide relief; in this way it is a good first-aid remedy, especially if the diarrhea is mild. Typically the *Podophyllum* diarrhea occurs in the morning, and the stool firms up by evening. The stools generally contain mucus. The diarrhea may be quite watery and gushing and may be brought on by bathing the animal. If the diarrhea persists, the anus may prolapse easily and the stools may become very putrid. Hot weather is an aggravating factor, unlike the cold and damp aggravation of the *Natrum sulph* morning diarrhea. The diarrhea often alternates with other conditions in these animals.

Pulsatilla

In animals needing *Pulsatilla,* the stools are ever-changing. Diarrhea may alternate with constipation. Eating tends to immediately bring on the diarrhea. Unfixed females may have bouts of diarrhea during the heat cycle. Nighttime often increases the diarrhea. *Pulsatilla* animals tend to be thirstless (unusual with diarrhea), and they desire lots of fresh air. They love affection.

Sulphur

These animals, like those needing *Nat sulph* and *Podophyllum,* tend to be worse in the morning, and the diarrhea may drive them out of bed. The stool is usually irritating, so the anus becomes very red and inflamed, creating burning discomfort. When the burning subsides, the anus may itch severely. These animals are often very thirsty and may not be hungry. They are generally lazy, hot, and unkempt.

Veratrum album

Like the vomiting when *Veratrum* is needed, the diarrhea is often severe, leading to weakness, coldness, and collapse. Vomiting and diarrhea often occur together, and intense purging may ensue from both ends. Straining can lead to exhaustion. Sudden onset and rapid deterioration is typical, so these animals will usually need veterinary care along with homeopathy.

Constipation

When digestive waste products do not move through the colon fast enough, constipation may occur. The colon continues to remove water from the feces, so they become drier, harder, and more difficult to expel. Additionally, as more waste continues to accumulate, the colon may enlarge to accommodate the extra volume, leading to a larger fecal mass that is even harder to evacuate. Not only does this complicate the current situation but also, over time, the colon may stay enlarged rather than return to normal once the feces are evacuated.

Many factors can contribute to constipation, including diet and inactivity. Regular exercise helps maintain regular bowel function, thus couch potatoes suffer more than their share of constipation difficulties. Poor diet is the most obvious source of trouble, however. Low-residue diets, such as high-meat and low-fiber recipes, are a major culprit. This is especially a potential with cats, as they need high-meat diets and may be quite resistant to inclusion of grains, vegetables, or other fiber sources. While wild or feral cats do eat a high-meat diet, consumed hair provides indigestible bulk, which assists passage of waste through the intestine.

Raw bones are a good food and calcium source for carnivores, but they may cause problems in some animals. Overzealous feeding may lead to hard impactions, so be sure these are used at supplemental levels only. I see problems with bone impactions in dogs on high bone diets, like Dr. Billinghurst's raw meaty bone diet. Many of these diets simply have too much bone in them. Splintering problems are also a potential with bones, but this occurs mainly with cooked bones, and the benefits of bones generally outweigh the risk, provided the amount of bones is reasonable. Chewing bones helps maintain healthy gums and teeth and is a great stress reducer as well.

Other factors that may contribute to constipation include chronic drug administration, aluminum sensitivity, and possibly vaccination. If you suspect a problem, avoid using aluminum cooking utensils and food bowls as well as aluminum pet food cans.

General Care for Constipation

If you believe your companion is constipated, try to determine the severity of the problem:

- Are you sure she is constipated? Intense straining may occur with an empty rectum and thus look like constipation, so be sure before initiating corrective measures.
- Is this an isolated incident, or is it a regular occurrence?
- Is there a lot of straining? Is it constant?
- Is he able to pass any stool?

- Is there any mucus, blood, or other material coming from the rectum?
- Is there vomiting, loss of appetite, or listlessness?

Have your companion checked right away:

- if you see blood or excessive mucus;
- if straining is constant or intense;
- if you notice vomiting or weakness;
- if you are unsure of the condition (constipation versus empty straining).

Have an examination soon:

- if home care does not resolve the problem within a day or two;
- if the condition is recurrent.

Acute Constipation

Fasting may be beneficial in constipated animals, especially if they drink plenty of liquids. Offer freshly prepared broth, even tuna broth, to encourage fluid consumption. Oils can be used as mild laxatives; vegetable oil may be mixed in a small amount of food. Butter (not margarine or butter substitutes) also helps, even in cats with hair ball problems; give one-quarter to one-half teaspoonful per ten pounds. You can also use vegetable oils like flax or olive oil. Give cats one dropperful every two to four hours, up to four doses in a day. For dogs, give one-half teaspoon per ten to fifteen pounds. Alternately, tuna packed in oil provides an easy method of encouraging oil consumption (canned tuna is not very healthy for long-term use, however). Do not try to administer mineral oil directly by mouth. The oil is so bland that it may not trigger a swallowing reflex, thus the oil can go down the trachea rather than the esophagus, causing severe (often fatal) pneumonia. Mineral oil is not healthy for consumption in any case; vegetable oils provide the same benefit without toxicity. The prepared laxatives in toothpaste-like tubes should also be avoided, especially for cats, as they are often preserved with sodium benzoate, a chemical that is poisonous to cats.

Herbal laxatives such as Swiss Kriss and Gentle Dragon are safe and sometimes work well in mild to moderate cases. Chickweed tea can help also in some animals. Be sure to get the affected animal out for exercise or play to stimulate a desire for a bowel movement.

Chronic Constipation

Chronic cases often will require medical treatment (preferably holistic), especially if they are of long duration, but proper diet and regular exercise will greatly improve success. Play with your animal daily; this will help bonding and minimize stress as well as assist bowel function. Additionally, many constipation problems can be eliminated by adding one or more of the following to the diet: water, fiber, and oils. Always add water to the food for constipated animals, and add fiber or oil as needed. For fiber, you can use bran or ground psyllium seeds, though bran is easier on the gut. Mix about one teaspoonful per meal for a twenty-pound dog; adjust for cats or larger dogs, then adjust as needed for each patient. More vegetables will also provide fiber. Cooked pumpkin or winter squash is a good fiber source. You can also add butter (not margarine or butter substitutes) or oil; add one-half to one teaspoonful per ten to fifteen pounds. Adjust as needed to maintain a healthy stool that is passed without difficulty. Feed a home-prepared diet if possible (see the Appendix for resources) with plenty of fiber foods. Add bran to these recipes if needed to improve stool consistency. Digestive enzymes provide support by encouraging complete digestion. Floressence may also help. See above, under "Acute Diarrhea," for dosage. Give this for one to three months.

For cats, be sure not to use the clumping cat litters. These sometimes accumulate in the cat's gut because they lick it off their paws. This can cause severe problems. An inexpensive litter can be made with sand and peat moss; mix to get the best consistency. Start with about two parts peat moss to one of sand. Peat moss is rather dusty, so it would work best in an area that can tolerate dust. Potting soil can work also and is a bit less dusty.

Homeopathic Medicines for Constipation

Alumina

The constipation of an *Alumina* patient can be very intractable, as all muscle functioning (including urinary bladder and skeletal muscles) is weakened. These animals may go for days without any desire for stool. When the urging finally comes, it is attended with much straining, often painful, starting well before the movement. Sedentary females are prone to this condition. The stool is usually dry, hard, and knotty and may be accompanied by blood. Along with the muscle weakness there is associated mental weakness, expressed as listlessness and poor memory.

Bryonia

The main keynote of *Bryonia*, aggravation from motion, may partially explain the tendency toward constipation in these animals. Even the motion of a bowel movement can be painful. The stools are large, hard, and dry, as if burnt. These animals may have diarrhea as well. Thirst is extreme, and they will drink large volumes of water frequently, preferably cold (these animals will drink from the toilet or sink, or when fresh water has just been poured into the bowl). They may be quite irritable.

Calcarea carbonica

While *Bryonia* is worse from motion, *Calcarea* is worse from exertion. Thus the *Calcarea* state predisposes to constipation in that the effort of moving the bowels creates more discomfort than the fullness. The strange-seeming result is that these animals feel better when constipated. The *Calcarea* patient is sluggish, obese, big boned, and very sensitive to cold, especially cold air. Stools are large and hard but often followed by pasty and then liquid feces. They may be whitish and sour, as is the entire *Calcarea* patient (pale and sour smelling).

Graphites

The stool in a constipated *Graphites* patient is large and knotty, and pieces are joined together by threads of mucus. Defecation is quite painful in these animals, and they may have cracks or fissures of the anus. Sluggishness predominates, and skin disease may accompany internal complaints. Like *Calcarea*, this remedy is often indicated for obese females.

Lycopodium clavatum

Lycopodium animals may have constipation alternating with diarrhea, usually accompanied by flatulence. When the animals are constipated, their stools are hard and small yet difficult to expel. Travel is always difficult for *Lycopodium* individuals, and they typically become constipated when away from home.

Natrum muriaticum

Dryness characterizes many complaints of the *Nat mur* individual—not surprising in the picture of a remedy made from table salt. These animals are thirsty and easily overheated, especially by the sun. Inactivity is common among those needing *Nat mur,* and this can lead to constipation. The stool is dry and crumbling and may alternate with diarrhea. Grief may initiate a *Nat mur* state, yet consolation is intolerable, even angering the animal. The fur may be oily, yet the skin will have a dry rash or dandruff.

Nitric acid

The constipation of these angry, chilly animals is very similar to that of *Graphites.* The anus is extremely painful, even long after a stool, and even soft stools are painful to expel. Cracks may form in the anus and mouth. The fecal mass is often hard, and much painful straining may be required to pass a stool. The anus may protrude, and the pain in the anus may be so intense that it affects walking.

Nux vomica

As with diarrhea in the *Nux* state, constipation is accompanied by frequent urging, which is often ineffective. Absence of all desire for defecation is a contraindication for this remedy. *Nux* is the first remedy to consider in cases of constipation arising from drug use. These animals are generally chilly and irritable, although they may be friendly when well (this is in contrast to the *Nitric Acid* patient, who remains cranky whether sick or well).

Opium

The *Opium* state is one of sluggishness and drowsiness, even stupor. All systems are affected, thus the constipation results from inactivity of the bowel. Constipation is persistent, with round, hard, black balls of stool. The keynote is that there is no desire to expel a stool, even with a very full rectum. The anus may remain open with dark bloody mucus oozing out. These animals can be very colicky. *Opium* is one of our best remedies for chronic, obstinate constipation, which otherwise is difficult to treat.

Unfortunately, the U.S. Food and Drug Administration currently places homeopathic *Opium* in the same category as the narcotic from which it is made, so this remedy is unavailable from U.S. homeopathic pharmacies. This ruling is confusing, as remedies above 12C or 24X have no drug in them, and even low potencies have extremely small amounts. The same ruling applies to *Cannabis sativa* and *Cannabis indica.*

Plumbum metallicum

This remedy (lead) is characterized by weakness, as are most metal reme-dies. The *Plumbum* state is similar to that of *Alumina*. Generalized muscle weakness leads to inactivity of the colon and rectum, resulting in constipa-tion. Like *Opium* patients, these animals are often colicky due to the obstruc-tion. Impacted fecal matter may cause vomiting of bile and small intestinal contents. The vomitus may look like feces (fecal vomiting). Generalized weakness will often accompany the constipation, so these patients may have difficulty walking.

Sepia

The *Sepia* state is very similar to that of *Nat mur*, except *Sepia* individuals are among the chilliest, as they are cold even in a warm room. They are indifferent to family members and intolerant of discipline. The constipa-tion may be severe, with large hard stools that are difficult to expel. The body produces a lot of mucus in an attempt to pass the stool; this mucus may ooze from the rectum and will glue itself to the feces. Gelatinous mucus may also follow passage of a bowel movement. Constipation during preg-nancy often points to *Sepia*.

Silicea (Silica)

Generalized weakness characterizes the *Silicea* condition. These chilly, del-icate individuals just do not have the power to move the bowels. The stools are emptied with difficulty and may recede back into the rectum before being completely expelled. There is a constant urging to expel a stool, but with poor result. As a major remedy for vaccine-induced disease, *Silicea* is often needed at some point in constipated animals. These animals are extremely sensitive to external stimuli, whether it is noise, brushing their hair, or correction.

Sulphur iodatum

This remedy is similar to the *Sulphur* state but the animal is even hotter and loves cold weather. Constipation can be persistent, and the stool is often bright yellow. These animals may have extreme anal itchiness, and you may see them scoot and lick constantly on the anus.

Bloat

An uncommon but life-threatening condition of dogs (very rarely cats), acute bloat generally occurs due to poor food digestion. This poor digestion leads to a rapid accumulation of gas in the stomach, which can cause closure of the esophagus and even rotation of the stomach and spleen. Shock then rapidly ensues, and the dog may decline and die within a matter of an hour or two. This is obviously an emergency situation, and veterinary care should be sought immediately.

If bloat develops in your companion, you may see that he is agitated and restless. He often attempts unsuccessfully to regurgitate. The abdominal distension is generally easily visible. He may become rapidly weak, and his gums may turn bluish or mud-colored. This is a critical situation. What to do:

- If you see any distension of the abdomen, take your companion for an *immediate* examination. This is especially urgent if the distension is sudden or shortly after eating.
- If you *know* the distension has accumulated slowly, you may not need to rush but you should still have an examination right away.

Acute Care for Bloat

Obtain immediate veterinary help.

Homeopathic medicine may abort the bloat or improve the condition and enhance survival. Try one of the remedies below while you are preparing to go to the veterinary hospital (and/or on the way). Walking may help in some cases. If you catch the bloating very early, you may try walking him for a few minutes to see if relief will follow.

Chronic Care for Bloat

Some animals can have a more chronic tendency to bloat. The severity of episodes in these dogs (or uncommonly cats) ranges from life-threatening to mild. I strongly suggest working with an experienced prescriber due to the potential for crises, but one of the remedies may provide relief when distension occurs.

Diet is often a triggering factor in animals that bloat. Dry foods with soybean meal have been implicated by some studies, although other studies have exonerated these foods. I believe the problem to be individual sensitivity to foods. Foods that are unnatural for carnivores (like soy-beans) are likely to cause problems in some individuals. Dry foods are overall the most problematic for bloat; the condition is rare on other diets. Animals who have had bloating issues should be on fresh, meat-based diets. Use food enzymes to aid digestion for the first few months until they stabilize. Low-dose slippery elm treatment can also reduce bloating tendency. Give about one-fourth teaspoonful daily for a ten- to twenty-pound dog; you can mix this in food or give it separately.

Homeopathic Medicines for Bloat

Note: Due to the intense nature of this condition, I have rated the reme-dies. Those with two asterisks indicate my top choices, those with one aster-isk are next, and those with no asterisk are lowest. This is not absolute, however. Choose the one that fits your companion's total picture the best. *Nux* is a great place to start, however. A friend who manages a horse ranch has stopped many colics in horses with *Nux*. If you are unsure, give *Nux* while you think about your choices.

*Argentum nitricum

These animals have more of a tendency to chronic bloating. They often crave sugar and sweets, and they have many fears. Belching and flatulence are common. The mouth may be full of mucus when this remedy is needed, and the animal may vomit mucus. The stomach and abdomen are gener-ally very painful.

**Belladonna

Sudden onset characterizes the *Belladonna* state, along with heat and red-ness. These animals are usually quite restless and agitated, and the mouth is hot, bluish-red, and dry. The pupils are typically dilated and may appear glassy. Lying down worsens the pain, so the dog remains standing. The heart is usually pounding. As you can see, this is an intense remedy state.

**Carbo vegetabilis

Usually the first medicine I grab for acute bloat, *Carbo veg* is helpful in many cases of poor digestion with flatulence, both acute and chronic. Typical symptoms include weakness, coldness, and blueness. Collapse frequently occurs in this remedy state along with a strong desire for fresh air in spite of the coldness. If the gums are blue and cold and the dog is weak or collapsed, give *Carbo veg* frequently (every few minutes).

*Colchicum

Key symptoms of *Colchicum* are intense nausea and intense abdominal pain. The pain is better when bending double. Even the smell of food induces retching. These animals often have a mucous jellylike discharge from the anus. They may be very thirsty.

Eucalyptus

This aromatic resin is irritating to mucous membranes, thus discharges frequently occur in the state associated with this remedy. Nasal, bronchial, and rectal catarrh (mucus) may accompany the gastric distension. Flatulence and belching of foul gas commonly attends as well. These animals, like those needing *Carbo veg,* digest foods poorly.

Lycopodium clavatum

This is another remedy for poor digestion, and *Lycopodium* patients are known for flatulence along with *Carbo veg* and *Eucalyptus* animals. These ravenous animals will often overeat, leading to distension and discomfort. *Lycopodium* is more for chronic bloating rather than the intense acute state. Urinary trouble often accompanies the digestive complaints.

*Magnesium phosphoricum

Cramping, colicky pains predominate in the *Mag phos* state. Pain is so sharp as to cause the patient to cry out. Twitching, muscle cramps, and stiffness of the legs may occur along with the bloating and abdominal pain. Teething seems to initiate the *Mag phos* state, so if a young animal experiences colic, consider this remedy.

Nux moschata

If your companion becomes drowsy, dreamy, and confused, and she is thirstless, this remedy is a consideration. Females need this remedy more than males. The condition may appear during pregnancy. These animals produce gas from almost all foods they consume.

**Nux Vomica*

Once again, *Nux* proves its value in our homeopathic medicine chest. The disordered digestion of the *Nux* state may easily lead to bloating. The unusual pattern, however, is that the distension occurs some time after eating, even several hours later. Vomiting (like the *Nux* straining at stool) is often ineffective, so the result is constant retching without bringing anything up. Successful vomiting usually relieves the patient but comes with much difficulty, if at all. These animals tend to be chilly and irritable.

Chapter Nine
RESPIRATORY SYSTEM, NOSE, AND SINUSES

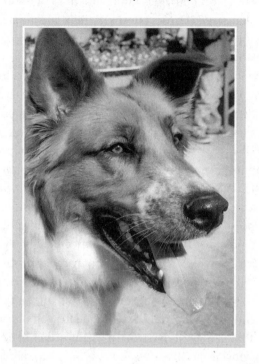

The Air We Breathe

Function

Sneezing and Nasal Discharge

Nosebleed

Coughing

Lung Problems

The Air We Breathe

Just as good healthy food provides nourishment to our bodies, clean fresh air nurtures our lungs and cleanses our spirits (*spirit* and *respiratory* derive from the same word root). Today, clean and fresh air may be difficult to find. While we may not be able to directly affect industrial air pollution on a day-by-day basis, we can be thoughtful in our decisions that contribute to the quality of our atmosphere. Drive less, use public transportation whenever possible, ask yourself if a contemplated trip is really necessary. Also, support governmental leaders who value quality of life over consumption and quantity-based standards. We all know what to do. It is simply a matter of priority.

Closer to home, the most obvious air pollutant is cigarette smoke, from tobacco as well as marijuana. The choice to smoke is appropriately an individual one. If you share your living space with others, however, smoke outside whenever possible. You will benefit as well. I have seen many respiratory ailments in animals that improved or disappeared when guardians took steps to improve air quality. Even incense may cause problems, so please be considerate. Practitioners of traditional Chinese medicine associate the lungs with grief; some believe that smoking is an attempt to fill a void or to mask the feeling of grief. Could this be true for you or for a friend?

Indoor air toxins may derive from a vast number of sources. Carpet, paint, finishes, vinyl floors, plastics, and common household cleaners and other chemicals are just a few products that off-gas dangerous chemicals. Environmental illness and "sick building syndrome" are becoming more and more common, especially with the modern tendency to build houses and offices with reduced ventilation in an attempt to reduce energy costs. While energy conservation is laudable, it should not come at the expense of health. The best solution is to use natural nontoxic products at every opportunity so the air quality is not diminished.

Open windows whenever possible, even on warm days. Turn off the air conditioning and breathe some fresh air. Clean those dusty lungs! If you use air conditioning or forced air heat, change the filter regularly. Reusable high-efficiency filters (HEPA filters) will not only do a better job than the disposable types, but they also save landfill space as well as money. Another option is a room air filter, though most filters remove particulate matter only. While this is sufficient for pollens, dust, and some smoke, it will not remove solvents like glue and paint fumes. For these, you must use a filter with carbon (activated charcoal) filtration in addition to particulate filtration (HEPA). Also be sure to change filters regularly. Carbon filters can reach their maximum quickly if used with new construction, paints, and so on.

Function

Like the digestive system, the respiratory system provides a necessary interface between our bodies and the outside world. While the former provides us with solid nutrients, the latter serves to exchange gaseous materials with our environment. A thin membrane within the lungs allows oxygen to enter the body, as carbon dioxide and other "waste" gases exit (of course, in the wonderfulness of our ecosystem, plants utilize carbon dioxide—it is not a waste gas to them). Respiration is virtually the entire function of this system. The rest of the system exists to support this gas exchange and provide a buffer between delicate lung tissue and the outside world. In a sense, though, our respiratory system is also a connection to the outside world, since we exchange energy (in the form of air particles, carbon dioxide, and oxygen) with every other being on the planet. This is an invisible but real energy exchange, linking us all together.

The long entryway comprising the nose, sinuses, throat, and trachea warms, moistens, and filters incoming air, lessening the shock to the lungs. Upon expiration, these same conduits cool the air and remove some moisture, conserving bodily resources. This is recycling at its most basic and efficient level. Additionally, the outflow expels dust particles that were trapped during inspiration.

Within the lungs, bronchi and bronchioles distribute the air movement to all sections, finally delivering air to the alveoli. Also known as air sacs, the alveoli provide the site for swapping oxygen and carbon dioxide. An alveolus is really nothing more than a tiny, balloon-like membrane that is intimately connected to equally tiny capillaries, which transport blood. The thinness of the membrane allows gases to freely pass through. Diffusion supplies the force: oxygen moves from oxygen-rich air to oxygen-poor blood; carbon dioxide moves from carbon dioxide–rich blood to carbon dioxide–poor air.

Many of the symptoms we view as disease are really only heightened activity as the body attempts to maintain a buffer and an open airway. The body produces nasal discharge, for example, by using mucus to trap dirt and debris. Small cilia (hairlike filaments) move the mucus outward, eventually forcing the discharge to the outside with the aid of sneezing and snorting. Increased mucus is thus a response and evidence of particles or bacteria in the airways that the body is attempting to move to the outside. Similarly, coughing removes particles from deeper in the airways through forceful air movement. The presence or absence of mucus establishes either a wet or dry cough, respectively.

Inflammation of the walls of the bronchi and bronchioles, as well as the alveoli, provides another layer of resistance to invasion. Thickening results from the inflammation, creating a more solid barrier. Up to a point, the bronchi and bronchioles remain flexible, but ultimately the thickening interferes with proper functioning. Similarly, thickened alveolar membranes still allow passage of gases up to a certain point, yet provide greater imperviousness to foreign materials.

As with all body systems, viewing symptoms as productive rather than destructive alters our approach to illness. Instead of trying merely to stop the symptoms, we prefer to aid the body in eliminating the need for them. A good example is the use of cold medicines in humans. These drugs tend to stop discharges and reduce coughing. While this may be beneficial in reducing discomfort, the consequence is reduced effectiveness of the self-cleaning capability of the airways. You may feel better for a time, but the cold lingers on due to the hampered immune response.

Rather than suppressing discharges, homeopathic medicines stimulate the immune system, thereby aiding the eliminative effort. In some cases this may mean an increase in discharges for a short time. In many instances, however, discharges and coughing do stop fairly quickly. Rather than acting to oppose symptoms, however, the medicines have changed the susceptibility of the body so that infections or foreign materials are readily eliminated. As a consequence, the body no longer needs to react with symptoms, and they no longer occur.

Sneezing and Nasal Discharge

As mentioned above, the body uses sneezing and discharges to expel debris and infectious organisms. It is important that we not artificially suppress these symptoms but instead boost the body's efforts to cleanse the airways.

General Care for Sneezing and Nasal Discharge

If your companion experiences sneezing and nasal discharge, first you must assess the severity of the problem.

- Is this an isolated incident, or does this happen regularly?
- What does the discharge look like? Is it thick or thin, what color (if any) is it, and is there any blood?
- Is the discharge foul-smelling?
- How frequently is it occurring? Is it constant, or does it come and go?
- Does the discharge interfere with breathing?
- Does the discharge irritate the skin around the nose—is the nose reddened?
- Is she weak and listless?
- Does the sneezing occur in fits? Is it violent?

Have your companion checked right away:
- if you notice weakness;
- if sneezing fits occur more than two to four times a day, especially for more than three days;
- if sneezing is violent;
- if you see blood (more than a few specks), or if discharge is foul-smelling;
- if discharge obstructs breathing.

Have an examination soon:
- if discharge persists for more than a week;
- if condition persists after home treatment;
- if you see acrid (irritating) discharges.

Next, try to determine patterns or circumstances. Are there triggering conditions such as:
- eating or drinking;
- smelling foods, cigarette smoke, and so on;
- times of day;
- stress or anxiety;
- are other animals in the household affected—thus, could the condition be contagious?

Acute Sneezing and Nasal Discharge

If sneezing begins suddenly, and especially if it is violent and one-sided, the problem may be a foreign body in one of the nostrils. This may be something innocuous like a piece of lint that can be expelled by the body, or it may be more serious. If you live in the western United States, foxtails present a threat. These are seed heads of grasses (*Alopecurus* spp.) that have sticky spikes on them. The spikes grab onto hair and may then propel the foxtail into body cavities, and even into the skin between the toes. Ears, eyelids, and nostrils are common sites of foxtail embedding. The foxtails can travel deeper and deeper due to one-way barbs, so the sooner they are removed, the easier the removal. Anesthesia is often necessary.

Cats occasionally get litter into their nostrils, though in most cases it is easily expelled. I have pulled blades of grass, food particles, and even a maggot out of my patients' nostrils at various times.

To assist in removal of foreign bodies, the remedies *Silicea* and *Myristica* have proven of great benefit. If you suspect a foxtail, however, do not delay in getting veterinary help.

Other causes of acute sneezing include upper respiratory infections and air pollution. Although homeopathic treatment is generally based upon the expression rather than the cause of disease, it is helpful to know the cause to prevent further illness, as well as to understand the severity and likely outcome.

Antioxidants such as vitamin C and vitamin E will reduce the intensity of the inflammation, as well as boosting the immune system. Use moderate doses: for vitamin C (natural C if available) give 10 mg per pound twice or thrice daily, and for vitamin E (mixed tocopherols) give 5 mg per pound once a day. If the nasal discharge irritates the skin around the nostrils, apply vitamin E, *Calendula* ointment, or aloe topically. If you believe your companion's health is depleted, an immune-boosting supplement such as echinacea, astragalus, cat's claw, *Cordyceps* (a mushroom), or DMG may be helpful. Herbs are best used in short stints, such as a week or two at a time. DMG is safe to give for much longer.

Keep in mind that these upper respiratory infections, especially in cats but including kennel cough in dogs, can be quite contagious. Wash well between handling other animals of the same species after exposure to a potentially contagious animal. Even changing clothes is a good idea. Within a household, you can separate the infected ones, though often exposure has occurred by the time you realize the cat or dog is ill. Again, change clothes (shoes too!) and wash well between handling infected and noninfected animals. You can use coveralls or an overcoat/gown if you must nurse an infected animal and then care for others.

Chronic Sneezing and Nasal Discharge

Have a thorough examination to assess the reason for the condition. If necessary, particularly if the discharge is one-sided, obtain X-rays of the nose and sinuses. A one-sided discharge may be due to an abscessed or decayed root of an upper canine tooth, as well as a tumor or a fungus infection, so a diagnosis is essential. Veterinarians typically recommend a bacteriological culture, though this is rarely of benefit, as chronic conditions are generally not primarily bacterial infections. These can be quite persistent, especially in cats with chronic upper respiratory viruses like calicivirus and rhinotracheitis virus (feline herpesvirus). If your cat suffers from a nasal discharge that does not clear up within a week to a month (depending upon severity), work with a homeopathic veterinarian.

Use antioxidants and immune boosters as above, and be sure the diet is high quality; home-prepared meals are best. Fasting can help some cats, as can cooking the food for a month or two if the cat is chilly or overweight.

Homeopathic Medicines for Sneezing and Nasal Discharge

(See also "Conjunctivitis" in Chapter 10, "Eyes")

Allium cepa

This remedy is made from a red onion, and its symptoms are just as you might expect: profuse watery eye and nose discharges, red eyes, and frequent sneezing. The left nostril is typically affected more strongly than the right. Curiously, the nasal discharge irritates and burns the nose and upper lip, while the eye discharge remains more bland. The *Allium cepa* state often arises during cold damp weather and in the spring, but the patient is worse in a warm room.

Arsenicum album

Once again, *Arsenicum* shows its merit, as the entire respiratory tract falls within the range of this remedy. Discharges tend to be watery, yet burning and irritating to the skin and mucous membranes. The nasal passages may be quite painful to touch. Discharging may start or be more severe on the right side.

The *Arsenicum* patient is generally restless, thirsty, and chilly, and often very fearful and skittish. Cleanliness is paramount to the *Arsenicum* state, so animals may expend much effort to clean the nose.

Calcarea sulphurica

A primary symptom of *Calc sulph* is thick, lumpy, yellow mucus discharges. These may occur anywhere, but most commonly we see them in the nose and eyes. Eye inflammation may occur in newborn or very young animals, so this remedy may be useful in kittens with rhinovirus or calicivirus infections (feline URI), and possibly in early cases of canine distemper. In the nose, the yellow discharge may be blood-tinged and often affects primarily the right side. The tongue may have a yellow coating as well, especially at the base.

Like those needing *Allium cepa*, these animals are worse in warm rooms, but the condition may arise in cold damp weather.

Hepar sulphuris calcareum

The *Hepar sulph* state generally occurs late in the course of an upper respiratory infection. As such, the inflammation has progressed to the point of sore, sometimes ulcerated nostrils and a foul discharge that smells like old cheese. Blood often accompanies the discharge. Any inflammation in a *Hepar sulph* state is usually quite painful to the touch. These animals tend to be very irritable as well, so touching the area may trigger a vicious bite or scratch response.

These chilly animals worsen upon entering cold air or drafts and are worse in winter and at night.

Hydrastis

While these patients have a thick yellow discharge similar to that of *Calc sulph*, the discharge is ropy rather than lumpy. Also, these animals are usually quite sick and depressed and often somewhat emaciated. The discharge is very acrid and very tenacious—animals have difficulty clearing it from the nose, and it collects in the back of the nasal passages as well as the sinuses. Cats with chronic sinusitis may benefit from this medicine. A headache often accompanies the sinus congestion, so affected animals may appear dull and listless.

These patients tend to be worse in cold air, causing the discharges to become quite profuse.

Kali bichromicum

A keynote of *Kali bichromicum* is the development of tough crusts that attach to the outer portion of the nostrils and are very difficult to remove. Pulling these crusts off usually tears the skin because of the strong adherence, resulting in a bleeding sore. The accompanying discharge is greenish-yellow and thick. Postnasal discharge may occur as well, and breathing through the nose can be very difficult if not impossible. Violent sneezing often results from the obstruction.

A sore throat typically accompanies the nasal congestion, so these animals may have difficulty swallowing, and their throats will be bright red. The *Kali bichromicum* state is worse in the morning and in cold, damp weather.

Kali sulphuricum

Like *Calc sulph*, this remedy state produces a lot of yellow discharges, though the *Kali sulph* discharges are initially watery, only becoming thick later in the illness. The pus may become greenish as it thickens. Another similarity to *Calc sulph* is a yellow coating at the base of the tongue.

These animals worsen in the evening and in warm rooms, improving while walking in cold air. This remedy may be needed after *Pulsatilla*, if *Pulsatilla* helps but does not cure the cold.

Mercurius (vivus or solubilis)

Mercurius is suited to a condition that closely resembles that of *Hepar sulph* in that the illness is rather advanced and destructive. Inflammation is often profound, producing intense redness, ulceration, corrosion, and nosebleed. The *Mercurius* discharge is foul, cheesy-smelling, and greenish, and it corrodes skin and mucous membranes upon prolonged contact.

These animals are also quite irritable, but unlike those needing *Hepar sulph*, these patients are worse in warmth and sunshine (sunshine incites sneezing). Consider also *Mercurius corrosivus* if *Merc v* or *Merc s* do not help and you still think *Merc* is the best remedy.

Mercurius corrosivus

I have seen good result with *Merc corr* in a household calicivirus outbreak in cats, with nasal symptoms as well as drooling and mouth ulceration. These were very ill cats, and *Merc corr* turned several around nicely.

Natrum muriaticum

Nat mur is said to be "infallible for stopping a cold commencing with sneezing," and I have had success in a couple of cases where sneezing was the first sign. Discharge is usually watery at first, or it may be watery alternating with dry. There may be ulcers or irritation on the nose itself, especially on the wings. *Nat mur* is probably best in these early stages before thick discharges arise.

Pulsatilla

When *Pulsatilla* is indicated, the animal will generally produce thick yellow or yellow-green discharges that obstruct the nose and fill the eyelids. These discharges tend to be bland. Often *Pulsatilla* is needed at the end of an illness, when inflammation has subsided but drainage continues to occur. The inflammation that should be present to eliminate the disease cannot manifest, and the body needs help in finishing the cure.

Classically, these sweet-natured animals are thirstless, avoid heated stuffy rooms, and like lots of attention and nurturing. They can be quite demonstrative in this need for attention. Discharges worsen while the animal is inside, and they improve upon going out into open air. The right nostril or eye will be affected more often than the left side.

Sabadilla

Sabadilla is useful in humans with hay fever (and thus in animals with similar symptoms), with red watery eyes, violent itchy sneezing, and fluent runny nasal discharges. The discharges are mucus, either transparent or thick and yellow-gray, rarely watery. It can be helpful in prolonged cases where other remedies have not helped. These patients are usually chilly, but may be improved in open air.

Sepia

While *Sepia* also produces a thick greenish discharge, these cats and dogs are nothing like those needing *Pulsatilla*. The *Sepia* state is one of indifference to others and sadness. Additionally, these animals tend to be quite chilly, and will hug the fire in an attempt to stay warm. The left side bears the brunt of disease.

Silicea (Silica)

Poor reaction highlights the need for *Silicea*, as these patients cannot mount a good immune response. Weakness abounds throughout the body, even in this inability to rid the body of illness. Thus those needing this well-known abscess remedy have as much difficulty eliminating nasal discharges and infections as eliminating infections from puncture wounds. And these animals often have a history of one infection after another, as well as poor skin, poor teeth and gums, and generalized lethargy.

Other *Silicea* hallmarks include chilliness, sensitivity to touch and noise, and a history of many vaccinations. Additionally, these animals may be thin, weak individuals.

Sulphur

As with most *Sulphur* discharges, nasal discharges tend to be watery, profuse, and irritating. Occasionally they become yellowish. Sneezing predominates, and animals may rub the nose and eyes due to the burning irritation. Redness develops as well, a *Sulphur* keynote—red eyes, red scabby nostrils, red anus, and so on.

Sulphur animals may be quite thirsty and often have poor appetites. Early morning is a time of worsening. Finally, these animals (and people) are known for a lack of concern for appearance, so dogs (and even cats) appear unkempt and unclean.

Sycotic co

This is one of the bowel nosodes, and it can be a great remedy for upper respiratory infections such as feline herpesvirus (rhinotracheitis) and calicivirus infections. It may be hard to obtain, as it is a prescription remedy, but it is helpful if you can get some. There is thick nasal mucus (catarrh), often with postnasal and sinus involvement, so these animals may have difficulty breathing through their noses. The nose may also be dry and crusted, with cracks. There may also be cracks in the angles of the lips, and ulcers in the mouth and on the tongue, with increased salivation.

Nosebleed

Bleeding from the nose, if separate from a respiratory condition, can indicate a bleeding disorder, so this should be investigated thoroughly. If it occurs as part of a nasal condition, however, it may be due to irritation of the mucous membranes. As long as the bleeding is neither severe nor persistent, you can feel safe treating this with homeopathy. If you see any evidence of anemia (lethargy, pale gums), however, if the bleeding is profuse, or if you see bleeding in any other location, have an examination right away. Pressure and cold applications may reduce or stop the bleeding.

Yunnan paiyao is a Chinese herbal formula that is often quite effective at stopping hemorrhage from any cause. It comes in capsules. Give one or two capsules (depending upon the intensity) for dogs over twenty-five pounds. For cats and small dogs, give one-quarter to one-half capsule. This dose may be repeated two to four times a day as needed. There is also a small red "safety pill" that may be administered in emergency situations. This preparation is generally for short-term use only.

See also "Hemorrhage" in Chapter Fifteen, "Therapeutic Indications by Condition."

Homeopathic Medicines for Nosebleed

Arnica montana

Primarily, *Arnica* will be indicated when the nosebleed follows an injury or a shock. The injury may not be directly to the nose. There may be much bruising, and these animals tend to be extremely painful, to a greater extent than the injury would warrant. Consequently they are very fearful of touch.

Ferrum phosphoricum

This remedy is often indicated when the nosebleed accompanies a fever. The blood is usually bright red. The animal may be rather thin and delicate, with pale gums. See also the description below, under "Homeopathic Medicines for Coughing."

Hamamelis

Hamamelis may be needed for long-lasting hemorrhage with soreness of the nose. There may be a foul odor as well, and the blood may be dark.

Millefolium

The blood will be bright red when *Millefolium* is indicated, and bleeding may occur after strenuous activity.

Phosphorus

Like *Ferrum phos* and *Millefolium*, this remedy is indicated when the blood is bright red. These animals are usually thin, active, graceful, and friendly. They often have a tendency to vomit, especially after drinking or after eating foods too quickly. The vomiting does not affect them much, however, and they quickly return to eating or other activity. See also the description below, under "Homeopathic Medicines for Coughing."

Coughing

As with sneezing, coughing provides a way for the body to remove foreign materials and infectious organisms from the respiratory tract. Forceful expulsion of air carries particulates out of the trachea and bronchi, thus mechanically cleaning the airways. Mucus may be produced here, as it is in the nose, to bind these particles and prevent them from moving deeper into the lungs. In this instance, coughing moves the mucus as well as the particulates it contains, resulting in a moist cough. A moist cough may also accompany circulation problems due to inadequate movement of blood through the lungs. Pooling of blood in the lungs can lead to seeping of fluid (plasma) through the alveolar walls into the airways. Coughing will then expel this fluid, allowing air to penetrate into the alveoli so that respiration can occur.

While the selection of a homeopathic medicine is not dependent upon which mechanism is producing a cough, obviously you need to know the cause. This determination will help decide what supportive measures may be beneficial, and it allows you to understand the severity and prognosis of your companion's illness.

General Care for Coughing

If your companion is coughing, try to ascertain the severity of the situation:

- Is this an isolated incident, or does it happen regularly?
- How long does the coughing spell last?
- Is the cough moist or dry?
- Is he bringing anything up—mucus, blood, pus?
- Is breathing hindered?
- Are the gums nice and pink, or are they muddy, dark, or bluish?
- Is she active, or lethargic?

Have an examination *immediately:*
- if breathing is hindered;
- if gums are not pink (gum color should be the same as yours—if your pet's gums are pigmented, you can look under the eyelids, or at the vagina if you have a female);
- if she is extremely weak.

Have your companion checked right away:
- if he is weak and lethargic;
- if the cough is moist, especially if any material is coughed up;
- if coughing is severe, or if spells last more than a few minutes;
- if cough is worsening.

Have an examination soon:
- if coughing persists for more than a few days (the more severe the cough, the sooner you should get an exam).

Next, try to determine patterns and circumstances.
- Are there triggering conditions such as:

- air pollution;
- dampness;
- going out into cold air;
- entering a warm room;
- drinking;
- lying down?

- What time of day or night does the cough occur?
- Are other animals in the household affected?

Acute Coughing

If your companion's energy is good and the condition seems mild, try some vitamin C (5–10 mg/pound, two to three times a day, natural vitamin C if available) and vitamin E (3–5 mg/pound, once a day, mixed tocopherols). If the cough doesn't resolve itself within a day or two, treat with one of the remedies listed below. For lung congestion, such as with upper respiratory infections, you can also try the following formula, from *Rosemary Gladstar's Family Herbal:* Using dry herbs, mix two parts licorice root, one part each of cinnamon, echinacea, and elecampane, and one-fourth part ginger root. Make as a tea, with one teaspoonful herbs to a cup of boiling water. Allow to steep, then remove herbs. Give one dropperful to small dogs (or cats, though cats do not take this formula well due to its taste), and one-half to one teaspoonful per twenty pounds for larger dogs. Give three to four doses daily. This is a great formula for colds that settle in the chest for humans, and for similar conditions in animals. Elecampane is the prime mover in this formula, but it has a strong aromatic taste. You can add a little honey for taste if that helps. Also see the remedy *Inula helenium* below for homeopathic usage of elecampane in animals who won't take this formula.

For drier coughs, including asthmatic and allergic coughs, give nettle tea at the same doses as the formula above. Cats will usually take this fine. It can help with any lung condition but is especially helpful with drier coughs. I have used nettle tea successfully with kennel cough also, though the elecampane formula might work better with wetter coughs. Dehydration is often a component of dry coughs and asthma, so adding more water to the diet, as well as encouraging broth consumption, often helps animals with these coughs. Use broth without added salt, and preferably homemade.

Chronic or Severe Coughing

For more severe conditions, I strongly recommend working with an experienced homeopathic practitioner. Veterinary monitoring is essential, as these conditions can be life-threatening. Obtaining a diagnosis is particularly important for the same reason. If you cannot work with a homeopathic prescriber, you can try one of the indicated remedies in addition to conventional therapy, though interpretation and response may be unclear. Herbal therapy such as echinacea or cat's claw for infections, or hawthorn for heart failure, may be of benefit, but a diagnosis is needed to know what to use. Gingko, nettles, and bromelain/quercetin may help asthmatic coughs. A holistic veterinarian can provide the best assistance.

Homeopathic Medicines for Coughing

Aconitum napellus
A sudden dry cough in an individual that has recently been chilled, especially in a cold wind, is a good indication for *Aconite*. These animals usually have a fever and a thirst for cold water. They may be quite anxious and fearful. Kennel cough may respond to it if the symptoms fit. The best responses occur when this remedy is administered early in the course of an illness.

Antimonium tartaricum
Antimonium tart is indicated in fairly serious respiratory affections, with copious amounts of mucus and a loose rattling cough. Although abundant, the mucus proves to be quite difficult to expel. These patients may be very weak, with poor respiration, leading to drowsiness and trembling. They

must sit up to breathe, and vomiting may follow coughing fits. Despondency and chilliness generally accompany the condition. Consider this remedy for canine distemper.

Arsenicum album

Arsenicum is often helpful with asthma, a major cause of coughing in cats, although other remedies are frequently needed for permanent relief. Nighttime aggravation is usually present, as are restlessness, thirst, and chilliness—all classic *Arsenicum* symptoms. The cough tends to be dry, although it may alternate with a loose cough; coughing may follow drinking.

Belladonna

Belladonna states generally arise suddenly and are attended with intense anxiety, sometimes aggression, and dilated pupils during periods of aggravation. The cough is dry and accompanied with fever, chilliness, and sweating (check the foot pads in cats and dogs). Coughing often occurs on slight motion and may occur in spasms. It may be indicated in kennel cough. These patients may be thirsty for cold water, or they may be thirstless.

Bryonia alba

The *Bryonia* cough is similar to that of *Belladonna:* a dry cough aggravated by slight motion, and fever with great thirst. Onset is more gradual, however, and the thirst is even greater, as this is one of our thirstiest remedy states. The *Bryonia* cough is aggravated upon entering a warm room. Motion is generally intolerable for these patients, even being carried around. They usually prefer to be left alone. Coughing and breathing may be quite painful, so rapid, short respiration may ensue. The animal may sit up to breathe more comfortably.

Cina

Infestation with worms can induce a *Cina* state, so it is more commonly needed in young animals. They tend to be moody, irritable, and touchy— to the point of biting or swatting at those around them. The *Cina* cough is gagging, hacking, and spasmodic, sometimes violent. The aggravation occurs in the morning when *Cina* is needed; this is different from most other remedies. It may also be worse at the full moon. This is another remedy to consider for kennel cough.

Drosera
Also a good choice for kennel cough, *Drosera* is indicated for violent, spasmodic coughing spells. The throat is very ticklish, so vocalization or touching the throat often incites a coughing spell. The cough may be worse when the animal lies down, an unusual symptom. Coughing is deep, as if it comes from the abdomen. Hoarseness and laryngitis may accompany the cough.

Dulcamara
Aggravation in cold damp weather or from lying on damp ground points to the successful use of this remedy. It is also commonly needed toward the end of summer, when days are warm and nights are cold. Frequently the cough is asthmatic and dry, although it may be loose. Coughing may be brought on after exertion. A common initiating cause of the *Dulcamara* state is rapid chilling after being hot, as after exercise on a cold damp day.

Ferrum phosphoricum
These patients tend to have low-grade inflammations with productive coughing. They may cough up blood or bleed from the nose. The cough is usually tickling and hacking and may be spasmodic. *Ferrum phos* is often indicated in earlier stages of infections and inflammations. Mentally these animals may alternate between depression and excitability, and they generally wish to be left alone.

Hepar sulphuris calcareum
One of the major croup remedies for children, *Hepar sulph* can also benefit animals with bronchial inflammation. Coughing is almost always productive when *Hepar sulph* is indicated, and a thick yellow pus is produced. These animals are chilly, and any time they become chilled the cough worsens. Cold drafts are especially troublesome. Mentally, irritability and violence often predominate, and touch may bring about a vicious response. There may be a history of abscessed wounds.

Inula helenium
This is elecampane, a wonderful herb for the lungs. Its homeopathic indications include dry tickling cough, productive cough with thick expectoration, and general languor and debility, possibly combined with weak digestion. It can be used in a low potency, as a semiherbal application, by

giving a 3X, 6X, 3C, or 6C dose, three or four times daily. This will support the lungs when there is congestion of a viral or inflammatory nature (as opposed to fluid buildup from heart or other organ weakness).

Ipecac

Coughing with nausea is a keynote for *Ipecac*. These animals will cough, usually violently, and then often vomit. Bleeding from the nose or mouth may accompany the cough. Asthma may be accompanied by skin disease, and it may be aggravated in damp weather. Breathing can be quite difficult, with violent wheezing; it is better in warm and open air but worse in cold air. *Ipecac* may be indicated when animals cough until they stiffen and pass out.

Phosphorus

This polychrest remedy centers its action in the lungs. Not surprisingly, then, many respiratory conditions will improve under its influence—if the individual is in a *Phosphorus* state. Bleeding often accompanies any *Phosphorus* condition. These animals may cough up blood-tinged mucus or bleed from the mouth or nose. The cough is typically dry and deep, and it is worse in cold air, especially upon leaving a warm room to go out into the cold. These animals may tremble when coughing and may cough more in the presence of strangers. They are generally chilly, thirsty for cold water, ravenous, and startle easily. Constitutionally, these animals are friendly and vocal, with long lean bodies.

Pulsatilla

The *Pulsatilla* cough is generally dry at night and loose in the morning. Heated rooms aggravate the *Pulsatilla* condition, while open air will relieve it. Sitting up will also provide relief, as will lying with the head elevated. This remedy is frequently needed near the end of a respiratory infection, when congestion has settled in the chest and the body needs to clear the discharges. Animals needing *Pulsatilla* are generally sweet, desire attention, and are not thirsty, even with a fever.

Rumex crispus

A characteristic of *Rumex* is tickling in the throat leading to coughing. This tickling is so severe that slight touch will elicit a cough. The other very important sensitivity is to cold air; every breath of cold air will initiate a cough. Any temperature change may also elicit a coughing spell. The *Rumex* cough tends to be dry and persistent. This remedy should be considered for kennel cough.

Spongia tosta

Spongia comes to mind for croupy, barking coughs. The sound of the cough has been compared (very aptly) to that of sawing through a pine board. Eating and drinking warm things will generally improve the cough; cold drinks may aggravate it, as may cold wind. Excitement usually worsens the cough. *Spongia* may be indicated in coughs from heart disease. These animals may be quite anxious and fearful, and often startle from sleep, moving into coughing or breathing difficulty. *Spongia* may be indicated for kennel cough.

Lung Problems

If your dog or cat has problems indicating more serious lung or heart problems, she should be under the care of a competent homeopathic prescriber, and close veterinary supervision is essential. Symptoms might include shortness of breath, rapid tiring upon minimal exercise, or severe wheezing. You might also notice gurgling or rattling sounds during breathing, indicating fluid accumulation. If you see any of these signs, obtain a thorough examination right away, and determine the extent of the problem. Any of these conditions may respond to correctly prescribed homeopathic medicines, but they are serious conditions and should be treated by someone with experience. If there is fluid buildup in the chest, as from heart disease, *Apocynum* can be a good remedy, but the animal should be under professional care.

Chapter Ten
EYES

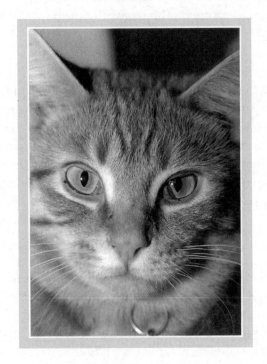

Overview

It is said that the eyes are a window to the soul. This is true for cats and dogs as well as for humans, but it is only part of the phenomenon of gazing into another's eyes. We also gain a rapid sense of the health of the individual, both physical and mental. Discharges, redness, glassy appearance, dullness—all of these tell us that sickness abounds inside our companion. Yet even without these obvious signs there is more—sadness, pain, discomfort, fear, anger, joy, excitement—in short, we know immediately and intimately the mental state as well, and we intuitively apprehend the state of the overall health from this glance into the eyes and thus into the soul. Mentally, our companion experiences and expresses the *feeling* of illness, while the physical aspect of illness alters the body. And mental expression often precedes physical expression, for what the soul perceives may solidify into illness if ignored. Daily eye-gazing is one of our best opportunities to know our companion animals. Not only does this provide an early warning of impending illness, but also it may help prevent illness by affirming the relationship and the value of these friends. Keep in mind, however, that most animals, by their nature, find intense eye gazing uncomfortable, so keep your gazes short and "light."

Function

Obviously, the eyes provide a window to the outside world, much as they give others a glimpse into our internal world. Without the benefit of vision, dogs wouldn't be dogs and cats wouldn't be cats, at least as carnivores dependent upon sight to find and catch prey. While vision problems sometimes can respond to homeopathic treatment, it is beyond the scope of this chapter to address treatment, as vision loss is generally the result of deep chronic illness. I'll focus instead upon superficial eye problems and injuries.

The eyelids provide protection and moisture retention to nourish the cornea (the clear front portion of the eyeball). In order to obtain more clarity, the cornea has no blood vessels (except following some injuries), so moisture and nutrients must move slowly through the corneal tissue from the sclera (the white portion of the eyeball). Tears assist this nutrient flow, and blinking moves the tears across the cornea regularly to keep it moist. Without adequate moisture, the cornea rapidly loses transparency, and without tears to lubricate and cleanse the cornea, it will develop abrasions and ulcers. If untreated, this can lead to a rupture of the cornea and loss of the eye.

Cats and dogs have an inner eyelid that provides further protection. This membrane is called the *membrana nictitans* (anglicized, the nictitating membrane) or third eyelid; *nictitation* is a fancy word for "winking" or "blinking," so this means a winking or blinking membrane. In cats especially, the third eyelid partially covers the cornea (we say it is elevated) when the cat is sleepy or not feeling well; this is an early symptom of illness in cats. This is not as pronounced in most dogs.

The conjunctiva (from Latin "to join together") are the pinkish membranes that line the eyelid and connect the sclera to the eyelid; it is really one membrane but separated by anatomists into these two divisions, thus the plural name. Together they form a pouch called the conjunctival sac (where all the sand and grit that gets into your eye ends up). There is an upper and a lower sac, corresponding to the upper and lower lid.

The iris is the colored part of the eye, and the pupil is the opening in the iris that allows light through. The iris dilates (enlarges) in low light and contracts in bright light. Iris conditions are always evidence of chronic disease and should be treated by a skilled homeopath.

Conjunctivitis

Because the conjunctival sacs catch debris, and because they are lined with a permeable membrane that is exposed to the outside world, inflammation is rather common. The inflammation may be a result of trauma, or it may be a symptom of disease. If illness is responsible, it may be either acute illness (similar to colds in people) or chronic disease. Acute conjunctivitis is common in young animals, especially in cats as a part of an upper respiratory infection.

Three primary infectious agents can cause upper respiratory infections in cats. In order of occurrence, they are feline rhinotracheitis virus, feline calicivirus (this is often mispronounced—the correct pronunciation is "*kay* li see virus," since the virus looks like a calix ["*kay* lix"]—a cup or chalice), and *Chlamydia psittaci*. Rhinotracheitis is a herpesvirus, though not the same one that humans get. All herpesviruses tend to recur periodically when the animal is under stress. This one is no exception, so infected cats will have occasional outbreaks until their immune system can handle the infection. These outbreaks initially can cause mouth ulcers and a nasty eye and nose infection, including eye ulcers, but as the cat ages the infection tends to center in the eyes as recurrent conjunctivitis. Calicivirus infection is hard to distinguish from rhinotracheitis infection in the initial stages, but recurrence is rare, so you won't see the repeated outbreaks of conjunctivitis in adult cats. Chlamydial infections are relatively uncommon but can cause nasty conjunctival infections; ulcers are not common with chlamydia, and the infection is limited to the eyes in most cases.

While dogs occasionally develop conjunctivitis, they don't have a comparable sensitivity and associated group of infectious agents as with cats. Most occurrences of conjunctivitis in dogs result from trauma, dirt, allergies, and chronic illness. One of the chronic causes of conjunctivitis in dogs is a condition known as "dry eye" or keratoconjunctivitis sicca (a Latin name that means dry inflammation of the cornea and conjunctiva), also known by the acronym KCS. This condition occurs more in small breeds of dogs and results when their tear production diminishes, sometimes to almost zero. Without tears, the eyes dry out and the cornea becomes irritated. In addition to homeopathic treatment, we use artificial tears (a solution designed to mimic tears) to rinse and lubricate the eyes. Veterinary ophthalmologists sometimes recommend a surgical procedure to transplant a salivary gland duct to the affected eye to provide permanent lubrication. This can be quite effective as a local treatment. KCS is a chronic illness, and homeopathic treatment is best left to experienced practitioners, though some of the remedies in this section may help.

If your kitten develops conjunctivitis, it is likely to be contagious and acute rather than chronic, so you can try home treatment, but see the precautions below. If an adult cat or a dog develops conjunctivitis, it may be acute trauma (like a scratch) or else it is probably chronic disease. Uncommonly, it may be an acute infection in cats, as some cats will still contract the acute upper respiratory agents, especially if they are immune-compromised. As with acute illness, you can attempt treatment, but if you don't see a timely response, you should seek expert help.

General Care for Conjunctivitis

If your companion develops conjunctivitis, you must first assess the severity the problem.

- Is this an isolated incident, or has she had it before?
- Is there a discharge? If so, what does it look like? Is it watery or thick, yellow, white, green, bloody? If it is thick, is it dry or wet?
- Are the eyes painful? Does she keep them closed?
- Are there other symptoms of illness?

- Is she eating? If mouth ulcers develop, she will likely stop eating.
- Is she weak and listless?

Have her checked right away:
- if you notice weakness;
- if discharge is thick and looks infected (yellow or greenish, sometimes brownish);
- if you see blood;
- if the eyes are painful, or if she keeps them closed;
- if the condition started from an injury like a cat scratch;
- if she is not eating.

Generally, I recommend an examination unless the conjunctivitis is obviously very minor (minimal discharge, eyes open, conjunctiva not too red). If ulcers form, they can *rapidly* worsen and lead to rupture of the eyeball and subsequent loss of the eye. Minor scratches can ulcerate quickly also, with the same result. *Don't take chances.*

Have an examination soon:
- if the condition worsens or other symptoms develop;
- if the condition persists after home treatment.

Next, try to determine patterns or circumstances:
- Are other cats in the household affected?
- Was the onset sudden—could it be from a fight?
- Does the discharge irritate the skin around the eyes?
- Are there other signs of allergy such as sneezing?

Acute Conjunctivitis

As I mentioned above, I suggest a veterinary examination to check for scratches or ulcers on the cornea. A veterinarian can use a special stain to detect small injuries to the cornea that cannot be seen without the stain. It is important to know if these are present, so that you can watch closely for worsening in case an ulcer develops. If an ulcer does develop or if the injury is severe, your veterinarian may recommend surgically suturing the third eyelid closed for a couple of weeks. This provides a natural bandage that protects the cornea until it heals; it is a good technique for serious problems and may save the eye.

The usual conventional prescription is an eye ointment or solution with antibiotics with or without steroids ("cortisone"). Steroids interfere

with the immune system and can greatly increase the likelihood of ulceration and eyeball rupture, so they should *never* be administered to an
animal with a cornea injury or ulcer. As most conjunctivitis cases are viral,
traumatic, or allergic, the use of antibiotics is usually unnecessary and
useless. In a few cases, a secondary bacterial infection occurs and the
antibiotics may help.

An eyewash often provides as much benefit as the drugs, especially if
you add herbs to the wash. For a basic eyewash, add one-fourth teaspoon
of salt to one cup of boiled water (to purify the water). Distilled or filtered
water is best. Allow to cool before use. You may add herb tinctures at the
rate of ten drops per cup. For teas, add one-half teaspoonful dry herb to the
cup of boiled water and salt, but filter it before use. Many herbs have healing and anti-infective properties. Goldenseal, eyebright, *Calendula,* and
Hypericum (St. John's wort) all fit this category. Use one or two at a time.
Marshmallow and calendula tea is a good combination here also, as it is
very soothing. The safest way to apply eyewashes is with a cotton ball; this
way you don't risk poking the eye if your patient jerks her head. And you
can flood the eye easily, which not only applies the herbal medicines but
also washes out some of the debris. You can keep the eyewash out of the
refrigerator so it is not so cold, but make it fresh at least every other day;
every day is even better.

Vitamins also help the body. Vitamin C (5–10 mg/pound, two to three
times a day, use natural vitamin C if available) and vitamin E (5–10
mg/pound, once a day, mixed tocopherols) help reduce inflammation and
stimulate healing. Vitamin A is a great stimulant for corneal healing. Use
cod liver oil and place one drop directly in the eye daily, then give about
one-eighth teaspoon per ten pounds daily by mouth.

Similisan homeopathic eyedrops may also benefit mild cases of conjunctivitis, especially allergic or minor traumatic cases. This product is a
combination homeopathic preparation for short-term use. It works well for
debris in the eyes or dry, irritated eyes. Don't use it for more than a couple
of weeks, though. If the condition persists, you should seek outside help
from a homeopathic veterinarian, if available. Although topical homeopathic medicines can theoretically interfere with oral homeopathic medicines, I have not found this product to cause a problem.

The following remedies may be of use, but don't delay obtaining help
for serious conditions, or even if you are unsure. Many of the remedies can

help even if there is ulceration, but you should have your companion under a veterinarian's care and use the homeopathy along with other appropriate treatments.

Remember also that the acute infections in cats can be very contagious, so use caution and common sense. Often, exposure has already occurred within a household by the time you see the symptoms, though it may be helpful to isolate the infected cats if you have more than one cat in the house. And don't forget to wash your hands and even change your clothes (and shoes) before going to another household with cats if you have been exposed to a cat with potentially infectious eye or upper respiratory conditions. (These often occur simultaneously.)

Homeopathic Medicines for Conjunctivitis

(See also "Sneezing and Nasal Discharge" in Chapter Nine, "Respiratory System, Nose, and Sinuses")

Aconitum napellus

Many acute infections and inflammations fall under the realm of *Aconite*'s effect. Usually the *Aconite* state comes on as a result of either intense fear or a sudden chill, often from a cold wind. Eye troubles may start from exposure to bright sunlight on a cold day with snow on the ground. Sudden inflammation following removal of a foreign body from the eye may require *Aconite*. The remedy may be useful with ingrown eyelashes. This remedy is best given during early stages of inflammation, when the condition is intense. The eyes will be intensely red, possibly swollen and bloodshot. There will be a profuse watery discharge in most cases. These animals are usually sensitive to light.

Think of this remedy with sudden onset, chill, fear, and intense fevers or inflammation in the early stage of illness.

Allium cepa

The onion provides us with another good remedy for minor eye inflammation. As you might imagine, the eyes water profusely when *Allium cepa* is needed—as if the animal had been cutting an onion. The tears in this case are very bland, although the eyes will feel burned and sore. There will often be a very irritating discharge from the nose, and it may be worse in the left nostril. These animals' symptoms are worse in a warm room and better in open air. The cold often progresses to laryngitis.

Apis

Swelling is a hallmark of the *Apis* state, so the eyelids and the conjunctiva may be intensely inflamed and swollen. The conjunctiva may even protrude somewhat due to the swelling, prohibiting complete closure of the lids; this state is called chemosis. The lids may be stuck together with a thick sticky discharge. Ulceration may occur. The cornea may be opaque or have opaque spots. This remedy may help with KCS (see above).

Apis animals are usually warm (they seek cool areas) and thirstless.

Argentum nitricum

This remedy is silver nitrate—the chemical we place in the eyes of newborn infants to keep them from developing syphilis in the eyes. An affinity to conjunctivitis in newborns is not surprising. *Argentum nitricum* is a good remedy to consider for young kittens with conjunctivitis. The discharge here is copious and purulent and is yellow to greenish. Like the *Apis* state, the eyes may be chemotic—intensely inflamed with swollen, protruding conjunctiva. Ulceration is common, and the eyes are often bloodshot. The margin of the lids may be inflamed and crusty. The left side may be worse.

The inflammation of *Apis* and *Argentum nitricum* is similar, but the latter is more moist and discharges more pus. Animals needing this remedy may have gassy diarrhea and even belching. They are very warm-blooded and fearful of new situations, crowds, narrow spaces, and heights.

Arsenicum album

Irritating tears may call for *Arsenicum* if you have a chilly, restless, thirsty patient. The conjunctivitis may be intense when this remedy is needed, with great sensitivity to light and a yellow or a watery discharge. The eyelids may be greatly swollen, even completely closing the eyes. The inflammation is hot and intense and the eyes quite painful, but warm compresses will relieve the pain.

Like *Apis*, *Arsenicum* may be indicated for KCS, as there may be a paucity of tears in some cases. Ulceration may occur here as well. The right side is generally worse than the left side.

Belladonna

Like *Aconite* states, *Belladonna* conditions appear suddenly, and the inflammation is intense. But whereas the mental state of *Aconite* is fear, that of *Belladonna* is violence and irritability.

The pupils are often dilated in *Belladonna* affections, so that the eyes look glassy. The conjunctivas are red and inflamed but usually dry. The inflammation may be so great as to roll the eyelids outward. The eyeballs themselves may protrude outward. This is another good remedy to consider for KCS.

Calcarea sulphurica

This remedy, like *Argentum nitricum,* has an affinity to conjunctivitis in newborns, so it may be useful for young kittens. The eyes discharge a thick yellow pus. The cornea may be smoky gray. The eyelids are often itchy. These animals dislike drafts and cold, but they also dislike warm stuffy rooms, so they seek the open air.

Euphrasia

This remedy is made from the herb that is known as eyebright. The discharges are the opposite of those of *Allium cepa* in that here the tears are extremely acrid, but the nasal discharges are bland. There may be thick, irritating discharges as well. Discharges, whether tears or pus, may leave a stain. The eyes water all the time. At night, the patient is very chilly and restless, like *Arsenicum.* The eyelids may spasm occasionally. The profuse irritating tears and chronic inflammation are the primary indications.

Mercurius (vivus or solubilis)

When *Mercurius* is needed, the discharges are very acrid but thin. There may be pus in the anterior chamber (the space behind the cornea), so you may see a whitish clot. The lids may spasmodically close, and they are usually red and inflamed. The nose is usually affected with a foul greenish discharge that irritates the nostrils.

These animals tend to be irritable, and they do not like to be disciplined or even given instruction; they may scratch or bite if moved off of a bed, for example.

Pulsatilla

Thick bland yellow discharges are the rule when *Pulsatilla* is needed. This remedy, along with *Sulphur,* is often needed at the end of an upper respiratory infection when the inflammation is not so intense, but it won't clear up. The eyes are itchy and mildly inflamed.

These animals are usually of sweet disposition, though they may demand attention. They tend to be thirstless.

Rhus toxicodendron

The pus here is also yellow and profuse (like *Pulsatilla*), but the inflammation is very intense. This remedy is from poison ivy, so as you might imagine, the eyes become red and swollen. Instead of itchiness, however, there is great pain. The cornea may be badly ulcerated, and the lids may become stuck together with gluey matter. The eyeball itself is often inflamed. The pain in the eye is intense, especially upon movement (all *Rhus tox* pains are worse from initial movement).

These animals are very similar to those needing *Arsenicum* in that they are chilly, restless (especially after midnight), and thirsty. Local inflammations may be more swollen and itchy when *Rhus tox* is needed. Nausea is generally worse with *Arsenicum*. Joint pains that are worse with initial motion and better with continued motion, if present, would suggest *Rhus tox*.

Sabadilla

Here the eyes are usually very red and watery, worse on going into the open air (though overall the patient may feel better in open air). Tearing is often profuse. The eyelid margins are usually red. Violent sneezing often accompanies conjunctivitis. It is similar to *Allium cepa*, but the eyes usually appear redder.

Sulphur

Sulphur, like *Pulsatilla*, typically comes into service as an upper respiratory infection is coming to a close, but the body cannot quite finish it off. In the *Sulphur* state, tears and discharges are acrid and the margins of the eyelids often severely inflamed. The cornea may be ulcerated as well. The eyes are usually itchy and burning, causing the patient to rub them a lot. The eyes may be dry while inside, but tears flow when the animal goes outside.

These animals are usually hot and thirsty, and the appetite may be minimal, especially in the morning. The appetite improves in late morning and may peak about an hour before the next mealtime.

Syphilinum

This is a deep-acting remedy that is available by prescription only. It really should be administered under the direction of a skilled homeopath. I list it here because it has proven successful in some chronic conjunctivitis cases that did not respond to other remedies.

Hypopyon (Pus behind the Cornea)

This condition often occurs following an injury or possibly following acute conjunctivitis. It is basically an intraocular abscess. Pus develops in the anterior chamber—the space between the iris (colored part) and the cornea. You will see a whitish cloudiness that is behind the cornea—not on the surface of the cornea. This condition is serious and usually treated with antibiotics. If you choose not to use antibiotics (and they may not be needed), don't wait more than a few days if you are not seeing improvement. Adhesions can easily develop, so an atropine eyedrop may be needed, even with the correct remedy. Preferably, you should work with a homeopathic veterinarian, or at least one that is cooperative with your treatment. You can also use the homeopathic remedy along with the antibiotics to speed healing.

Homeopathic Medicines for Hypopyon

Hepar sulphuris calcareum
When *Hepar sulph* is needed, the eye will be extremely painful, and the animal will usually be irritable and snappish, especially with any attempt to examine the eye. There may be pimples surrounding the eye, and the eye itself may be extremely inflamed. The cornea may be severely ulcerated. *Hepar sulph* is very similar to *Mercurius*.

Mercurius (vivus or solubilis) and Mercurius corrosivus
See the description above under conjunctivitis. When the infection goes deeper, the iris color may appear muddy. These remedies are similar, and you may need *Mercurius* for females and *Mercurius corrosivus* for males, though this is not always true. Don't give these remedies before or after *Silicea*.

Silicea (Silica)
As a major abscess remedy, *Silicea* is often useful for hypopyon. The main indications are poor immune response and general weakness. There may be conjunctivitis as well, but the pain is not nearly as intense as the *Hepar*

sulph state. The eyes are sensitive to light, and there may be a sluggish ulcer (indolent ulcer) on the cornea. *Silicea* conditions move slowly as a rule.

Thuja occidentalis

Thuja is most commonly used in veterinary medicine for the damaging effects of vaccination, so if hypopyon develops shortly after a vaccine, consider *Thuja*. *Silicea* is another major antivaccinosis remedy. With *Thuja*, the conjunctiva are not usually as inflamed. Indolent (poor-healing) ulcers may also respond to this remedy.

Corneal Ulcers

Ulcers are very serious and should be under the care of a veterinarian, but one of the following remedies may help heal the ulcers. The remedies are discussed in either the "Conjunctivitis" or "Hypopyon" sections, so no description is given here. Use vitamin A (cod liver oil) topically in the eye (one drop daily) as an aid to healing.

Indolent ulcers occur in animals that have poor delivery of nutrients to the eyes. These often occur in dogs whose eyes bulge out.

Homeopathic Medicines for Corneal Ulcers

Apis mellifica, Argentum nitricum, Arsenicum album, Hepar sulphuris calcareum, Mercurius, Mercurius corrosivus, Rhus toxicodendron, Silicea, Sulphur, Syphilinum, Thuja.

Indolent (poor or slow healing) ulcers—*Silicea, Thuja.*

Entropion (Inversion of the Eyelids)

Entropion occasionally occurs as a growth defect. It is mild, but the eyelashes can badly irritate the cornea, resulting in constant tearing and redness. Many remedies are possibilities, but two stand out. If these do not work, you could consult a homeopath for other possibilities. If you don't see a response, surgery is indicated.

Borax

Besides the entropion, the characteristics of animals needing this remedy have two main features. One is extreme sensitivity to noise, especially a gunshot, even at great distance. The second peculiarity is a fear of falling, so these animals may avoid going down stairs, and if picked up, they may be frightened at being put down. An animal needing this remedy may also have mouth ulcers.

Calcarea carbonica

This remedy is good for a lot of developmental problems, including entropion. These patients tend to be soft and flabby and may be big boned. They may also be rather clumsy. The eye inflammation may be less than when *Borax* is needed.

Injuries to the Eyes

Any serious eye injury should be checked by a veterinarian, but there are a few remedies that can help speed healing. As I mentioned above, a minor injury to the cornea can quickly deteriorate, so have a veterinarian assist you in monitoring progress.

Arnica montana

Arnica is good for bruising anywhere, generally from blunt injuries. The eye muscles may be partly paralyzed after the injury. The eye may be bloodshot. When *Arnica* is indicated, the pain is such that the patient is extremely afraid of touch. *Arnica* may stimulate reabsorption of blood that is in the eye due to an injury (*Hamamelis* may be better). This remedy may be useful for a cataract that follows an eye injury, though *Conium* is usually the first choice.

Asarum europaeum

Can be useful for painful lacerations to the eye. The eyes tend to be burning, with watery tears, when *Asarum* is needed. Can be used following surgical incisions of the eye. See also *Staphysagria*.

Calcarea sulphurica

This remedy is useful for infections or inflammations as a result of splinters in the eye.

Calendula officinalis

Calendula is a good remedy for infected wounds. In eye injuries, it is helpful for inflammation with pus that follows an injury. You may use the remedy in a potentized form or topically. For topical use, boil a cup of water; as the water cools, add one-fourth teaspoon of table salt and ten to twenty drops of *Calendula* tincture.

Conium maculatum
If your companion develops a cataract after an injury, *Conium* may resolve the cataract (consider *Arnica* also).

Euphrasia
Consider *Euphrasia* for corneal opacity following an eye injury.

Hamamelis
This remedy is similar to *Arnica* and is helpful for bruising eye injuries with intraocular hemorrhage.

Ledum
Ledum is good for eye bruising also. The specific indication is bloodshot eyes with leakage of blood into the tissues, so there may be blood just under the surface of the eyelids, conjunctiva, and sclera as well as possibly into the anterior chamber (under the cornea).

Millefolium
This antihemorrhagic remedy can be of service with bleeding into the anterior chamber (between the cornea and the iris). This may occur with trauma, but if it occurs spontaneously, there may be a bleeding disorder. Some drugs, like those used for high blood pressure, can cause bleeding in the anterior chamber.

Staphysagria
Any laceration may heal better with this remedy, especially if the laceration is painful. Corneal lacerations fit this category, so use *Staphysagria*, but have the eye examined for safety.

Symphytum
This is the first remedy to consider for eye injuries, especially those from a blunt object. I have also used *Symphytum* successfully for corneal abrasions. A friend had a chronic abrasion from getting dirt under a contact lens a few years before. The inflammation periodically recurred, but a couple of doses of *Symphytum* stopped the problem permanently.

Chapter Eleven
URINARY SYSTEM

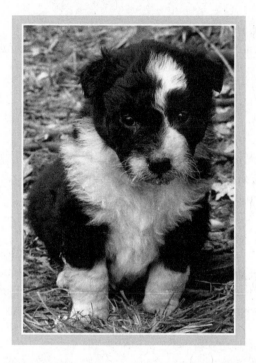

Function

Urinary System Disease

Cystitis (Bladder Inflammation)

Urethral Obstruction and Catheterization

Decreasing Kidney Function (Kidney Disease, Kidney Failure)

Urinary Incontinence

Incontinence from Injury

Function

The primary functions of the urinary system are excretion of toxic (or otherwise unneeded) substances and maintenance of the body's water balance. The kidneys also produce hormones that affect the circulatory system.

Metabolic by-products may be eliminated through the intestines, liver, skin, lungs, and kidneys. Excretion via the kidneys occurs by two main mechanisms: filtration and secretion. Filtration occurs as the blood passes through a network of clusters of tiny blood vessels (glomeruli) in the kidney. Many molecules can slip through the blood vessels into a kidney cell that transports the molecule into small tubes (tubules) that ultimately connect to the ureters; the ureters are the tubes that transport urine from the kidneys into the urinary bladder. This is a somewhat passive system in that the molecules move out into the urine in relation to their concentration in the blood and the amount of blood that moves through the filtration network.

Secretion is an active method of transfer; certain substances are pumped by the body out of the blood and into the tubules. This process allows more control over their excretion rate. In actuality, many substances are both filtered and secreted. Additionally, many substances are reabsorbed after filtration, thus allowing the body to conserve resources by reclaiming useful substances and letting others pass into the urine. This conservation allows the body to filter the blood about sixty times in a day.

Water is also regulated by these same mechanisms of filtration and reabsorption. By regulating the amount of water excreted, the kidneys maintain a constant volume of blood plasma, and this keeps blood circulation and blood pressure at effective levels. If blood pressure should drop due to water loss or inadequate water intake from which these methods cannot compensate, the kidneys secrete an enzyme called renin that initiates the production of another substance (angiotensin), which constricts the blood vessels and restricts sodium and water excretion; this increases blood pressure and thus improves circulation. A hormone, erythropoietin, is also produced in the kidneys and stimulates production of red blood cells. In chronic kidney disease these chemicals are usually diminished. Thus kidney disease directly affects blood volume and circulation as well as toxin elimination. The kidneys are organs that we simply cannot live without.

The urinary bladder is primarily a storage sac for urine. After production in the kidneys, urine is transported to the bladder via the ureters. When the bladder is full, it sends a signal to the brain, and the animal finds an appropriate spot and empties the bladder via the urethra. This is done by contracting muscles in the bladder itself as well as by contracting abdominal muscles. Until the time for emptying, muscles in the urethra (sphincter muscles) stay contracted to retain urine. Upon contraction of the bladder muscles, the urethral muscles relax and allow passage of urine. The bladder is normally emptied two to four times a day.

Urinary System Disease

Essentially, disease of this system occurs either in the production of urine or in the elimination of urine. Production problems result from kidney malfunction, while elimination problems are mostly bladder related. Most kidney diseases are slow to occur and difficult or impossible to cure, whereas most bladder problems show up quickly and can be cured. Untreated or improperly treated bladder diseases may progress to kidney diseases, so prompt attention is essential. Conventional medicine suggests that progression occurs by ascension of bladder infections up the ureters to the kidneys. Conventional veterinarians prescribe antibiotics for bladder problems based upon this theory in order to prevent kidney disease.

Homeopathic veterinarians, however, believe that the disease moves into the kidneys as the body weakens and that this movement has nothing to do with bacteria, rather that the disease simply increases in strength. If the urinary system is the disease focus in a given individual, it is likely that, as disease deepens, the body will shift the focus of illness from the bladder to the kidneys. Additionally, if the bladder symptoms are suppressed, this deepens the illness and thus may shift disease to the kidneys. We thus believe that antibiotic treatment of most bladder diseases may in fact cause this shift rather than preventing the movement. Most bladder problems are not infectious (urine is usually sterile even when the bladder is inflamed), and even when there is bacterial growth, it is usually secondary to the bladder disease rather than causative. See Chapter Two, "The Nature of Disease," and Chapter Three, "The Nature of Cure," for more information about disease.

Since kidney disease is so difficult to reverse, prevention is virtually the only medicine. As with all systems, diet is critical. A fresh-food diet with raw meats provides the best possible nutrition. This is essentially what carnivores are designed to eat, and it works best. Dry food places the most stress on the kidneys because most animals drink inadequate amounts of water, thus the kidneys must work harder to maintain the water balance. Cats are especially subject to kidney disease since they evolved in an arid environment, and they do not normally drink water. They typically meet their water intake needs from the bodies of their prey, and a healthy cat on a healthy diet may take a sip of water every couple of weeks. Cats (and most dogs) who live on dry food are almost always somewhat dehydrated. To gain an idea of the impact of dry foods, try placing some dry food in a bowl and adding water. You will be amazed how much water is necessary before the food is saturated.

The other stressors on the kidneys are toxins and vaccination. Many toxins directly damage kidney cells. As the body has very limited capacity to replace kidney cells, each damaged cell results in decreased function. While we cannot do much about pollution outside the home (though we can limit our contribution to pollution), we can take steps to minimize household poisoning by using natural, nontoxic cleaning materials, limiting the use of paints and finishes, and buying natural rather than synthetic products.

The first time I clearly recognized the impact of vaccinations was in a cat with recurrent "bladder infections." Fluffy, a female Persian, kept returning to my clinic for urinary straining. The condition would surface again and again for several months before it would abate. Then, after only a few months of respite, her bladder problem would return. I finally saw that the recurrences followed her yearly vaccinations by a month or two. All doubt was erased when I stopped giving her these boosters, as she never again had a bladder "infection." Later, as I understood homeopathic theory better, I saw that this was predictable according to the theory.

According to homeopathic principles, there are several categories of disease. These are not syndromes in the conventional sense, nor are they considered diseases. They are simply general types of bodily reactions. One of these categories is sycosis. The general reaction of sycosis is an overreactivity. One of the main systems impacted by sycosis is the urinary system (urogenital systems, to be more precise). And a major initiator of sycosis is vaccination. Vaccinosis, disease caused by vaccination, is a subcategory of sycosis—thus it is not surprising that vaccination can incite bladder inflammation.

Once the urinary system is diseased at any level, no matter the cause, it may progress to a kidney disease. Since antibiotic or other suppressive treatment of bladder disease may lead to kidney disease, and since bladder disease is more treatable and more obvious than kidney disease, I'll cover bladder problems first.

Cystitis (Bladder Inflammation)

Veterinarians may refer to this condition as a urinary tract infection (UTI) or lower urinary tract disease (LUTD). The latter name is newer and recognizes the noninfectious nature of most cases.

When the urinary bladder becomes inflamed, the first symptom is usually *frequent attempts to pass urine.* Affected animals will often urinate in unusual or inappropriate locations such as carpets, rugs, chairs, sinks, newspapers, and so on. The animal may be unable to rest because of the repeated straining. It is not that there is extra urine, but that the inflammation mimics the feeling of fullness in the bladder, so the patient constantly feels like she needs to urinate. From humans with cystitis, we know that this is a very uncomfortable feeling.

Another clue that occurs occasionally is that there is an odor associated with the bladder inflammation. The odor is imperceptible to humans, but males of the same species as the affected animal find the odor attractive. Thus, if you see that males are hanging around a spayed female or a neutered male, that animal may have cystitis. (She may also have vaginitis, an inflammation of the vagina, as this can also produce odors that attract males.)

Cats have more problems with cystitis than dogs as a rule, and females have cystitis more frequently than males, especially in dogs. (I use the word *dog* to denote male or female canines, not a male canine—for that I will specify "male dog.") In cats, the balance is more even, but in males the risk is immensely greater than in females (see below).

Urine examination substantiates the inflammation because the urine typically contains many white blood cells (inflammatory cells). Infection is uncommon, however, though often assumed. Sometimes there are crystals in the urine, and these may create problems. The most common type of crystal is one we call triple phosphate crystals (also called struvite crystals) because they consist of three phosphate compounds. These crystals form in alkaline urine. Carnivores normally produce acid urine because of the digestive by-products of meat consumption. Cereal-based commercial foods, however, tend to produce alkaline urine, and this is a major factor in crystal formation. If there is a primary infection, the bacteria often excrete alkaline substances, which can cause the same problem. Additionally the bacteria grow more readily in alkaline urine, so I suspect that diet is a primary factor even when there is a secondary infection.

In females, the urethra is short and has a comparatively wide diameter, so the crystals usually pass easily, though they may irritate the urethra and bladder. In males, the urethra is longer and relatively narrow as it passes through the penis, and this is where problems arise. Fortunately for male dogs, this is rare, but male cats suffer greatly from this problem. It is all too common that the urethra of male cats becomes plugged and blocks urine output. *This is a dangerous situation and can easily be fatal if the obstruction is not quickly removed.* If the obstruction keeps him from urinating, the pressure from the urine in the bladder will back up and stop the kidneys from functioning until the obstruction is cleared. It is as though his kidneys have shut down. *This can be fatal in as little as twenty-four to forty-eight hours. If this condition occurs, you must seek veterinary care immediately.* This can happen in male dogs also and very rarely in female cats or dogs. If you do not believe him or her to be passing urine or if you cannot tell, get an examination.

It can be difficult to know if urine is passing because the frequent straining may keep the bladder empty and thus he may pass only a couple of drops. Cats sometimes will urinate in a sink or bathtub, apparently (in at least some cases) to let their guardian know about the problem. If so, you can see the drops of urine. Frequently, there may be some blood in the urine, and it may be pink to red.

Cats may also avoid the litter box because of association of pain with the box. This may result in a cat that refuses to use a litter box even after the cystitis has cleared. Some apparent behavioral urination problems may be cystitis or may have begun with cystitis.

If you can't see any urine, try to feel for a full bladder. In cats, this is rather easy—if there is an obstruction, the bladder will feel like an orange or even a grapefruit in the rear of the abdomen. This is very uncomfortable, and even the most friendly cat may growl and try to get away. Don't try to squeeze the bladder—it is possible to rupture a urinary bladder in an obstructed animal. Once again, if you are unsure, see a veterinarian.

If there is an obstruction, the cat will quickly deteriorate and become lethargic, the breath may smell sharp, somewhat like urine, and he may vomit. This is because the kidneys cannot excrete toxins. The toxins make him feel sick, and the body tries to excrete them through the saliva, vomitus, and skin in a desperate attempt to preserve life. If you find this condition, do not wait to seek veterinary help, as death could come in a few hours.

In a few animals, the crystals consolidate and become stones either in the bladder or in the kidney. These must sometimes be removed surgically, although medical treatment and diet changes may dissolve the stones. This must be diagnosed by a veterinarian, usually by radiographs or ultrasound, though we can sometimes feel the stones. In these situations, however, often the animal suffers from recurrent bouts of cystitis. If your companion keeps returning to urinary straining, be sure to get an examination, and obtain X-rays or ultrasound as needed. If the crystals are oxalates, magnesium citrate can help dissolve them. Use about 20–25 mg per ten pounds, based upon the magnesium content, daily.

General Care for Cystitis

If your companion develops cystitis, first you must assess the severity of the problem.

- The first and most important question, especially in males, is whether or not he is passing urine. This is critical.
- If he is passing urine, is the urine volume small or large? (If he is passing a large volume of urine, the problem may not be cystitis but may be a kidney problem, diabetes, or another illness.)
- Does the breath smell sharp or urine-like?
- Is he vomiting?
- Is this an isolated incident, or does this happen regularly?
- What does the urine look like? Is there blood or mucus in it?
- How frequently is it occurring?
- Is he straining hard, or is the straining prolonged?
- Is he weak and listless?
- Is he dehydrated? (To check for dehydration, pick up some skin over the back and let it drop. It should return to its original position immediately. Any slowness of return indicates dehydration. Compare the response with a healthy animal if possible.)

Obtain a veterinary examination immediately:
- if you are unsure about urination and he is listless or depressed;
- if he cries out as if in pain (there is a mournful cry that cats make

when their urethra is obstructed. Many veterinarians can diagnose an obstruction by the sound of the cry. The cry may be associated with straining to urinate, but it may also appear unrelated);

- if he vomits at all.

These conditions especially pertain to male cats because of the frequency and severity of the condition in these animals.

Have your companion checked right away:

- if you notice weakness or dehydration;
- if urination is especially frequent and painful;
- if he has ever been obstructed before (obstruction is more likely in cats that have been obstructed previously);
- if you see blood or mucus in the urine (a pinkish urine is not so urgent and you can try home treatment for a day or so if he is otherwise OK);
- if frequent straining persists even with fasting (see below).

Have an examination soon:

- if the condition persists for more than a couple of days after correcting diet and after home treatment;
- if he has had the problem before, especially within the past few months.

Next, try to determine patterns or circumstances. Are there triggering conditions such as:

- eating;
- recent vaccination;
- fighting with other cats, especially being bullied;
- times of day (morning, before breakfast, night, etc.);
- stress or anxiety in the house?

Acute Cystitis (without Obstruction)

If his energy is good and *you are certain he is not obstructed,* fast him for twenty-four hours on broth. Often this will diminish the intensity of the straining. You may continue the fast for two to three days if he remains in good spirits. Fasting reduces the load on the kidneys by lessening the byproducts of digestion that the kidneys must eliminate. Additionally, the extra fluid from broth helps to flush out the bladder. You can give broth by syringe or dropper if he does not drink it on his own. Extra vitamin C (10 mg/pound, two to three times a day; sodium ascorbate is best here) will help acidify the urine, dissolving any crystals and inhibiting bacterial growth. The amino acid D-L-methionine is a good acidifier also and can be given at the dose of 5–10 mg/pound, two to three times a day. If you cannot find this form, you can use L-methionine; this is readily available at health food stores. Cranberry juice is helpful also, though it is hard to administer. Some people have success using capsules of cranberry concentrate. Cranactin is one brand; give about one-quarter to one-half capsule per ten pounds, two to three times a day.

Tinkle Tonic, an herbal preparation by Animal Essentials/Animals' Apawthecary (www.animalessentials.com), is a good herbal support for urinary problems if homeopathic treatment is not successful. It is in a glycerin base, so animals take this better than alcohol-based tinctures due to glycerin's sweetness. You can also make an herbal tea, or use tinctures, with corn silk, nettles, red clover, dandelion, and marshmallow root. Use equal parts (dried herbs) of all five and make a tea with one teaspoon herb to one cup water. Give one-half ml (cc) per ten pounds, three or four times daily. With tinctures, mix equal parts of each herb, then give four to six drops per ten pounds, three or four times daily. With tinctures, you may need to put the drops into a small amount of broth with honey to mask the taste. Finally, sometimes apple cider vinegar in the drinking water can help by acidifying the system. Add only a small amount, or he won't drink any water. I have little experience with this but have heard of good reports in some cases. Bearberry can be helpful as well, but should only be used for a week or two. See *Uva ursi* below.

Homeopathic Medicines for Acute Cystitis

Aconitum napellus

In cystitis, as in other inflammatory conditions, *Aconite* is best used early in the course of illness. Often, no symptoms arise other than the primary complaint of frequent attempts to urinate. The animal may be restless and fearful. Aconitum states often arise following exposure to cold, often windy conditions.

Apis mellifica

These animals have burning at the end of urination and are generally thirst-less and warm. They may be restless or listless and indifferent to others. The indifference, if present, differentiates *Apis* from *Pulsatilla*.

Arsenicum album

Arsenicum is a good remedy to consider, especially if the frequent urination worsens after midnight. These patients will often be very restless with the cystitis, and they may be worse when alone.

Berberis vulgaris

Barberry is useful for cystitis when the kidneys are also affected. There will be burning in the urethra and bladder, during and after urination. Characteristically, however, the kidneys are also quite painful in *Berberis* complaints. The slightest touch in the region of the kidneys (on the back, on either side of the spine, just behind the last ribs) is painful. Sometimes this even affects walking with the rear legs. See *Eupatorium purpureum* also. Jarring motion worsens the patient needing this remedy.

Cantharis

This remedy has the reputation as the best choice for cystitis in humans, and presumably this would apply in cats and dogs as well. It can be help-ful, but don't just give it without considering other remedies. Straining is frequent and may be severe with great pain in the urethra and kidneys. There may be involuntary urination after straining stops. The urine may contain blood. There may be blisters inside the vagina (visible with an instrument for internal viewing such as an otoscope) or in the mouth.

Equisetum

These animals have pain at the close of urination, and cats may bolt from the little box as they finish urinating. They can have constant urging and straining with little output. They may also leak urine. The bladder area (lower abdomen) may be painful to touch.

Eupatorium purpureum

Eupatorium purpureum (don't confuse with *Eupatorium perfoliatum*), like

Berberis, is indicated when there is kidney pain as well as bladder pain. Here the pains often follow exposure to cold. They are less sharp and acute than deep and dull, so the patient may be less frantic or intensely painful and more lethargically painful. The urine may contain mucus or even appear milky. Desire to urinate is constant, though that is a common symptom. Like *Berberis*, the patient may have difficulty standing due to the pain, which can be intense. Stools may be loose and greenish. Any motion can aggravate the *Eupatorium purpureum* condition.

Lycopodium clavatum

A keynote for *Lycopodium* is urinary and digestive disturbances. I find this a good guide to using the remedy. Not all cases with a history of both urinary and digestive symptoms need *Lycopodium*, but if this is present, I would consider the remedy. These animals often have a history of diarrhea, frequently with gas—but typically the diarrhea and the cystitis occur as separate bouts of illness. *Lycopodium* patients are often timid in new situations but bossy when they feel comfortable. They know their position in the hierarchy of the family and are submissive to those they know are above them but very bossy to those below. This is a good remedy in many cats with LUTD.

Mercurius (vivus or solubilis)

This is a good remedy to consider for cystitis when there is concurrent diarrhea, with urging/straining to urinate and defecate simultaneously (*Lycopodium* more often has them at separate times). Straining may be intense and may continue after the urine or stool has been expelled. There may be mucus and/or blood in the stool or urine. These animals can be quite irritable, especially when disciplined. As with other complaints needing *Mercurius*, males may do better with *Mercurius corrosivus*.

Nux vomica

Nux is a good remedy to consider for cystitis with lots of straining and frequent attempts to urinate with little success. There may be blood in the urine (though most cystitis cases have blood, so this is a common symptom). These animals may have a history of a lot of conventional drug treatment. *Nux* is good to use for patients who have had prior bouts of cystitis treated with antibiotics, but the cystitis keeps returning. They tend to be irritable and even quarrelsome, though not usually so much as those need-ing *Mercurius*. They may be worse in the morning or in open air.

Pulsatilla

Pulsatilla is another good remedy for cystitis, especially in females. The urging is often worse when they lie down. Another common indication for *Pulsatilla* is a tendency to urinate involuntarily when startled or excited. Although hard to observe in animals, this symptom is a good pointer to *Pulsatilla*. These animals are generally sweet and need lots of attention, they like open air, and they drink little. This remedy, like *Nux*, may be useful for patients with a history of conventional drug use.

Sarsaparilla

All urinary symptoms are worse at the end of urination: blood or mucus may pass after the bladder has emptied, and there may be intense pain as urination ends. The pain may be so intense that the patient cries out in anticipation of urination or at the close of urination. A peculiar symptom in people is difficulty urinating unless the person is standing; these animals may find it difficult to urinate in a squatting position. The *Sarsaparilla* state may come on after the patient is chilled, especially during damp weather.

Solidago

This remedy is good for chronic kidney and bladder inflammations. The urine is foul-smelling, reddish, and bloody, sometimes with mucus and crystals. The kidneys may be painful here, like *Berberis* and *Eupatorium pur-pureum*. If your cat or dog suffers from chronic inflammation of the urinary system, a course of *Solidago* 6X, two or three times daily for a month or two, might help remove the tendency by cleansing the system.

Staphysagria

Staphysagria can be helpful in bladder inflammations. There is burning pain during and after urination, which can be worse at night or worse when cold in bed. (Contrast with *Aconitum*, which is worse with exposure to cold, usu-ally outside in cold windy conditions.) The urine may be bloody and scanty. These animals may be sweet like *Pulsatilla* but often have some resentment or anger, especially in reaction to other animals getting attention or a feel-ing that they don't get enough attention themselves.

Thlaspi bursa pastoris
This remedy is almost organ-specific in that its main symptoms are in the urinary bladder. Chronic cystitis with a tendency to phosphate crystals may respond to *Thlaspi*. It even has a reputation for unblocking urethral obstructions. The sediment often looks like brick dust.

Thuja occidentalis
I have had good success with *Thuja* in cystitis, probably because of the connection of vaccination and bladder inflammation. The urethra may be swollen, and the bladder may be mildly paralyzed, making urination difficult. These cats may seem obstructed, but when a catheter is passed, no blockage is found. There may also be mucus that collects at the urethral opening.

Urtica urens
This is another good remedy for cystitis with very frequent urging and little urine passage. These poor cats find little rest because of the constant urging. There may be crystals in the urine or even bladder stones.

Uva ursi
Uva ursi has great irritation, spasms, and sometimes mucus clots, blood clots, or pus. The mucus is tenacious—tough—and hard to remove. This is bearberry (kinnick kinnick), and it is helpful in cystitis as an herbal tincture but irritating to the bladder if used for more than a couple of weeks.

Urethral Obstruction and Catheterization

See above (under "Cystitis") for precautions and general information. When an animal has a urethral obstruction, it is impossible to urinate, and *this is a life-threatening situation.* Generally, you should seek immediate veterinary care to relieve the obstruction. A few remedies have occasionally relieved an obstruction without catheterization, so I will list these. However, do not delay seeking veterinary care—you should see results within ten to fifteen minutes if the remedy will work. Repeat each remedy every few minutes for three doses. If you see no response from this, the remedy will likely not work. You may try another remedy if the cat is in good health and good spirits, but excessive delay is unfair to him and could be risky.

Urinary catheterization is not without risk, however. While passing a urinary catheter is often the only option when a cat becomes obstructed, damage to the urethra may occur, and this leaves him more likely to have a reobstruction in the future. Immediate reblockage may occur due to urethral swelling, and later reblockage may occur as a result of scar tissue that forms after the urethral trauma. Scar tissue is a big problem, as it narrows the urethral diameter, making passage of tiny crystals and sediment even harder.

Many cats undergo a painful and drastic surgery called a perineal urethrostomy because of recurrent obstructions. In this surgery, the penis and scrotum are removed up to the perineum (the area just below the anus) to create a shorter, larger diameter urethra—essentially like that of female cats. The surgery may be necessary in some cases, but it is brutal. Be sure the surgery is necessary before agreeing to the procedure. Obtain a second opinion if possible.

Many times, the necessity for the surgery is created by trauma from urethral catheters. In my opinion and experience, most problems occur when the catheter is left in place rather than used to unblock the obstruction and then removed. The longer the catheter is left in place, the greater the irritation to the urethra. Overzealous catheterization is another problem—sometimes the obstruction is difficult to remove and the attempts to clear it are too rough.

Homeopathic Remedies for Urethral Obstruction

Coccus cacti, Nux vomica, Thlaspi bursa pastoris, Uva ursi, Solidago
Try each remedy for three doses at five- or ten-minute intervals, but don't wait more than an hour or so to take him in to a veterinarian, and only try this if the cat is bright and alert. The indications are essentially the same, so use your intuition or use whichever remedy you have available. All of these except *Nux,* and maybe *Uva ursi,* are hard to find, so unless you have them already you probably won't find them quickly enough. *Thlaspi* is also known as the herb shepherd's purse; perhaps a few drops of the tincture or infusion would work if you are lucky. *Thlaspi* is indicated for heavy crystal formation, sometimes like brick-dust. It can be useful for spasmodic retention, like *Staphysagria. Coccus* has the specific indication of a urethral obstruction from a blood clot, so if you see this and *Coccus* is available, try it first. *Uva ursi* has great irritation, spasms, and sometimes mucus clots, blood clots, or pus. The mucus is tenacious—tough—and hard to remove. This is bearberry (kinnick kinnick), and it is helpful in cystitis as an herbal tincture but irritating to the

bladder if used more than a couple of weeks. Finally, *Solidago* (goldenrod) can have thick sediment, blood, mucus, and crystals. The urine is foul-smelling. It is said to "sometimes make the use of catheter unnecessary."

As these are all uncommon remedies, you likely will not have them on hand. Use their herbal tinctures if these are available *(Uva ursi, Thlaspi, and Solidago)*. And if you have a cat who has obstructed before, I suggest having these on hand, as well as some of the remedies listed under cystitis. This way you will have them if your cat obstructs again.

Follow-up Treatment if Catheterization Is Required

If your cat has had a urethral catheter used, give the homeopathic remedy *Staphysagria* afterward. This remedy will help reduce the inflammation from the trauma. Many cats immediately reobstruct because of swelling and spasms secondary to the trauma to the urethra. This looks like a sediment blockage, but it is not. *Staphysagria* (or *Thuja* in some cases) may relieve this condition. *Thlaspi* and *Magnesia phosphorica* may help here as well.

If your cat is urinating fine but seems in pain, try the *Staphysagria* for this as well. If it is of no help, try also *Magnesia phosphorica*, which can help with bladder pain following catheterization.

To help reduce scarring from obstruction and catheterization, you can give the remedy *Thiosinaminum* in low potency. This remedy helps minimize scarring and adhesions anywhere in the body. Give a 6X potency two to three times daily, preferably in water, for two to four weeks. This can help with scarring that occurs post–perineal urethrostomy as well, if your cat is unfortunate enough to need this procedure. (See "Dosage: How to Handle and Administer Remedies" in Chapter Five, "Using Homeopathy at Home" for information on liquid dosing). The remedy *Petroleum* is also mentioned for strictures from chronic urethritis, though I have not used it for this myself. It may help with a cat who has had recurrent bouts of cystitis and recurrent catheterization. Here I would use a 30C potency, but it is probably best to do this under the care of your veterinary homeopath.

Decreasing Kidney Function
(Kidney Disease, Kidney Failure)

When the kidneys have lost 50 to 75 percent of their cells, we say that kidney failure has begun (a harsh term, though this *is* a critical situation). This is because the kidneys generally have little to no capacity to regenerate tissue, thus lost kidney cells are lost for good. Up to this point, however, the kidneys can keep up with the demand, so the loss is undetectable. (Conventional texts generally state that kidney failure begins when 75 percent of the cells have died. This is the point at which the blood indicators rise definitively into the abnormal range. I believe we can recognize early diminishing function when the kidney blood values creep into the high end of the normal range, however. I consider persistent high-normal values—those at the high end of the accepted normal range—indicative of early kidney disease. This is especially true in cats, as I think the accepted high end of the normal range is incorrect—it is too high. Animals on raw-meat diets, however, have higher values, which must be interpreted within the context of raw-fed values. Once we begin seeing blood levels climb, the animal is on a downward path, though the time it takes to deteriorate to life-threatening illness is quite variable.

The main symptoms of kidney disease are weight loss, poor appetite, and increased thirst with increased urine output. (In some cases, especially acute [sudden] failure, there may be no thirst and no urination.) As the illness progresses, you may see signs of toxicity such as ulcers in the mouth. The latter is a very critical sign, as the kidneys are unable to keep the animal alive without help for more than a number of days when ulceration has begun. The early symptoms are not definitive, though, so blood testing is necessary to confirm the diagnosis, although most experienced veterinarians can recognize the disease from clinical observation.

The main blood values associated with the kidneys are the blood urea nitrogen (BUN) and creatinine. BUN is a breakdown product of protein digestion and is primarily eliminated by the kidneys. If kidney function is reduced, the level of BUN increases rather rapidly. Creatinine is a by-product of muscle energy use in the body and is also excreted by the kidneys. The creatinine blood level also increases in kidney disease, but it does so more slowly than the BUN. Creatinine is thus a more stable indicator of kidney function. Normal values for any blood component vary with the laboratory that performs the testing, but normal BUN is about 10–25 mg/dl in dogs and 10–30 mg/dl in cats. Normal creatinine levels are about 1–2 mg/dl. For animals on raw meat based diets, the BUN may be five to ten points higher, and creatinine may also be slightly higher than published normal values.

Cats suffer much more from kidney disease than dogs for a number of reasons. First, having evolved in arid climates, cats are very efficient at conserving water. Their kidneys work hard to retain as much water as possible, which not only puts extra stress on kidney cells but also produces concentrated urine, predisposing to bladder issues and crystal formation. Secondly, cats are skittish and fearful by nature, as they are prey as well as predators. As primarily solitary animals, they must rely upon themselves alone to detect predators, unlike herd animals, and this has swayed their evolution toward being easily startled animals. In traditional Chinese medicine theory, the emotion associated with the urinary system is fear. Thus the constant guardedness that some cats experience can predispose them to kidney and bladder illness. Finally, recent studies at Colorado State University have shown a link between panleukopenia (cat distemper) vaccination and kidney damage. Dr. Michael Lappin at CSU suspects the kidney tissue culture cells in the vaccine, as the virus is grown on these cells for vaccine production. The panleukopenia virus, however, has a great affinity to the kidneys, and can persist in kidney cells for up to a year following infection. This is why kidney cells are used to propagate the virus, and I suspect that the vaccine virus itself damages the kidneys because of this affinity.

As a consequence of the much greater prevalence of kidney disease in cats, the following treatment section focuses more upon them than dogs, though the same principles apply to dogs. It is easier to give subcutaneous fluids to cats than dogs, though (see below).

General Care for Kidney Disease

Any time kidney disease is present, you should work with a veterinarian, as diagnosing and monitoring the disease is difficult, at least in the beginning. If your companion develops signs that could be kidney failure, take him in right away.

Have an examination immediately:
- if you see ulcers in the mouth or if the mouth odor is strong, along with other symptoms of possible kidney failure;
- if your companion stops drinking and urinating;
- if she is weak and listless.

Have an examination soon:

- if you see increased thirst or urination, or any other signs of possible kidney disease.

Although kidney disease is ultimately fatal, the course of illness is not always rapid and can often be moderated quite a bit. Homeopathic remedies may be very useful, and it is best to work with a homeopathic veterinarian if possible. The supportive care outlined below is greatly helpful also. If your nonhomeopathic veterinarian is cooperative and willing to assist you, the remedies listed here may work well along with the supportive care.

Acute kidney failure is an exception in that it is highly fatal and the only chance for recovery is with intensive fluid therapy and hospitalization. The listed remedies may help but are not to be used in lieu of veterinary care. Furthermore, in rare cases, a stone in the ureter (the tube between the kidney and the bladder) can obstruct the ureter. This can cause acute kidney failure. It is surgically treatable, though a very difficult surgery. It would be wise to investigate this possibility if your companion develops sudden (or even fairly sudden) kidney disease.

General support for kidney failure includes proper food, supplements, and regular administration of fluid therapy. Fluid therapy in this situation is not related to dehydration of the patient; rather it is a way to maintain good blood circulation so the body tissues are well nourished. It also helps remove body toxins by increasing blood flow to the kidneys and by increasing the excreted urine. It does not matter that your cat is not dehydrated. The fluid therapy is essential, so do not let your veterinarian dissuade you from this if she believes your cat is not dehydrated. Your success depends to a great degree upon successful utilization of this tool. I will give some guidelines for home use as I have a lot of experience and many veterinarians express discomfort with home administration and therefore have little experience with this aspect of home care. Some animals, however, simply never adjust to administering subcutaneous fluids at home, and consequently the procedure is quite stressful. In these situations, I believe the cat has spoken, and it is best not to force this treatment. The reason for this treatment, as with any medical treatment, is quality of life, and any life extension is secondary to improved quality. Treating an animal against his will violates this principle. If your companion continues to struggle with this or any other treatment, and especially if the struggle heightens over time, you must reevaluate your priorities.

The fluids are designed to be given intravenously (by direct injection into the veins), but veterinarians commonly use them subcutaneously (injected under the skin). This is rather easy to do, and it works best if the guardian learns how to do this at home so it can be done regularly. Taking a cat (or dog, but this condition is much more common in cats) to the veterinary clinic frequently is too stressful. Your veterinarian will need to show you how to give the fluids. It is not difficult, but it does take some practice. Some veterinarians are resistant to the idea of home use of fluids, but it is too valuable to ignore. If your veterinarian will not assist you, then ask him for a referral to someone who will help. You will also need to get the fluids through your veterinarian (some pharmacies also stock fluids which are less expensive, but you will need a prescription).

We usually give fluids daily or every other day, although the frequency may vary from once a week to twice a day. This procedure works better in cats than dogs although it can be used with dogs. The volume of fluids to be given is usually approximately 100 milliliters (100 cc) per cat. This is usually adequate (some veterinarians recommend more, but I rarely find more to be helpful). Adjust frequency rather than volume to regulate the dosage. For some cats, even 60–75 ml is sufficient, at least in the early stages. For dogs, use about 100 ml per fifteen pounds, and you must change locations if giving more than about 150–200 ml.

It is critical that the fluids be warmed prior to administration. Cats in kidney failure are almost always cold, and fluids will sap their heat further, even if they are at room temperature. Additionally, they dislike the cold fluids. Unfortunately, many veterinarians do not warm the fluids. If you take your cat in for subcutaneous fluid therapy, insist that the bag of fluids be placed into warm water for about ten to fifteen minutes prior to use. Additionally, the tubing that carries the fluid to the needle can be put in a bowl of warm water, as the fluids may cool off during the transit through the tube. Check the temperature of the fluids by running some of the fluids onto the inside of your wrist, as you would check a baby's bottle. Fluids should be about body temperature, or a little warmer.

I also prefer smaller needles than most veterinarians dispense. The most common size is an eighteen gauge, which may be in a green plastic case. While the fluids run through this size more quickly, I find it to be more discomforting to the animal, especially a small cat. Twenty or twenty-one gauge needles (pink or purple case) seem much more comfortable, and the extra time involved (not a lot) balances the discomfort with the larger needles.

I usually start with daily administration (occasionally twice daily) until the cat improves, then taper the frequency to the amount needed to maintain good energy and appetite. In early stages this may be once a week; as the disease worsens it may be needed once or twice a day. Most cats learn to tolerate the fluid therapy well. Warm fluids feel good to a cold cat, and a treat afterward helps entice him into cooperation. Many guardians observe that their feline companions seem to learn that they feel better after the fluids are given and thus willingly comply.

Diet is the second facet of home care, and it is equally critical. Many veterinarians and guardians do not understand diet needs in kidney disease. As in all conditions, I believe fresh, home-prepared foods with raw meat to be the best option for prevention and maintenance of health. Some animals with kidney disease do not handle raw meats as well for some reason, though. These are usually older animals. I always recommend a gradual transition to the raw-meat diets, and this is especially critical in older animals. Many animals can handle the raw meat well, so I recommend giving these diets a try; just do it slowly, and if your companion cannot digest the raw meat, then prepare the diets with cooked meat.

Protein requirements for animals with kidney disease are generally poorly understood. It is commonly thought that when there is any evidence of kidney disease, the protein level should be reduced. This is not correct for most animals. Protein reduction has little impact upon the progression of kidney disease. In fact, reducing the protein level in the diet may reduce the effectiveness of the kidneys. This is because the amount of blood filtered through the kidneys (the glomerular filtration rate) is tied to protein in the diet, and reducing the protein reduces the filtering, thus decreasing the excretion of toxins. (In rats, extra protein induces excessive glomerular filtration, and restricting dietary protein prevents progression of renal failure.[1] Although this has not been shown to occur in dogs or cats, this data is used to support protein restriction in these animals. I believe this is not correct, as dogs and cats are carnivores, whereas rats are primarily herbivores; this difference would account for different protein needs.)

Some of the toxins that the kidneys excrete (like the BUN) are a by-product of protein metabolism, so the body steps up filtration as protein increases; this improves filtration of all toxins. Normally, this compensates for the increased protein intake. Only when the kidney function has reduced beyond a certain level is this inadequate. Reaching this level has little to do with protein intake, though it does affect excretion of toxic by-products. *Protein reduction is necessary only when the kidney function has diminished to the point that these toxins build to a level that affects health.* Even then it is only to minimize a symptom of kidney disease, not to minimize the impact upon the kidneys. When the body cannot properly eliminate the protein by-products, these may cause nausea, mouth ulcers, poor appetite, and so on. Reducing the protein and improving the quality of the protein will then lessen the toxicity.

When should the protein level be reduced? Essentially we only reduce protein when its toxic by-products cause illness, and this varies from animal to animal. Practically there are some guidelines according to blood testing. Protein should not be reduced until the BUN reaches about 80 mg/dl, the creatinine reaches 2.5 mg/dl, and/or serum phosphate levels increase. Testing should be done when the animal is well hydrated, as dehydration can falsely elevate these values.[2] As each case is different, the clinical symptoms give the best indication. The point is that you should not restrict protein at the first sign of kidney disease.

More important than the total amount of protein are two related factors. The first is the quality of protein, and the second is the available calories in the diet from nonprotein sources. As you now know, it is the by-products of protein digestion that build to toxic levels when the kidneys cannot excrete them adequately. But the formation of these by-products depends upon the efficiency of the protein digestion in the first place.

Higher quality protein sources, such as eggs, provide proteins that are easy to digest and break down completely with few by-products. The other important consideration is providing adequate calories in the diet from nonprotein sources. The body generally breaks protein down into amino acids (the building blocks of protein) so these can be incorporated into proteins the body needs. The body recombines these amino acids into new proteins once they have been absorbed. This produces relatively little waste. If the diet is low on calories from carbohydrates and fats, the body then uses proteins to provide calories; comparatively this is a wasteful process and leaves a lot of work for the kidneys.

In early stages of kidney disease you want to use high-quality protein and extra fat and carbohydrate. Members of many Inuit tribes formerly subsisted on virtually all-meat diets without suffering because they also consumed large quantities of fat. Without the fat, they sickened rapidly and sometimes would die because of the high toxin production that occurred from obtaining their huge calorie requirements from proteins.[3] High-quality protein sources include eggs, cottage cheese, milk, and yogurt. Meats are of lesser quality, but turkey and chicken are somewhat better than red meats.

Finally, supplements can help nourish the body and the kidneys. Since the kidneys depend upon the bicarbonate ion for part of their function, the addition of baking soda (sodium bicarbonate) to the food may help many animals. Excessive urine flow washes the bicarbonate ions out of the kidney tissue, and the baking soda replenishes the ions. Just a pinch in the food daily is enough for a cat; use up to one-fourth teaspoon for dogs. Calcium is important as the serum phosphorus level tends to be high and calcium binds some of the phosphorus. Elevated phosphorus can damage the kidneys. Be sure the diet has adequate calcium, but don't add too much. Follow recipes accurately if you home-prepare foods, and don't use bone meal as a calcium supplement (with kidney failure), as there is phosphorus in the bone meal. Boron can also lower blood phosphorus. The human dose is 3 mg per day, so with cats you would give about one-tenth of this amount.

Herbs such as alfalfa, red clover, nettles, marshmallow root, and dandelion are especially good for kidneys. Parsley and mullein can reduce blood phosphorus levels, so these can be very helpful as well. Make a tea from one or more of these and give about one-half dropperful per ten pounds, three times a day. If she will take them in food, you can mix some of these plants in food (a pinch of each, up to edibility tolerance). Bee pollen, royal jelly, and ghee (Indian-style clarified butter) help nourish the stored kidney energy according to ayurvedic principles. Use just a pinch of the bee products and about one-fourth teaspoon daily of the ghee. The ghee also provides extra fat for calories. If you purchase ghee, be sure it is fresh, as it can go rancid on the shelf.

You can make ghee by taking unsalted butter and boiling it over low to medium heat until the water portion evaporates and the milk solids settle out. This takes about ten to fifteen minutes. The butter will foam once after a few minutes, then the foam will subside. It will foam again late in the process, at which time the settled milk solids will turn a golden brown. Remove from heat immediately and allow to cool. Strain through cheesecloth or a strainer into a jar, but don't get any of the milk solids into the jar. This will keep in the refrigerator for a few months, and it can be frozen for long-term storage. Ghee is a good cooking oil, as it does not burn at high heat. (See the *Sundays at Moosewood Restaurant* cookbook, published by Fireside/Simon & Schuster, for more detail.)

Chamomile tea baths can help skin detoxification, which assists the kidneys. Make the tea with a tea bag, or use one teaspoon chamomile per pint of boiled water. Allow to cool, then sponge on your cat with a cloth. Chamomile can antidote some homeopathic remedies, however, so if your remedies are not working, this may be an issue for your cat. Finally, glandular support products like Renafood and Feline Renal Support, from Standard Process, often prove very helpful. These are primarily available through veterinarians and other licensed health care practitioners, though you may find them online as well.

Acute Kidney Failure

Although it is rare, the kidneys sometimes suddenly stop working. Usually the kidney tissue swells and will not allow passage of urine through the tissue. When this happens, the kidneys stop producing urine, and the animal stops drinking water. He also becomes profoundly sick. This can be spontaneous, a drug or vaccine reaction, or it may be from antifreeze poisoning. Antifreeze (ethylene glycol) is highly toxic to the kidneys, and animals often like the taste. Its effects are irreversible, although if you see an animal drink the antifreeze, it is possible to save him with immediate veterinary care. Ethylene glycol is an alcohol-like substance; acutely intoxicated animals will appear inebriated. If your outdoor cat or dog appears inebriated, take him immediately to a veterinary clinic. *Do not waste any time with other treatment if your companion drinks antifreeze—take him directly to a veterinarian.*

There are safer alternatives for antifreeze now, so the next time you have the radiator flushed, ask for a propylene glycol antifreeze. Sierra is the first company to market propylene glycol antifreeze; Prestone also makes a propylene glycol formula. Fortunately also, many companies now put compounds in antifreeze to diminish palatability. Propylene glycol is still a safer compound for the environment, however, so use this if you can.

Acute kidney disease is usually diagnosed by a veterinarian. Treatment must be done at a veterinary hospital with aggressive fluid therapy and diuretic medications. The following homeopathic medicines can help, but they should be used in conjunction with veterinary care rather than in lieu of proper care. This condition is very difficult to treat in the best of circumstances, so don't take chances. As I mentioned above (in "General Care for Kidney Disease"), in rare cases there may be a stone in the ureter, which can be treatable with early intervention.

Homeopathic Medicines for Acute Kidney Failure

Use one of these remedies in the highest available potency, and repeat every two to four hours until your companion begins producing urine. These animals should be under veterinary care receiving intravenous fluid therapy along with homeopathic treatment.

Apis mellifica

This remedy is good for swelling anywhere and is also good for autoimmune diseases, so it is a good possibility and is usually available at health food stores. These animals are not thirsty, but they are hot and seek cool spots.

Apocynum cannabinum

Said to be a chilly *Apis,* this remedy can be good for kidney shutdown where the urine output diminishes and results in fluid accumulation in the abdomen, chest, or elsewhere. Nausea and vomiting may be profound when the kidneys are affected. They may vomit food immediately upon eating. Unlike *Apis* patients, these animals are thirsty.

Arsenicum album

Arsenicum has great affinity to the kidneys, and though I use it more for chronic kidney failure than for acute kidney failure, it is a consideration here as well. It is commonly available, and this is a plus since acute kidney failure is a very urgent condition. These animals are usually thirsty, chilly, and restless, and their symptoms may worsen after midnight. They may become thirstless as the disease progresses, and they are usually weak at this time.

Eucalyptus

This remedy may be indicated if a kidney inflammation accompanies an infection elsewhere in the body. There will usually be mucus or pus in the urine when *Eucalyptus* is needed.

Nitri spiritus dulcis

This remedy has a reputation for success when kidney failure occurs in humans following scarlet fever. If your companion develops kidney failure after any disease that produces a fever, this remedy is a good choice. You will have to order the remedy unless you have a good homeopathic pharmacy in your community. This is a limiting factor with this remedy as well as the next one.

Picric acid

This remedy may be useful for animals whose kidneys have stopped producing urine. They will be very weak and easily exhausted, and if they move much, it will be as if their legs are extremely heavy.

Serum anguillae (Eel serum)

If you can obtain this remedy quickly, I suggest it as the first choice as eel serum has a specific effect upon the kidneys, causing acute shutdown. The homeopathic remedy thus may reverse acute kidney disease and has been used successfully in many human cases. A differentiation between *Apis* and this remedy is that with *Apis* there is likely to be swelling somewhere (usually the limbs or the face), whereas if eel serum is the remedy there is usually no visible swelling.

Chronic Kidney Failure

In chronic kidney disease, the animal may be treated at home as described above under general care. Use one of the following homeopathic remedies to help maintain kidney function.

Homeopathic Medicines for Chronic Kidney Disease

Apocynum

This remedy is indicated for uremic vomiting, so it may be useful for fairly ill animals who vomit frequently. *Apoc* may help them feel well, but if they are vomiting a lot and this does not improve, it may be time to let them go.

Arsenicum album

Arsenicum proves its vast application once again by its usefulness in kidney disease. The thirst and chilliness of kidney failure are key parts of the *Arsenicum* picture. These patients will usually be restless as well, and worse after midnight. Cats needing *Arsenicum* often hang their heads over their water bowls without drinking. They are thirsty, but drinking probably creates nausea. These animals also show a similar relationship to eating. They act hungry but eat very little.

Berberis vulgaris

Berberis, or barberry, is a good kidney tonic and detoxification agent. Use one to three drops of the tincture, or use a low potency like a 6X to 6C. Administer three times a day. Oregon grape root is *Berberis aquifolium* and has similar properties. It is easier to find, though not as good as *B. vulgaris.* This can be used along with a remedy that matches the symptom picture, as it is more local support. See also *Solidago.*

Bioplasma

This is a combination of all the Schüssler tissue salts (cell salts), so it is not an individual remedy. I have seen at least one case, however, where this really helped support a cat with kidney disease. Most health food stores sell tissue salts and can get this if they do not have it on the shelf. You could also try the Phosphate combination cell salts, especially if high phosphorus levels persist. You can use these alone or in conjunction with more "constitutional" remedies.

China (pronounced "keena")

A key indication for this remedy (made from a tincture of the quinine-containing bark of the Peruvian *kina-kina* tree) is prostration because of loss of body fluid, so this fits the kidney failure picture nicely. I have found better success with the following remedies, however, which are compounds of quinine.

Chininum arsenicosum

As a combination of arsenic and quinine, this remedy covers many aspects of chronic kidney failure, and I have found it very helpful in many, many cases. Usually the picture resembles that of *Arsenicum,* but the patient does not respond to *Arsenicum,* so I use *Chininum arsenicosum.* Without other indications this would often be my first choice, especially in cats. I have seen several cats live comfortably for a long time with this remedy.

Chininum muriaticum

This remedy is even less common than *Chininum arsenicosum*, so it may be very hard to find. It would be similar to the latter remedy as well as similar to *Natrum muriaticum*. If *Natrum mur* seems correct but provides no benefit, consider this remedy. *Nat mur* (table salt) has great affinity to kidneys, as does *Arsenicum album*, so this remedy may also prove useful, though I have less experience with this compound than *Chin ars*.

Chininum phosphoricum

As with the other *Chininum* remedies, if your animal seems a *Phosphorus* type, you could try this salt.

Chininum sulphuricum

The combination of the mineral sulfur with quinine gives us this remedy. I choose it similarly, in that if *Sulphur* seems indicated but does not work, I consider *Chininum sulphuricum*.

Ferrum muriaticum

This is one of the few remedies listed for chronic interstitial nephritis, the primary "disease" affecting cat kidneys. These animals have common symptoms like anorexia and unquenchable thirst, though they can be thirstless. They can have stomach pain, which may show as discomfort upon touching the abdomen or picking them up. There may be a history of cystitis with blood, the spleen may be enlarged, and they may be prone to quarrels and probably are more likely males.

Mercurius (vivus or solubilis)

Mercurius may benefit many animals when the disease has progressed to the point that mouth inflammation accompanies their other symptoms. There may be ulcers on the gums. These animals are often irritable and may wish to be left alone.

Natrum muriaticum

This remedy, made from table salt, is another good remedy for animals with kidney failure. Eating salt makes one very thirsty, so by the "like-cures-like" principle *Natrum mur* is very useful for thirsty animals such as those with kidney failure. These patients are more likely to be warm than cool, and they avoid the sun. They also tend to want to be left alone rather than wanting petting or other attention.

Solidago

This is goldenrod, and it has a nice affinity to the kidneys. As with *Berberis*, above, use this in low potency, even down to 3X, two or three times a day. You can use this in conjunction with another remedy that fits the symptom pattern. There may be soreness around the kidneys and back; urination may be difficult and scanty, with blood, mucus, and protein.

Sulphur

As the greatest of polychrests, *Sulphur* can benefit many situations. It is a good remedy to consider for kidney failure when the animal is sluggish and very unkempt. These animals generally care little for their appearance, so they make little effort at cleaning themselves. This is especially striking in cats. While *Sulphur* patients are generally warm, those in kidney failure are often cold, so don't rule *Sulphur* out if your cat seeks heat. He may not be as chilly as a cat needing *Arsenicum* (who will hug the heat vent), but he may avoid cold areas. These animals will be thirsty but often have poor appetites. They are usually friendly, relaxed, and easygoing.

Urinary Incontinence

Some animals (mostly dogs) cannot retain their urine in the urinary bladder when they relax—usually when they lie down or sleep. This happens primarily in female dogs after they have been spayed. It is thought to be due to the lack of estrogen, because giving estrogen compounds will usually control (not cure) the problem. The hormone that has usually been used is diethylstilbestrol—the infamous drug known as DES and associated with cervical cancer and many other problems as a consequence of administration to pregnant women. Obviously, this drug should be avoided. Another newer drug that works in most cases is phenylpropanolamine, a diet drug that is available over the counter. If you cannot get relief from homeopathy or acupuncture, this drug is much preferable to DES if medication is necessary. Ask your veterinarian for dosage and instructions for use rather than using the drug on your own (she will probably prescribe the drug herself). Phenylpropanolamine is not without problems, however, and has been withdrawn from human medicine. Try plantain and buchu as herbal supplements, as these have been reported to help in humans. Use one-fourth the human dose per twenty-five pounds.

Estrogen deficiency may indeed be the problem, although most spayed female dogs do not suffer with urinary incontinence. There must be other factors, though we do not know. Possibly spaying too early is a problem, but I don't know of studies that make this connection. I am concerned about the tendency to spay and neuter animals at six to eight weeks of age rather than at six to eight months of age. I don't agree with this policy, and I wonder if urinary incontinence will increase along with a host of other troubles if this trend continues (see also Chapter Fourteen, "Reproductive System").

According to traditional Chinese medicine, there is an energy meridian that runs up the front midline of the body. This acupuncture meridian is called the conception vessel because it strongly affects the urogenital systems. When we spay an animal, we make an incision right on the conception vessel, very near points that can be used to treat urinary incontinence. Perhaps the disruption of the conception vessel at a vulnerable age creates an energy blockage that contributes to incontinence. Whatever the cause, acupuncture is a good option for treatment before considering drug use.

General Care for Urinary Incontinence

Have a veterinarian examine your dog to see if there is another problem or reason for the incontinence. Sometimes the urine output has increased, and this is the reason she can no longer hold her urine all night. The cause should be determined, as appropriate treatment for this may eliminate the incontinence.

If it seems to be incontinence only, it is not a health threat except for the occasional dog who may get urine burns around the vulva from constant exposure to urine. Be sure to change her bedding frequently and keep her clean. *Calendula* ointment is protective and soothing to the irritated skin. Plantain and buchu can help as well; see above in the introduction to urinary incontinence.

Constitutional treatment is the best bet for curing the incontinence, but you can try one of the following remedies first. If her mental state fits the chosen remedy, your chance of success is best.

Homeopathic Medicines for Urinary Incontinence

Bryonia

When *Bryonia* is needed, almost all complaints are worse from motion. If your dog leaks urine while walking (most incontinence cases occur when resting), *Bryonia* might be helpful.

Causticum

Causticum is by far the most common remedy prescribed for urinary incontinence. It is generally good for any situation when there is muscle weakness and fatigue and the animal is chilly. It is good for old broken-down constitutions, so it is more likely to help in older, weak animals.

Equisetum

Here the incontinence may be accompanied by or alternate with cystitis. There may also simply be a history of cystitis, with pain at the end of urination. Involuntary stools may also accompany the urinary incontinence.

Kreosotum

This is a major remedy for bed-wetting in children and may occasionally be useful for urinary incontinence in dogs, although the conditions are not really equivalent, as bed-wetting is more an emotional problem than a hormonal one. If there is a possibility that your dog's problem is stress or emotional, consider *Kreosotum*. The urine tends to be irritating when *Kreosotum* is needed.

Nux moschata

This remedy is especially useful in patients with mental confusion; they may easily get lost in familiar surroundings. *Nux moschata* also has an affinity to female organs and hormonal problems, including incontinence. These dogs tend to be thirstless with a dry mouth, so they may hang around the water bowl without drinking.

Pulsatilla

Pulsatilla patients have very weak urethral sphincter muscles, so they easily spill urine. In humans, they might leak a few drops of urine when startled or when laughing hard. Dogs may leak urine when excited. They may also leak urine when resting or sleeping. Like *Nux moschata* and *Sepia*, *Pulsatilla* is a good remedy for female organs. These dogs are typically sweet, and they love attention.

Sepia

Sepia animals tend to be rather distant and indifferent to attention. They are also extremely chilly. They may develop incontinence as well, and since *Sepia* is a good remedy for female hormonal problems, it can be useful for urinary incontinence of hormonal origin.

Incontinence from Injury

Occasionally, an injury to the spine will lead to incontinence. This especially occurs in cats with an injury known as a tail avulsion. An avulsion is when a nerve has been pulled away from the body, causing a paralysis (sometimes temporary). Tail avulsion occurs when the tail is pulled sharply, injuring the terminal end of the spinal cord where urethral and anal muscle nerves come off the cord. It often occurs when cats just get away from a car but the wheel runs over the tail; the forward momentum of the cat causes the tail avulsion.

Hypericum perforatum

This remedy is excellent for nerve injuries, and I have seen occasional good results in these cases (tail avulsion) with return of control over urine and bowel retention.

Chapter Twelve
MUSCULOSKELETAL (LOCOMOTOR) SYSTEM

Function

General Care for Musculoskeletal Problems

Arthritis, Hip Dysplasia, Spondylitis

Intervertebral Disc Disease (Slipped Disc)

Conditions of Growing Animals
    Panosteitis
    Hypertrophic Osteodystrophy (HOD)
    Osteochondritis Dissecans (OCD)
    Rickets
    Legg-Calve-Perthes Disease

Injuries to the Musculoskeletal System
    First Aid for Broken Bones
    Sprains and Strains
    Torn Muscles

Function

The locomotor system gives us mobility, and this provides a major differentiation between plants and animals. Mobility gives us a great advantage in many ways. If we cannot find food or shelter, we can go in search of them. What we gain is balanced somewhat by the loss of rootedness; we must go in search of foods rather than sinking deeply into the earth for sustenance. Because of this, we depend upon the musculoskeletal system for our lives, or at least we have until the very recent past.

Cats and dogs are no different. When living on their own, the optimal functioning of this system means as much to their survival as any system. No mobility means no food. Since domestication, this system is somewhat less important for survival, though working animals still depend upon good legs to keep a job. For those whose main job is companionship, the health of the locomotor system means painless movement and freedom to run and play. Unfortunately, for many companions movement is painful and limiting. Hip dysplasia, arthritis, and other musculoskeletal ailments have become all too common along with other chronic maladies. While these are the result of deep-seated illness and should be treated by an experienced homeopathic practitioner, there are some remedies that can provide relief from some of the pain. I will give some general guidelines for using homeopathy to help those companion animals who suffer from chronic musculoskeletal pain.

Dogs are affected by musculoskeletal problems to a much greater degree than cats, though this is changing somewhat—or possibly we simply recognize painful joint issues in cats better than in the past. Cats are very stoic, especially since, as solitary animals by nature, their only option when in pain was to lie low until things improve, or tough it out and go on with their lives. They did not have others to help with food or comfort. Most of the conditions in this chapter pertain to dogs, but remedies and treatments can generally be applied to cats as well. General care for most musculoskeletal conditions is pretty much the same, so I will start the chapter off with recommendations that apply across the board. Specific information that applies to only one condition will be given under the section for that condition.

General Care for Musculoskeletal Problems

With the exception of injuries, most musculoskeletal conditions are relatively benign and create more pain than threat to life, so immediate examinations are not generally necessary. If pain is intense, however, have an examination right away to determine the problem. This is especially important if the pain is in the neck or back or in a young animal, or if it has arisen suddenly.

For other than intensely painful conditions, exercise is generally helpful, though it should be mild, not strenuous. Exercise helps because most problems are skeletal rather than muscular, and strengthening muscles provides greater support, relieving bone stress. Massage often helps also by improving circulation and flexibility. Warm bathing or applications may help as well. Chiropractic adjustments and acupuncture are very good treatments for musculoskeletal problems of any sort. If you know a veterinarian who can provide these services, I recommend either approach. Some chiropractic physicians who usually work on humans are willing to help four-legged people as well. While many veterinarians and veterinary medical organizations oppose this, I see no problem with it and have known of animals who benefited greatly from such assistance.

Supplements may lend relief for these aches and pains, as most conditions are inflammatory. Antioxidants provide very good support. Vitamin C (5–15 mg/pound, two to three times a day, use natural vitamin C if available) and vitamin E (5–10 IU/pound, once a day, mixed tocopherols) are safe and indicated in all cases. Other stronger antioxidants include pycnogenol (1–2 mg/pound, two to three times a day), coenzyme Q_{10} (1–2 mg/pound, two to three times a day), and superoxide dismutase (SOD). For SOD, each tablet usually contains 2,000 IU or 125 micrograms of elemental SOD; give one-half tablet per ten pounds twice daily. Start with vitamins C and E plus one of the other antioxidants. You may double the dose of any of these supplements if necessary, but I recommend you try adding another one rather than increasing the dose. If you use two or more of the stronger supplements, you may even be able to decrease the dosage on each one. Boron may help in some cases as well; give about 0.25 mg (that's ¼ of a milligram) per ten pounds daily, or 1 mg per forty pounds.

If you still have no relief, you may try one of the following supplements in addition to antioxidant support. I find response to these to be very individual. One dog may respond nicely to a supplement that is minimally helpful in another dog. Try them individually at first, and if you see no benefit, try another one. You may combine them if necessary. Glucosamine sulfate is widely available and often helpful. Use 5–10 mg/pound twice a day.

Chondroitin sulfate is another compound that is sometimes helpful; it is often combined with glucosamine. If you use chondroitin sulfate, give 5–8 mg/pound twice a day. There are many brands available with glucosamine and chondroitin; I have found Cosequin, Inholtra, and Nutriflex helpful, though these are by no means the only effective products. D-L-phenylalanine, an amino acid, may relieve pain in arthritis as well as other bone and joint conditions; use about 5–10 mg/pound, two to three times a day. Turmeric (the spice) helps a lot of people with joint and muscle pains, and it may help dogs and cats as well; use approximately one-eighth to one-fourth teaspoon per ten pounds daily. Finally, the combination of bromelain and quercetin may help another group of animals with arthritis. Give 5–10 mg/pound, two to three times a day.

As with all conditions, diet is important to provide good immune system support. Fresh foods, including raw meats, are the best for cats and dogs, but the diet should be balanced. Chlorella or spirulina (blue-green algae) can help with support by providing a good mineral base. Use one tablet or one-eighth teaspoonful per 5–10 pounds daily. See the appendix for resources for home-preparing foods.

Arthritis, Hip Dysplasia, Spondylitis

Although these conditions are different in origin, their treatment is essentially the same according to homeopathic principles, so I am including them in the same section.

Arthritis is inflammation of a bony joint; the inflammation usually creates pain upon movement of the joint. A joint is a junction of two bones in a manner that generally allows movement. (By contrast, there are junctions between bones such as those in the head and the pelvis where the bones fuse together to form a solid unit. In the latter situation the bones essentially act as one bone, so most of us treat them as such and prefer to leave the technical description of fused bones to anatomists.)

In a joint, the bones are generally attached together with ligaments. These are fibrous tissue that attach to bone at each end. Tendons are essentially the same material as ligaments, but tendons attach a muscle to a bone. Thus, the Achilles tendon attaches the calf muscles to the heel, while the anterior cruciate ligament (the one in the knee that is often torn in dogs and human athletes) is one of four ligaments that attach the femur (the thigh bone) to the tibia (the leg bone or shin bone).

Connection by ligaments allows the bones in a joint to move in one or more directions. The knee joint essentially allows front-to-back movement only, while the shoulder joint allows circular movement. Each joint is somewhat different according to the species to which it belongs and the needs of that species.

Since there is movement of bone against bone in a joint, two adaptations have developed to ease the motion. Cartilage lines the surface of the bone in the joint as well as providing cushions in the knee joint due to the great force borne by that joint. Cartilage is similar to bone, but it is much smoother and softer and thus reduces friction and impact stress. Each joint also has fluid in the space between the bones; this fluid is thick and slippery, thus it lubricates the cartilage surface and reduces friction to a bare minimum. The joint fluid is retained within the joint by a layer of fibrous tissue we call the joint capsule.

Most joint pain occurs due to damage or loss of either the cartilage or the joint fluid or to deposition of bone within the joint. Any of these situations leads to bone rubbing against bone, and this is very painful. A tissue layer called the periosteum lines the outer surface of most bones. This tissue has a lot of nerves, and thus abrasion of the periosteum creates intense pain.

Joints exist not only in the legs (knee, elbow, ankle, wrist, shoulder, hip, etc.), but also in the spine between the vertebrae and in the mouth. Arthritis is inflammation of a joint in any location, though we generally think of it in relation to the limbs. There are two main types of arthritis: rheumatoid arthritis refers to an autoimmune disease wherein the body attacks the joint tissues, causing inflammation and pain; and osteoarthritis is an age-related degeneration of the joint cartilage. Osteoarthritis is also called degenerative joint disease and is partly nutritional as well as the result of chronic trauma to the joints. The chronic trauma often results from poor physical conditioning, since good muscle tone bears much of the stress on a joint. Autoimmune factors may play a part in osteoarthritis also.

Hip dysplasia is a poor development of the hip joint in dogs. The joint is a ball-and-socket type, with the socket being on the pelvis and the ball on the femur (thigh bone). In hip dysplasia, the socket is shallow and the ball is flattened. This creates an unstable joint, and the instability leads to inflammation (arthritis) and to calcium deposition in an attempt by the body to stabilize the joint. It is thought to be inherited, though good breeding practices do not always eliminate the condition from a given breed.

Large breeds are affected much more than small breeds, and cats are very rarely affected. As a developmental problem it occurs as dogs grow, and it cannot be ruled out in an individual until the age of two. Treatment is generally the same as for other causes of arthritis, although uncommonly severe cases may require surgical correction.

Vitamin C is especially important during pregnancy and for the first six months of a puppy's life if there is a risk of hip dysplasia. The vitamin helps strengthen the ligaments around the hip and encourages formation of a deep ball-and-socket joint.

Spondylitis (spondylosis) occurs in the vertebral column and is essentially an arthritis of the spine. In this condition, the body builds up large calcium deposits on the vertebrae in an apparent attempt to fuse the intervertebral joints. Spondylitis occurs more commonly in large breeds, though smaller dogs and cats are affected also. The cause is unknown, though as with other arthritic conditions, joint trauma and deterioration is one factor. Some holistic doctors suspect that it may reflect internal organ disease. Spondylitis can make the back very painful and stiff. Treatment is essentially the same as for arthritis in the limbs.

Homeopathic Medicines for Arthritic Conditions

(Including hip dysplasia and spondylitis)
Arnica montana
When *Arnica* is needed, the pain is intense and feels like a bruise. The dog is usually in so much pain that he is extremely afraid of touch for fear of being hurt. He usually prefers to lie still.

Belladonna
Conditions that require *Belladonna* often come on rapidly. In arthritis, the lower limbs and hips are more often affected, and the right side more than the left. The pain is so intense that the legs move constantly, as the motion relieves the pain. Walking may also help. The extremities may be cold though the patient is often hot overall. The dog may be quite irritable or even aggressive because of the pain.

Bryonia
In the *Bryonia* state, the pain is intensified greatly by motion, so these dogs refuse to budge. The affected joints are often swollen and hot. These patients are usually thirsty and may be irritable; they generally prefer to be left alone.

Calcarea carbonica

Calcarea is often indicated for big-boned, flabby dogs who tend to be clumsy. They move awkwardly and stumble easily. Cold and dampness are intolerable for Calcarea individuals, as these conditions worsen the pain and the animals' comfort in general. Even the affected limbs may feel cold and damp. The legs are often weak and weary; this may lead to trembling.

Calcarea phosphorica

This remedy is similar to Calcarea carbonica in the awkwardness and generalized weakness. Animals needing Calc phos tend to be thin rather than heavy, though. These dogs are rather delicate and spindly, and it seems their legs cannot hold them up. There is also a tendency for the animals to experience front-leg pains. These patients are worse in cold weather and at changes of weather.

Colchicum

This remedy is useful for arthritis where the joints are extremely painful. Motion is difficult, and the joints hurt so much that merely touching them causes the poor dog to cry out in anguish. It is easy to confuse this pain with that of Arnica, but when Colchicum is needed you may see stomach distress as well. Nausea is common, especially at the sight or smell of food. Colchicum conditions tend to arise in autumn.

Colocynthis

I have found Colocynthis helpful in some dogs with hip pain. A keynote is pain when rotating the leg inward.

Eupatorium purpureum

Herbalists know this remedy as gravel root. In tincture form, this herb often helps humans with arthritis, especially that in small joints like the finger joints. In this case, we apply it topically to the joints. While this is impractical for most animals, especially with arthritis in large joints, it may help with arthritis in toes or even with spondylitis. Apply once or twice daily.

Guiacum

This remedy is related to Rhus tox, and sometimes works when Rhus does not. Motion aggravates these patients (as with Bryonia), who may be quite stiff. Cold applications lessen the pain, while warmth worsens it, so these animals may choose to lie on tile floors or outdoors. Neck stiffness is common also, as is swelling of the affected joints.

Phosphoric acid

This remedy is more often indicated for spondylitis than for other arthritic conditions. These animals may also have a history of growing pains. Weakness is often a component of the picture when *Ph-ac* is needed, and there may be a tendency to dullness or lethargy, even a noncaring state. Spondilitis is more commonly in the neck when this remedy is indicated, though it can also help with lumbar spondylitis. Movement usually helps, as does warmth.

Pulsatilla

When *Pulsatilla* is needed, the pains are usually in the rear limbs, and unlike the pain with most animals, the pains here are worse from heat and better with cold. *Pulsatilla* is similar to *Rhus tox* (see below) in that the pains worsen upon first motion but improve upon continued movement. There is a tendency in *Pulsatilla* patients to constantly stretch the legs. These animals are often intolerant of closed, warm, and stuffy rooms. They are sweet and can be insistent upon getting attention.

Rhus toxicodendron

Rhus tox is a major remedy for musculoskeletal aches and pains. The classic sign that points us to the remedy is that the pains are aggravated when the animal first moves, but continued motion relieves the pain. This is not the only remedy that has this modality, but it is the most common one. *Rhus tox* patients are generally chilly, and the cold worsens their pain. Additionally, they are very restless, as lying at rest also worsens the pain.

Ruta graveolens

This remedy is probably second to *Rhus tox* in effectiveness for joint pains. *Ruta* may have greater effect when the pain originates from an injury, but it can be helpful in some cases of arthritis. The affected joints are stiff, and the animal is often restless from the pain. *Ruta* may be useful for spinal arthritis (spondylitis). Overexertion is often a cause of aggravation when this remedy is needed. As with the *Rhus tox* state, these animals are worse when sitting or lying and improve when moving about.

Sabina

In the *Sabina* state, the joint pains are worse from motion and worse from heat. Open air improves the pain. Nighttime aggravation is also a *Sabina* condition. The local symptoms may be confused with those of *Pulsatilla*, but motion usually improves *Pulsatilla* patients. Those needing *Sabina* tend toward deep sadness, and while sadness may also be a part of the *Pulsatilla* picture, it is not usually so profound. The *Sabina* state may be brought about by vaccination.

Silicea (Silica)

As another vaccinosis remedy, *Silicea* is useful in many arthritic patients whose symptoms start or worsen following a vaccination. These animals are usually weak and sluggish, though they may be mentally bright. They may appear delicate and fragile. You may observe that their toenails are distorted, often brittle or thickened. These animals tend to be very chilly and intolerant of cold. They may have a history of a lot of vaccinations; they may also have a history of repeated infections or abscesses.

Intervertebral Disc Disease (Slipped Disc)

Intervertebral disc disease occurs primarily in small breeds of dogs with long backs. Dachshunds are the stereotypic example of susceptibility. It usually occurs in middle-aged dogs, starting from about five years, since the ligaments that stabilize the vertebrae and hold the discs in place begin to weaken and become less flexible as the dog ages. The discs normally sit between vertebrae to cushion the joints, but when they slip, they often press upon either the spinal cord or upon nerves as they exit from the cord through spaces in the vertebrae. This creates intense pain and sometimes paralysis. Poor diet and possibly autoimmune disease are partially causative, as these may weaken the ligaments. Additionally, many dogs simply do not get enough exercise, which not only leads to mental and behavioral stress, but also stresses the body. In this case, inadequate exercise means the muscles around the spine are not as strong as they normally would be. Since muscles around any joint support the joint, along with ligaments, weaker muscles shift a greater burden to the ligaments, and failure risk is heightened. Furthermore, the elongated back in predisposed breeds leads to extra stress on the spinal column, as the forces upon the ligaments and muscles that support the joint are greater than in dogs with more normal conformation. Thus, a smaller, long-backed dog who does not get enough exercise and who does not get good food is ripe for developing intervertebral disc disease.

The first symptom of disc disease is usually pain in either the back or the neck. If the neck is the site of the damage, the pain may appear to be in the shoulder. As a guardian, you might observe that your dog is reluctant to use steps or to jump onto furniture. The onset is usually rather sudden, and there may or may not be an incident that triggered the disease. The trigger need not be very traumatic—something as benign as jumping down from a step is enough since the weakness has been building over time. You might hear your companion cry out, but often no incident is noted; instead you just see the dog in pain.

Disc disease can occur at several levels, from mild pain to severe pain to paralysis. Although most dogs experience pain only, irreversible paralysis of the lower limbs is possible, so don't ignore the condition.

General Care for Intervertebral Disc Disease (Slipped Disc)

If you see indications of disc disease, you must first assess the severity of the condition:

- How intense is the pain?
- Is there any limitation of movement of the legs?
- Is there any difficulty with urination or defecation?

See a veterinarian immediately:

- if there is paralysis or any limitation of walking, urination, or defecation;
- if pain is intense.

Have an examination soon:

- in all but the mildest cases. It is always best to confirm the diagnosis and obtain expert help with care. X rays may be needed to determine the risk for worsening, but if the case is mild, you may opt to wait.

Treatment Recommendations

If there is paralysis along with pain, especially if the paralysis came on suddenly, surgery may be suggested by your veterinarian. While surgery is risky in many situations, it can be helpful in others. It is most helpful when the dog suddenly develops paralysis, but there is still a deep pain response. Deep pain is essentially pain that is triggered by pressure on the bone; *this test should be done by a veterinarian.* If there is no deep pain, the prognosis for recovery of walking is poor and surgery is not often helpful. I have seen recovery in these cases with acupuncture, however.

In my experience, acupuncture and chiropractic care are the best choices for treatment of disc disease. Homeopathy can be helpful also, but may not be as consistent as the above modalities. If my companion were affected, I would use homeopathic remedies, but I would also use one of the other modalities. Surgery is a viable option also, but only if there is paralysis and the onset is sudden would I consider surgery first. I would use other methods in almost all other conditions. I recognize that often there is a small window of opportunity for surgical correction in sudden cases; if this is the situation with your dog, then you may need to opt for surgery, but get a second opinion if possible.

The conventional nonsurgical approach is steroidal therapy to reduce inflammation of the spinal cord. This method can be effective in many animals and should be considered if other methods are unavailable or not helpful. This method is generally recommended in less severe cases when other modalities (acupuncture or chiropractic care) may be equally beneficial with less risk. The high doses of steroids may cause intestinal ulceration and bleeding.

Once a disc begins to shift out of position, there is a fairly high risk that it may move further and cause paralysis, so no matter which treatment you choose, it is imperative that you limit your companion's activity for a couple of weeks or more. This is especially true if you use drugs that block the pain because there is no feedback to the body telling the dog to take it easy. Let her out for urination and defecation only on a leash for the first week or two. Next you may take her on short, nonstrenuous leash walks for another week or two. Only then, if she is free of pain, should you allow her to resume normal activity *gradually.*

In addition to therapy, use the suggested supplements above in the section "General Care for Musculoskeletal Problems." Superoxide dismutase (SOD) and bromelain/quercetin may be especially useful.

Homeopathic Medicines for Intervertebral Disc Disease

If the condition has not progressed to paralysis, one of these remedies may alleviate the problem, but you must restrict your companion's activity as described above.

Hypericum perforatum

This remedy is excellent for nerve damage and nerve pain. It may be useful in many cases of slipped disc. These dogs show rather severe pain. *Hypericum* may be the best choice for cervical (neck) disc disease.

Natrum muriaticum

If your dog develops disc disease following the loss of a close friend (canine or other), try this remedy. Grief often brings about illness, and *Natrum mur* is especially useful with slipped discs following grief.

Nux vomica

Nux is often my first choice for disc disease. It helps a good number of dogs when the condition is mainly causing pain. The onset is sudden (as with most cases), and the dog may be irritable. *Nux* would also be good to give along with drug treatment should you decide to opt for this (*Nux* can help reduce side effects of the drugs).

Conditions of Growing Animals

There are a few other less common conditions that affect the musculoskeletal system. These conditions generally arise in young growing dogs. The cause is unclear in most cases, but poor bone growth is the mechanism of damage. The time of onset breeds suspicion of vaccine damage.

For any of these conditions, use the supplements given above in the section "General Care for Musculoskeletal Problems" in addition to homeopathic medicines.

Panosteitis

Panosteitis is an inflammation of the inside of long bones in the legs; it occurs primarily in young growing dogs that are between six and twelve months old. It is generally a condition that heals on its own, but it can cause a lot of pain for a month or two. The bones are generally sensitive to pressure, so squeezing on the middle of the bones causes the dog to flinch. The femur (thigh bone) and the humerus (upper arm bone) are most frequently affected, but the tibia (shin bone) and rarely the radius or ulna (forearm bones) may be affected as well. Definitive diagnosis is by X-ray, but clinical diagnosis is usually sufficient.

Homeopathic Medicines for Panosteitis

Eupatorium perfoliatum

Known to herbalists as boneset because of its good work with broken bones, *Eup-per* has "violent, aching, bone-breaking pains." These animals are restless from the pain, so they will keep moving about, though the movement does not help their pain. They may moan with the pain due to its intensity, and they may be worse in the morning around seven to nine o'clock.

Mezereum

This remedy is close to a specific for panosteitis, as it has the symptom of tearing pain in the long bones. I have seen some good results with this remedy. It is also a good remedy for complaints after vaccination. These patients tend to be chilly and are especially worse in cold damp weather; they are also worse at night. Although the remedy has some affinity to pain in the tibia, I have found it useful for pain in other bones as well.

Ruta graveolens

Ruta is a good remedy for panosteitis as well. These patients also have pain deep in the long bones; the pain drives them to walk about as the motion relieves the pain. See above under "Homeopathic Medicines for Arthritic Conditions" for a more complete description.

Sabina

If the panosteitis is centered in the thighs, *Sabina* might be the correct remedy. As with *Mezereum*, dogs who need *Sabina* are worse at night, but unlike *Mezereum* patients, they are worse with heat.

Syphilinum

This remedy should only be used under the guidance of an experienced homeopathic practitioner, but it has an affinity to long bone inflammation and may be of help in cases that do not respond to other remedies.

Theridion

This is made from a spider, and it has an affinity to bones. It is listed for "pain in bones as if broken," as well as for "scrofulous [tubercular] diseases of bones." Pains are sharp here, though this is somewhat common with panosteitis. I have cured one dog's panosteitis with this remedy. Profound noise sensitivity is common when this remedy is needed, though it was not present in the dog who responded so well, exemplifying the general rule that not all symptoms of the remedy need be present in a patient, only that the patient's symptoms be present in the remedy.

Hypertrophic Osteodystrophy (HOD)

Hypertrophic osteodystrophy occurs in young dogs also, most commonly at three to six months of age. This is an inflammatory calcification on the outer surface of long bones near the ends. It used to be mostly associated with inflammation in the chest in older dogs, but these days it has been connected with vaccination in some cases. Weimaraners, Great Danes, Irish setters, mastiffs, German shepherds, and Doberman pinschers are among the breeds most commonly affected.

Clinically, the condition arises rapidly. Puppies suddenly cannot walk, or if they can, it is with great pain. They may also have a high fever and loss of appetite. Sometimes the bones are permanently disfigured. Most puppies live, although a few die, and some guardians opt for euthanasia because of the pain. There is no conventional treatment that is effective (to my knowledge). Pain control is the only conventional aid.

Homeopathic Medicines for Hypertrophic Osteodystrophy

In addition to the remedies listed for panosteitis, consider the following:

Asafoetida
Consider this remedy for scruffy, bloated, clumsy puppies. The bones are quite painful, and the pains are worse at night and with rest, and better with motion and in open air. They may be irritable, but they may also desire sympathy.

Phosphoric acid
This is also a remedy that can help when there is inflammation and great pain on the surface of long bones. There is great debility with stumbling and weakness. The pains are generally worse at night but better as morning approaches. The *Phosphoric acid* state may come on because of grief. The patient is often as listless and weak mentally as he is physically.

Silicea (Silica)

This remedy state is characterized by weakness and fragility in a delicate individual. The wrist may be the most painful area. Many of these dogs will have skin eruptions and allergies as well as the bone inflammation.

Thuja occidentalis

This is the only remedy listed in the homeopathic literature for the specific condition of HOD. As a major vaccinosis remedy, this remedy should be considered along with *Silicea* for those cases with a clear connection to puppy vaccines. In humans needing *Thuja*, the legs feel wooden and dead, so there is stumbling with difficulty controlling or sensing the location of the legs. Presumably, the same sensation occurs in nonhuman animals. These animals tend to be chilly.

Osteochondritis Dissecans (OCD)

Osteochondritis dissecans (dissecting inflammation of the joint cartilage) usually affects the shoulder joint, though it may also affect other joints. If the shoulder is affected, the pain is most easily detected upon extension of the joint by pulling the leg forward while holding a hand against the shoulder. A limp is also obvious when the dog is walking. In OCD, the joint cartilage develops a weak painful spot. Sometimes the cartilage pulls away from the bone and creates a flap of bone; surgery is often necessary if a flap forms. If there is no flap, the lesion may heal without surgery. Homeopathy and acupuncture may be helpful. OCD, like panosteitis and HOD, primarily affects young growing dogs. In this case the dogs are usually six to twelve months old.

Homeopathic Medicines for Osteochondritis Dissecans

In addition to the supplements recommended above in the section "General Care for Musculoskeletal Problems," you may try one of the following homeopathic remedies:

Calcarea phosphorica

Calc phos is a very good remedy to use to encourage bone healing. It is a specific remedy for this along with *Symphytum*. In either case, I suggest a low potency such as 6X or 6C, two or three times a day. Use either remedy if there is no clear indication for *Silicea* or *Syphilinum* (see below). You may even use one of these remedies in low potency along with infrequent doses of the indicated constitutional remedy in high potency. This is not classical homeopathy, but in the case of poor bone healing, it sometimes works.

Silicea (Silica)

This remedy is a good one for animals that have poor healing power. They are usually chilly, and they may be weak and frail. They may have a history of a lot of vaccination or a lot of abscesses and infections (or both). Many animals benefit from a dose of *Silicea* because of prior vaccinations.

Symphytum

This remedy, along with *Calc phos,* is great for encouraging bone healing. *Symphytum* may rank slightly higher. It also helps with bone pain after an injury. See the recommendations for *Calc phos* above.

Syphilinum

This is a deep-acting remedy that is available by prescription only and should be used under the guidance of an experienced homeopathic prescriber. I list it because it is the only remedy listed for dissecting osteochondritis. It may be of great benefit in the right cases.

Rickets

This condition occurs in very young dogs or cats and is essentially the result of a poor diet that is low in calcium. These animals have poor bone formation, and their joints become enlarged and painful. Rickets is rather uncommon these days, but it does occasionally occur. Successful treatment depends upon correcting the diet, but homeopathic medicines may help speed recovery. The new diet must provide adequate calcium, but oversupplementing with calcium is not helpful. Slight calcium addition for a month or so is appropriate. After this, a properly balanced recipe is enough. Added vitamin D helps the body utilize the calcium, so you may give about one-eighth to one-fourth teaspoonful of cod liver oil daily for a few weeks.

Homeopathic Medicines for Rickets

Asafoetida

As with HOD (see above), this remedy is good for scrawny, bloated, clumsy puppies or kittens with enlarged joints. Along with the abdominal distension, they may pass a lot of gas or have foul, forceful diarrhea. They may prefer open air to a warm room.

Calcarea carbonica
The calcium homeopathic remedies support the proper utilization of (the mineral) calcium in the individuals that fit the picture of the remedy. *Calc carb* animals tend to be big-boned, fat, chilly, and lazy. Their walk is often clumsy. They may also have a tendency toward constipation.

Calcarea fluorica
This remedy state is perhaps the most serious of the calcium remedies. Rickets is common in animals needing *Calc fluor,* and even newborn animals may be affected; this is uncommonly early for rickets. Their conformation tends to be unbalanced, with one side larger than the other—their faces may even be asymmetrical. These patients also tend to have problems with their teeth because of poor enamel formation.

Calcarea phosphorica
This remedy is somewhat similar to *Calc carb,* but these patients are lean and frail rather than stocky. They may be somewhat hard to please. Their bone pains are often worse at night and with any change of weather.

Phosphorus
Like *Calc phos* animals, those needing *Phosphorus* tend to be thin. *Phosphorus* animals are generally better proportioned and more agile. They tend to be friendly and vocal with great thirst for cold water. They also have a great appetite, though they may easily vomit if they eat too quickly.

Silicea (Silica)
These animals will generally be delicate and somewhat weak. There may be a history of recurrent infections, perhaps eye or nose problems or skin eruptions. Cold is usually intolerable for these patients.

Sulphur
These animals may be similar to those needing *Asafoetida* in their scruffy appearance and diarrhea. They don't usually have the bloating and irritability that is common with the *Asafoetida* state, however. *Sulphur* animals tend

to be laid-back and friendly, and their thirst is often greater than their appetite. They may be host to a lot of fleas.

Legg-Calve-Perthes Disease

Although this condition affects the legs, this is not the derivation of the name; it is named for the various people who first described the disorder. Animals with this disease develop a problem with the circulation to the head of the femur—the ball component of the ball-and-socket joint that forms the hip. To my knowledge there is no known treatment, and many of these animals must have surgery to remove the remainder of the femoral head, allowing the body to develop a "false joint" of scar tissue.

According to homeopathic principles, this disease is possibly treatable if the condition is caught early enough. The main remedies for the condition are *Tuberculinum* and *Vaccin atténué bilié*, both deep-acting remedies that are available by prescription only (see the *materia medica)* and should be used under the guidance of an experienced homeopathic practitioner. *Bacillus Calmette-Guerin vaccine (BCG vaccine)* is essentially the same remedy; I have used this with a cat who had already had surgery years prior for this condition, and *BCG vaccine* helped him. This is available from Helios (see the appendix) and possibly elsewhere. Other remedies to consider include *Phosphorus* and *Silicea*. See the descriptions above under rickets and in the *materia medica* for the latter two remedies. I suggest you consult a homeopathic veterinarian for this condition, as there is not much time to waste if the joint can be saved.

Injuries to the Musculoskeletal System

First Aid for Broken Bones

Any possibly broken bone should be treated by a veterinarian, but there are some remedies that can help. At the time of the accident, give *Arnica montana* until the swelling and the soft-tissue pain subsides—usually for the first day or two. Give the *Arnica* in higher potency such as 30C (higher is OK if you have it) every fifteen to thirty minutes initially, then every hour to every few hours as the animal improves. Rescue Remedy (the Bach flower remedy or its equivalent from another company) is helpful also for shock and trauma. Next, use *Symphytum* to encourage the bones to knit together quickly and strongly; this remedy also helps alleviate bone pain. Give this in 30C potency one to three times a day at first until the pain lessens (usu-ally up to a week), then use 6X or 6C twice a day for three to six weeks. If you believe the bones are still not healing well, you may substitute *Calcarea phosphorica* for the *Symphytum* or alternate the two remedies, one morning and one evening. *Eupatorium perfoliatum* (boneset) is another good remedy for bone pains and may help, especially in the early stages, if none of the above remedies help with the pain. Animals needing *Eup per* tend to be quite restless with the pain.

See also the remedies listed below under "Homeopathic Medicines for Sprains and Strains" for other possibilities. *Ruta graveolens* may reduce the pain if none of the above remedies help.

Sprains and Strains

A sprain is an injury to a joint, usually involving the ligaments, while a strain refers to an injury to a muscle. Thus, we might sprain our ankle and strain our hamstring muscle in the same fall. Treatment of either injury is similar. Immediately after the injury, the general recommendation is to ice the part to limit swelling. Wrap ice in a towel or use an ice pack if available, but don't put the ice directly on the skin as you may burn the skin. Starting about an hour or two after an injury, the best treatment is alternation of warm and cold packs. This encourages circulation to the area, allowing the body to begin repairing the damaged tissue.

Most practitioners recommend staying off of the injured leg for a few days, but I do not fully agree. While I think this is correct for a muscle strain, I believe a sprained joint should be moved. The movement seems to dimin-ish swelling and stiffness. Probably the improved circulation along with movement limits swelling and thus retains flexibility. If a ligament is badly torn, the joint should be treated and rested, but otherwise I find movement very helpful. I first discovered this by personal experience. I have relatively weak ankles even though my physical condition is good. I enjoy hard exer-cise, so through the years I have sprained my ankles numerous times. I pre-viously rested them after a sprain, but I sprained my ankle a time or two while out running, far from home. With no choice but to walk home, I found that, although the first few steps were very painful, the pain improved after a short time. During the ensuing days, I noticed that the extent of the injury was greatly lessened compared to similar sprains. I began treating further sprains the same way and have had much less trouble than with prior injuries. I now recommend mild activity after any musculoskeletal injury unless there is evidence of serious damage.

The supplements listed above in the section "General Care for Musculoskeletal Problems" will aid healing, as will one of the homeopathic remedies listed in the following section. Manganese is especially helpful with sprains and strains. For the first week or two, give one milligram per two pounds (or one kilogram) twice daily, then give one milligram per ten to fifteen pounds daily for another two weeks if needed. There is a tissue salt combination remedy from Hyland's, called Biochemic Phosphates, that can be a good relaxant and can help if none of the listed remedies does. Calcium-magnesium, in a two-to-one or one-to-one (Ca:Mg) ratio can also help alleviate pain by relaxing the muscles. Give about 5–10 mg/pound of the calcium (and 2.5–10 mg magnesium) as needed. This will calm her as well as help with pain. You can find formulas with calcium-magnesium in one capsule or tablet in these ratios. They may have other minerals like phosphorus or zinc; this is fine.

Homeopathic Medicines for Sprains and Strains

Arnica montana

Arnica is the first choice for injuries to muscles and joints. It is arguably the best-known homeopathic medicine for its wonderful effect upon sprains and strains. When Arnica is needed, the pain is usually so severe that the patient is fearful of touch. This remedy is often helpful and is a good place to start.

Bellis perennis

Bellis is the daisy and is related to Arnica. Its use and indications are similar to Arnica as well. With Bellis conditions, the injury may be much worse with hot applications and better with cold applications. Motion may improve either state, but the improvement is more pronounced in Bellis, as many Arnica patients desire rest.

Hamamelis

This remedy, made from witch hazel, is another good remedy for bruises, sprains, and strains. This state is typically better from rest and worse from motion.

Rhus toxicodendron

Rhus tox is not only a good remedy for chronic joint pains as with arthritis, but it is also good for many sprains. It has better action on joints than on muscles. You will often (but not always) see the typical *Rhus tox* symptom of worsening with initial motion but improvement with continued motion. Cold usually worsens the pain, while warmth ameliorates pain when this remedy is indicated.

Ruta graveolens

Last but not least, *Ruta* may be helpful in many joint injuries as well. Like *Rhus tox,* this remedy has greater influence in joint sprains than in muscle strains. *Ruta* follows *Arnica* well and is a good remedy for the later stages of injuries. It may also lessen the pain in fractures. Motion and warmth lessen the pains, and cold and rest may worsen the pain when *Ruta* is indicated.

Torn Muscles

When a muscle is torn rather than just strained, the pain can be quite intense. The tear is rarely complete, but if it is, your companion may need surgery. In all other cases, try the homeopathic remedy *Calendula officinalis* in oral form (not topical). Use a 30C if available. I have seen very good responses to muscle tears with *Calendula*.

Injuries to the Spine

See Chapter Thirteen, "Nervous System."

Chapter Thirteen
NERVOUS SYSTEM

Function

Degenerative Myelopathy (DM)

Coonhound Paralysis

Tick Paralysis

Vestibular Syndrome

Convulsions (Seizures)
   Tail Chasing and Back Quivering

Aggression and the Rabies Miasm; Ketamine-induced Aggression

Injuries to the Brain and Spinal Cord

Function

The nervous system provides two general functions. The first is sensory, in that the nerves allow us to detect and understand the world around us. Input from any of our five senses is carried to the brain by the sensory nerves. The brain is basically a giant mass of nerve tissue that processes the information, and once the information is analyzed, the brain initiates appropriate action in response. Information directing the bodily response (the second function) is delivered to the appropriate location by motor nerves; these nerves carry an electrical impulse away from the brain that directs a part of the body to carry out a needed action. This action may be movement of a muscle or a set of muscles, or it may be a glandular secretion of a hormone that then directs other organs to react. For example, if you put your hand on a hot stove burner, your sensory nerves quickly respond and give your brain the message, *hot,* and then your motor nerves initiate two actions: you jerk your hand away, and at the same time you probably yell "ow!"

The nervous system is quite complex, since it is basically the computer that runs our body. No action or sensation is possible without this system, making it an essential system for life. By the same token, its potential for malfunction is equally vast. Most of these conditions are beyond the scope of this book, so I have chosen to focus this chapter upon a few disease syndromes and upon injuries.

Degenerative Myelopathy (DM)

This is a syndrome that mainly affects dogs and most commonly affects large breeds. The condition first appeared in German shepherd dogs, but these days most other large breeds are affected as well. The primary picture is one of a paralysis of the hind legs that grows progressively worse with time. Ultimately, the dog may lose control of bladder and bowel function. There is no pain, as the problem is a loss of function of the spinal cord due to destruction of the cord tissue. It is thus easy to differentiate between this condition and other conditions that may cause weakness or stumbling, such as a slipped disc, hip dysplasia, or arthritis.

The cause is not known, but it is an autoimmune disease, so I suspect vaccinations as a cause or trigger in some cases. Distemper vaccination is a likely possibility, as it is in the same virus family as the measles virus, which has been connected to multiple sclerosis (MS) in humans. MS is basically the same disease as DM. Whereas the disease occurred primarily in older dogs when I first graduated from veterinary school, today it often affects young dogs and occasionally even cats.

If you suspect your dog may have this problem, have a veterinarian check her to verify the diagnosis or to see if there may be another problem. The condition is not urgent or life-threatening, but obtain all the information you can before deciding upon treatment.

General Care for Degenerative Myelopathy

There is no conventional treatment, and to my knowledge even holistic therapies provide minimal help. There are some homeopathic remedies, however, that may help slow the progression of the disease if not reverse the symptoms. I recommend seeking expert help if possible, but I will list some remedy choices for those without access to help. Antioxidants may help minimize the damage, though they won't reverse or stop the disease. Give vitamin C (5–10 mg/pound, two to three times a day, use natural C if available), vitamin E (5–10 mg/pound, once a day, mixed tocopherols), and vitamin A (75–100 IU, once a day). Other antioxidants include coenzyme Q_{10} (1–2 mg/pound, one to two times a day), superoxide dismutase (SOD),(2,000 IU or 125 micrograms per ten pounds daily), and pycnogenol (1–2 mg/pound, twice a day). Use one or two of these in addition to the above antioxidant vitamins. Lecithin may help maximize the transmission of nerve impulses; give one-half to one teaspoon per ten pounds daily. Phosphatidylserine may also help; here give 1–2 mg per pound, two or three times daily.

Homeopathic Medicines for Degenerative Myelopathy

Alumina

Aluminum has been implicated in many conditions, including nerve damage. The homeopathic remedy is called *Alumina*, and it has a reputation for helping some paralyses, especially if there is constipation accompanying the weakness. The stool is often very dry, and there is little urging. The skin may be dry as well, and you may see flakes of skin under the coat. These animals may improve and then worsen on a daily basis.

Argentum nitricum

Argentum nitricum is another remedy made from a metal compound (silver nitrate), and it may also be of assistance when there is a paralysis of the hind limbs, especially if the limbs tremble. Animals needing this remedy often have diarrhea with a lot of flatulence. They crave sugar and sweets, but sugar may worsen their ailments. They are often prone to anxiety and fears and may prefer to stay at home rather than go for a walk, although they prefer cool, open air and dislike warmth and warm rooms. They may also have difficulty with their tongues, and food may fall from their mouths while eating.

Cocculus
Animals needing this remedy may have a lot of trembling and even some spasms in their legs. They may have a history of car sickness, and riding in a car will often worsen the paralysis of the legs. They may have abdominal pain and bloating as an accompanying symptom. They often become nauseated easily, especially when seeing or smelling foods. These dogs tend to be mentally very slow and dull, or they may become so as the condition develops.

Conium maculatum
This remedy is made from poison hemlock, the substance Socrates drank as his death sentence. Poison hemlock causes painless paralysis that starts in the legs and moves upward until the arms are paralyzed and ultimately the respiration and heartbeat are stopped. In animals needing this remedy, we see a similar effect, as the weakness begins in the rear legs but slowly moves upward. These animals may have severe nausea that comes on as soon as they lie down (all conditions tend to be worse when *Conium* animals rest). This is a good remedy to consider for degenerative myelopathy, especially in older animals.

Gelsemium
Weakness, heaviness, tiredness, and sluggishness in various parts of the body suggest *Gelsemium*. Even the eyelids may droop on these dogs. There is mental dullness as well, though there is also anxiety. These dogs may be quite fearful of going out and may develop diarrhea easily as a result. They often prefer to be left alone. The weakness often comes on after a bout with another illness, though it may also result from grief.

Kali phosphoricum
Potassium salts are often helpful in nerve weaknesses, and *Kali phos* is the

"great nerve tonic." Other indicators are nervous system weakness and general nervous system malfunction. These animals may also be easily startled, like *Phosphorus* patients. There is stumbling and awkwardness in the rear limbs, often with fidgetiness. There may be mild pain in the feet or the thigh. The feet may be cold, and there may be cracks in the pads, similar to the acute distemper foot-pad affection. If *Kali phos* fits constitutionally, use as indicated, but it may help also in low potency, like 6X or 6C, as a tonic. The tissue salt can work well here.

Lathyrus

Lathyrus is considered to be almost a specific remedy for polio in humans. The paralysis is often profound, though there is no pain. When this remedy is needed, the reflexes are usually exaggerated, even though the nerves are weak. The walk is often spastic. *Lathyrus* is most commonly needed in males. Cold damp weather aggravates the condition.

Oleander

This poisonous plant produces hind-leg paralysis, so the remedy may alleviate this condition if the other symptoms fit the case. When *Oleander* is indicated, the legs are very weak and usually cold. The front legs may tremble, especially when the dog eats. These dogs are ravenous and cannot seem to eat fast enough. The food often passes through undigested, and there is a resultant diarrhea. Flatus accompanies the diarrhea, and stool often passes involuntarily along with the expelled gas.

Picric acid

The *Picric acid* state is similar to that of *Conium* in that there is a paralysis that starts in the rear legs and ascends upward. In this case, however, the disease progresses much more rapidly. Any exertion is extremely exhausting for these dogs. The left rear leg may be worse than the right, and if the paralysis progresses to the front legs, the right is generally worse. The dog may have persistent (sometimes painful) erections of the penis as an accompaniment.

Plumbum metallicum

This is another metal remedy, made from lead. Lead poisoning typically causes anemia, colic, and paralysis of extensor muscles (those that extend rather than flex a joint). Dogs needing *Plumbum* often have weak, floppy paws. In contrast to the typical condition with degenerative myelopathy, these dogs may have pain in their legs, though absence of pain does not exclude the remedy. Overall, these dogs are often in poor condition and very scrawny. Their stools may be yellow and soft, or they may be extremely foul-smelling.

Thuja occidentalis

Dogs needing *Thuja* are often easily chilled, and they may have a lot of warts or other skin nodules. Their rear legs are stiff and awkward because they may feel wooden to the dog. They may have always had a weak, lax, flabby body. Cold and dampness is intolerable and may worsen their condition.

Note to veterinarians and homeopaths: Any heavy metal is a possible remedy for DM, and the Lanthanide series may be even more specific. I have seen a couple of reasonably good responses to *Erbium phosphoricum* in DM dogs, for example. See *The Secret Lanthanides* by Jan Scholten.

Coonhound Paralysis

This condition is rare. It is not limited to coonhounds, but it is thought to be a virus infection that is transmitted from a raccoon bite, though not all cases have a definite history of a bite. In coonhound paralysis, the dog (cats are not affected) develops a gradually ascending paralysis that starts in the hind legs and moves upward. This may take several days. Most dogs recover, though it may take a few weeks. Rarely, the paralysis ascends to the nerves controlling respiration, and the dog may die. Coonhound paralysis is very similar to tick paralysis (see below), but the latter condition is much more rapid in onset and recovery and is not fatal.

If you suspect this condition, have a veterinarian examine your dog to get a diagnosis. Then, try one of the remedies listed above for degenerative myelopathy. *Conium, Lathyrus,* and *Picric acid* are especially good choices, though any one of the remedies may be correct. If you see no response, seek help from a homeopathic practitioner.

Tick Paralysis

The brown dog tick causes this condition, and though uncommon, it occurs regularly in areas that these ticks frequent. The southern United States is most affected. An occasional tick secretes a toxin that can paralyze a dog. The onset is rather quick (a few hours), and the paralysis ascends quickly from the hind legs to the front legs. Bodily inspection will reveal a fat tick, usually on the head and neck area. One tick is sufficient, as it is not the number of ticks but the one that secretes the toxin that is important. Treatment is simple: remove the offending tick, and the dog recovers as fast as he was affected. No other treatment is necessary.

Vestibular Syndrome

This is primarily a cat problem, and it occurs mostly in older cats. Affected cats suddenly begin stumbling and falling as if intoxicated. They sometimes cannot even stand, and this usually occurs without warning and rapidly. It is almost like flipping a switch—they seem fine, and the next time you see them they cannot stand or they are wobbly. They may cry out in distress, because they can be quite dizzy to the point of nausea. If you look at their eyes, in almost all (but not all) cases their eyes move rapidly back and forth, faster to one side than to the other. This is called nystagmus. This is what happens when you spin in circles several times and then stop, and the world seems to keep spinning. These cats experience a similar sensation, though much more intensely. Nystagmus can occur with other conditions as well. In vestibular syndrome, however, there are not usually any accompanying problems like ear infections, so the diagnosis is a rule-out of other possibilities. *Arsenicum album* and *Phosphorus* are often helpful here. Try *Ars* first. I have also seen *Nux vomica* work in one cat. The condition tends to relapse, so you may need to keep redosing with the remedy as needed, sometimes for a few months. In my experience, most cats recover within a few days, though some take longer and relapse several times.

Convulsions (Seizures)

If your companion animal experiences problems with convulsions, you should seek veterinary care to diagnose the problem. Sometimes seizures occur as a result of an underlying condition that may be serious or for which there may be a treatment. If there is no obvious cause for the convulsions, we say the dog or cat has epilepsy. It is best to find out the cause or rule out other causes before assuming the condition is limited to convulsions. As with many neurological conditions, vaccinations can be a cause. I have recognized rabies vaccines as causative in a few cases, for example, even in animals diagnosed by neurologists as having "idiopathic epilepsy" (epilepsy of "unknown" cause). Once you have a diagnosis, I suggest having your companion treated by an experienced homeopathic prescriber rather than attempt home treatment.

In this section, I will list some helpful supplements and two homeopathic medicines that may stop or prevent a convulsion that is imminent.

General Care for Convulsions

The B vitamins help brain function and thus are important for any animal with possible brain malfunction, including epilepsy. Give a human multi-B vitamin and use one-fourth of the human dose for cats and small dogs (under twenty-five pounds), one-half dose for medium dogs (twenty-five to sixty pounds), and a full dose for large dogs (over sixty pounds). In any animal with convulsions, the amino acids L-taurine and L-tyrosine can reduce the number of seizures by increasing the resistance to seizures. Use each one at a dose of 5–10 mg per pound, one to two times a day. The amino acid L-tryptophan has brain-soothing effects and may be of help also. The scare a few years ago about this substance being poisonous was based upon misinformation, and it is in fact quite safe; there was a contaminant in one batch that was toxic, not L-tryptophan itself. The contamination occurred because the batch was prepared using genetically engineered bacteria, and the bacteria apparently produced another toxin. This was well known, but for some reason the FDA pulled L-tryptophan off the shelves for awhile, though I understand that it is becoming available again. You may dose this at the same rate as for L-taurine and L-tyrosine. Finally, the antioxidant oils such as flax oil (one-fourth teaspoon per ten pounds daily), evening primrose oil (5–10 mg/pound daily), and borage oil (5–10 mg/pound daily) may benefit the animal by reducing inflammation and degeneration of brain tissue. Use either the borage or the evening primrose oil (in addition to the flax oil), or reduce the amounts by one-half and use both.

If your animal is having a convulsion, is in between a series of convulsions, or is about to have one (you may recognize preconvulsive behavior such as anxiety or restlessness), you can use the Bach flower essence called Rescue Remedy (or a similar product by another company), and this will often calm him. It will sometimes stop a convulsion. Calms Forte, by Hylands, may also help. You can put a tablet or two into an ounce of water, then give this by teaspoonfuls for a few doses. If he is biting and gnashing his teeth, be extremely careful because he may bite you seriously (though inadvertently). You can put the remedy onto the skin of his ears or on his nose if the mouth is too dangerous. Homeopathic remedies may be administered the same way if in liquid form (dissolve a couple of pellets in water if necessary). The herb valerian root is very calming (it is similar to Valium) and will reduce the seizure tendency, but it must be given while the animal is not in a convulsion, as anything that must be swallowed is too risky for dog and guardian to be administered during a convulsion.

Homeopathic Medicines for Convulsions (Seizures)—First Aid Only

Try either of these if your companion is in the midst of a convulsive period. Use the highest potency available and repeat every few minutes to every couple of hours. You should see a response by the third or fourth dose.

Aconitum napellus (Aconite)

This medicine is good for many acute conditions, and convulsions surely qualify. These animals are often fearful and anxious during or around the time of the convulsion, though absence of this does not rule out *Aconite*.

Belladonna

This is the other major remedy for sudden conditions such as convulsions. Animals needing *Belladonna* may have a tendency toward aggression rather than fear, and their pupils often dilate. They may have red ears or other parts of the body.

If your companion does not stop the seizure within a few minutes, take him to a veterinary clinic for medication. Whereas short convulsions are not too damaging, longer ones may increase the brain damage and worsen the epilepsy.

Note to veterinarians and homeopaths: If your patient is in "status epilepticus," wherein she just keeps convulsing, you may consider any of the following remedies, if you have them at hand: *Absinthium, Aconitum, Bufo, Helleborus,* and *Oenanthe.* Also, *Cresol* 7C is considered a specific for convulsions by Julien if other remedies do not alleviate the condition. I have also had some success using remedies made from vaccines as part of reversing seizures. These remedies should be used by experienced homeopaths.

Tail Chasing and Back Quivering

This is often considered a type of convulsion due to its rather obsessive, driven aspect. It occurs in cats and dogs. Affected animals chew at their tails, or more commonly, circle around as though they are chasing their tails. Sometimes the skin along their backs will quiver also, as though there is some sensation along the spine that is bothersome. We have assumed this to be like a seizure in that we assume there is some neuropathy that either causes the sensation (i.e. affecting sensory nerves) that drives the back quivering and tail chasing, or that directly causes the activity (i.e. affecting motor nerves). Recently I have seen a few cases that appeared to be caused from ketamine anesthesia, probably because of a ketamine-induced neuropathy. I have successfully reversed these using *Ketamine* as a homeopathic remedy. See the next section for more information on ketamine adverse effects.

Aggression and the Rabies Miasm; Ketamine-induced Aggression

Veterinarians who have practiced much longer than I tell me that aggressive animals are much more prevalent these days than ever before; I also have seen this in my three decades of practice. Just why this is the case is unclear, but many of us in the holistic field suspect vaccination as the culprit in a large segment of cases. Violence often increases after a rabies vaccination; sometimes this is short-lived, and sometimes it becomes a permanent state. In homeopathic medicine, we refer to a generalized tendency toward certain disease symptoms as a miasm; these are not syndromes as we understand in conventional medicine but rather patterns of disease expression. One of these is called the rabies miasm because it seems to be associated with the disease or with the vaccine for the disease. Human cases have been recorded in the homeopathic literature, and animal cases far outnumber those in humans—most likely due to all of the rabies vaccinations we give our beloved companions. This does not mean these animals have active rabies, but rather that they have what we might call chronic rabies, a noninfectious (in a conventional sense in that no live viruses exist in the body) disease that is similar to active rabies but on a less intense scale.

I am not suggesting that all cases of aggression in animals occur because of rabies vaccination; this is too uncertain. But I am convinced that a significant number, perhaps the majority, are connected to this cause. In many cases, it is obvious that an animal changes after a vaccination. Due to the possibility of long lapses between cause and effect (including vaccination of the parent affecting the offspring), however, we simply cannot always tell. What I see with rabies vaccine–induced aggression may be simple violence, but often there is a fear component. The "fear biter" is a good example. Dogs and cats may also become fearful without aggression, but the fear has an intensity that is beyond timidity. These animals suffer as a result of vaccination, and though some are simply more sensitive to vaccine damage than average animals, for some the problem results from excessive vaccination.

While rabies vaccines may be necessary in some situations, current policy, requiring constant boosters every one to three years, does not reflect our immunological understanding. Vaccination for rabies usually confers lifetime immunity; if not after one vaccine, it almost certainly does after the second one in most animals (about 95 percent). *Further revaccination is a fear-based legal requirement with no medical justification.* Additionally, many animals (indoor-only and city animals, for example) have no likelihood of exposure, thus vaccination for them is all but pointless. We need to work to change the laws so we are not required to do this to our companions. (See Chapter Sixteen, "Vaccination," for more information and for documentation.)

A second type of aggression can arise as a consequence of anesthesia with ketamine (Ketaset) or tiletamine (Telazol). These chemicals are in the same family of drugs as phencyclidine, also known as "angel dust," a hallucinogenic and highly disturbing street drug. Ketamine and tiletamine are also hallucinogens, and they work by inducing an altered brain state wherein the consciousness is somewhat separated from bodily sensations, though they do not always block these sensations from perception. They are called "dissociative anesthetics" because of this disassociation of consciousness. Unfortunately, they immobilize the patient without consistently affecting his pain perception. This can become a "bad trip" in the lingo of the drug culture. Imagine being in an altered mental state, one where you are totally out of control of your body and, to some degree, of your emotions. Then imagine having someone begin to cut open your body, and you can feel the pain but cannot react physically and do not have the ability to protect yourself from the emotional and mental trauma that ensues. This is torture, as bad as it gets. The result is a post–traumatic stress disorder (PTSD). Unfortunately, I have recognized many cases in animals. Cats suffer much more than dogs, as these anesthetics have been used much more with cats than dogs. Sadly for dogs, though, this has shifted in the past two decades, especially as some other anesthetic agents are no longer available.

This ketamine-induced PTSD is even worse in some ways than the rabies miasm fear and aggression. Because of the torture aspect, these animals often appear tortured, in the sense that their fear and aggression is much more primitive, much deeper. Animals with rabies vaccine issues can be fearful and aggressive, but their aggression is more defensive, almost more an exaggeration of normal protective behavior. When they do not perceive a threat, they may behave fairly normally and seem little affected. When ketamine or tiletamine PTSD occurs, however, the animals suffer continuously; there is little respite for them. They are living the terror, like the flashbacks that occasionally followed LSD use in the 1960s and 1970s. This is not uncommon with hallucinogenic medicines, and ketamine and tiletamine are no exception.

Why, you may wonder, does anyone use these drugs? I think most veterinarians simply have not observed the causation. We have been taught that these drugs provide good pain response, but unfortunately this is untrue. They were formerly used in children; one pediatric surgeon, who defended their use, decided to have a hernia repaired under ketamine anesthesia. He stopped using the drug immediately upon recovering from the procedure, as he felt every scalpel cut. He had also been under the impression that ketamine provided good pain control. His personal experience showed otherwise.

I have had some success treating these PTSD animals with *Ketamine* in potency, in other words, with a homeopathic medicine made from the drug. I have seen cats who previously could not be touched, but they climbed into their guardians' laps following treatment. There is hope. I have also helped some rabies vaccine–damaged animals with remedies made from the vaccine, though they often need other remedies as well. In either case, treatment is best carried out by a veterinarian with experience in these cases.

Regardless of the cause, many of these animals can be helped with homeopathy. Supplements such as B vitamins and L-tryptophan may help calm them as well (see the section above on "General Care for Convulsions" for dosage and discussion of these supplements). While I strongly recommend that serious aggression be treated under the care of a homeopathic veterinarian, mild aggression may be treated at home. Use great caution, though.

It is not worth having another being (child, adult, cat, dog) injured as a result of carelessness. Seriously aggressive animals, especially large dogs, may be too dangerous to keep around. As a veterinarian I always advocate for the animal, and I am not acting differently now, but we must use some consideration and "big picture" vision when we consider risking the safety of others. Please seek guidance if you have any uncertainty here.

Homeopathic Medicines for Aggression

These are some of the major remedies for aggression, though there are many others. If none of these seems correct, you may need to seek help from a homeopath.

Belladonna

Aggressive animals needing *Belladonna* often become suddenly violent, flying into a rage with dilated pupils and a glassy-eyed look. They may have red, hot ears or eyes. They are often quite destructive and may tear up bedding, furniture, and so on (this is also a symptom of rabies). There may be vertigo as well.

Hepar sulphuris calcareum

These animals are very irritable and contradictory, thus their aggression is often triggered by the one upon whom they vent the aggression. The triggering incident is typically minimal and does not seem to warrant the rage it receives. *Hepar sulph* animals are chilly and sensitive, and they may have an accompanying wound that is infected and extremely painful to touch.

Hyoscyamus

People needing *Hyoscyamus* often show lewd and lascivious behavior in addition to aggression; animals may also be hypersexual. This is often seen as masturbation, even in a neutered animal. Suspicion is a great part of this picture as well and may be seen as excessive sniffing or as an animal that seems to mistrust everyone. Jealousy is also common. Convulsions may accompany the aggression.

Lachesis

When *Lachesis* is needed, the animal may be very jealous and suspicious (like *Hyoscyamus*), but their aggression is usually not so intense. These animals are mostly passive, although they may be a bit edgy. Their aggression usually comes about as a response to a perceived threat, and they then respond viciously rather than in a manner consistent with the threat. (This remedy is from the bushmaster snake, so think of a snake striking—the venom is deadly.) These animals tend to be worse after sleeping; be wary of a just-awakened *Lachesis!*

Lyssin

This remedy is a prescription item, as it is made from the saliva of a rabid dog, though it is not infectious. Licensed practitioners may consider this remedy for those animals who do not respond to other aggression remedies, as this one sometimes opens the door to treatment.

Mercurius (vivus or solubilis)

These animals often experience both physical and mental ailments. They tend to be rather unapproachable in the sense that they don't seem to care about others, including their guardians. They hate to be ordered about, so they may bite and snarl when disciplined. Gum diseases are common in these animals.

Nux vomica

Nux animals are usually not really violent; rather they are irritable and snappish, especially when they are physically ill. They tend to have diarrhea or constipation with tremendous straining. These animals have often had a lot of medications.

Stramonium

In my experience, this remedy is one of the better ones for post–rabies vaccination aggression. These animals are very fearful, and this triggers aggression. If they hear something outside that they perceive as threatening, they may become anxious and agitated, and then they may attack the nearest animal (two- or four-legged). This is not the only remedy with this predilection, but it is a strong one. The animal may be fearful of the dark or of bright lights. *Stramonium* is made from a highly hallucinogenic plant, so this behavior is not so surprising.

Note to veterinarians and homeopaths: As I mentioned above, if indicated, sometimes a remedy from either ketamine or a rabies vaccine may be needed to unlock these cases. It is best to consult with someone with experience in these cases for guidance.

Injuries to the Brain and Spinal Cord

Obviously, any injury such as this needs veterinary attention to determine if surgical treatment is indicated. Many times, however, there is little to be done except wait for the body to heal itself. In these cases, homeopathy may provide additional help for healing. And in all injuries, the remedies may help, even if conventional intervention is indicated. Give *Arnica* at the time of the injury and for the first day or so, depending upon the symptoms. If surgery is needed, continue the *Arnica* until the day after the surgery unless another remedy is clearly indicated. Once the initial stage has passed, the symptom picture may guide you to another remedy.

For animals with a slipped disc (intervertebral disc disease), see Chapter Twelve, "Musculoskeletal System."

Homeopathic Medicines for Injuries to the Brain and Spinal Cord

Arnica montana
As in almost all injuries, this remedy is the first one to consider, as it may prevent further damage and it can speed healing. The symptom picture of *Arnica* is one of excessive pain such that the animal is quite fearful of touch or even the approach of others for fear of further injury. The pain is such that they cannot get comfortable, and even a soft bed feels hard.

Cicuta virosa
Cicuta is more effective for brain injury than for spinal damage. These animals often develop problems with ocular muscles after a concussion, leaving them either cross-eyed or with divergent strabismus (the opposite of cross-eyed—the eyes point to the sides rather than the middle). They often avoid company and prefer to remain hidden.

Conium maculatum
Conium is related botanically to *Cicuta*, but *Conium* is better for spinal injuries. These animals are often paralyzed in their lower legs, and the paralysis tends to move upward after a time. If your companion's injury starts out just affecting the rear legs and later affects the front legs, consider *Conium*.

Helodrilis

This is a remedy made from the earthworm. The provings suggested that it could be very useful for spinal trauma, and it has been very successful in at least one case. The remedy is indicated for paralysis with numbness and tingling in the legs after trauma, even very severe trauma.[1] Helodrilis is only available (as of this writing) from Hahnemann Laboratories (see the appendix).

Hypericum perforatum

Hypericum is the major remedy for injuries to nerves anywhere, especially when there is a lot of pain as with the tips of the fingers. This remedy provides great benefit in both spine and brain injuries, though it is used more often for spinal damage. The pain in the spine (or head) is quite intense (with Helodrilis there is more numbness than pain), so that any movement causes the animal to cry out. The animal may scream out upon approach, similar to Arnica animals, but the pain comes from the nerves rather than the muscles and bones. If Arnica does not relieve this terrible pain, try Hypericum.

Natrum sulphuricum

When this remedy is indicated, the animal has often experienced a change in his mental state following an injury to the brain or spinal cord. There is intense pain at the base of the brain and the back of the neck; this pain leads to depression and irritability. The remedy may still work months after the injury if these symptoms are present. Photophobia (discomfort of eyes in sunlight or bright light) may accompany the head pain.

Ruta graveolens

Ruta is similar to Arnica in its use for alleviating the pain of fractures and dislocations. For spinal injuries where there is much pain and restlessness, this may be the remedy. The rear legs easily give out upon standing or after exertion. The animal often cannot keep the legs still while lying, as movement diminishes the pain.

Thuja occidentalis

This remedy is useful for spinal injuries when there is not so much pain as numbness and awkwardness in the rear legs. There may be accompanying urinary problems.

Chapter Fourteen
REPRODUCTIVE SYSTEM

Overview

Most veterinarians today do not contend with many intact animals and their problems. Overpopulation, along with the inconvenience of living with unneutered animals, has brought us to this scenario, as most companion animals are spayed before puberty. Certainly there is a large community of people who breed animals, but as a part of the whole picture of animal companionship, this is still a small fraction. In my practice I have very few clients who breed animals, so perhaps my perspective is somewhat different than the norm, but probably not vastly different.

Considering breeding and neutering (spaying females and castrating males—*neuter* is not gender-specific) animals involves ethical questions that are sometimes difficult to resolve. Any discussion of these topics tends to bring out strong opinions and can be inflammatory. With this acknowledgment, I shall nonetheless delve into these areas, as they are ones that cannot rightly be ignored, or perhaps it is simply that I too have opinions regarding these matters. The perspectives that I present are not finalized, nor are they intended as directives; rather they are designed to inspire contemplation on your part. Each of us must decide for ourselves the appropriate choice when faced with any decision, including one involving other beings in our care. I only ask for your thoughtfulness in the process, and suggest cultivating an I-thou relationship when deciding for those other beings.

To me, the underlying question is, "Whose needs are we serving?" Whether we are considering breeding or neutering an animal in our care, we must ask this question. Furthermore, we must ask whether our actions may even harm or limit the animal, physically or emotionally.

In my opinion, if our actions don't serve the animal, then they are not the best choice. Not everyone will agree with this. Some will take the position that it is acceptable to make a choice that serves the needs of the human (in this case the word *guardian* is not quite accurate) rather than those of the animal. If these needs are met at some expense to the animal, however, I suggest examining the decision closely to see if there is virtue in the outcome. See also Chapter Seventeen, "The Bigger Picture," for an overview of our relationship to companion animals.

Neutering

To return to a more concrete examination of the issues at hand, I'll first discuss neutering. Generally, we neuter animals for two reasons: we don't like the behavior of (reproductively) intact animals, and we have concerns about animal overpopulation. From an ideal perspective, I do not believe we really have the right to neuter another being without his or her consent (recognizing that obtaining consent in this case is essentially impossible), no matter the reason. Yet this position is rather impractical, and the problems of animal overpopulation affect animals to at least as great a degree as they affect humans. More animals would suffer if we stopped neutering, so neutering is probably in the best interest of the species, at least for now. Furthermore, many people would not keep and care for an intact animal because of behavior issues, so neutering to alter behavior may even be good for the individual, assuming there is a value to the animal in having a home with humans—which, for the foreseeable future, is probably true, though I think we must reconsider animal-keeping in the larger picture.

Now, there are still those who would argue that an animal has the right to be intact, and many of these are quite willing to keep intact animals and keep them from breeding so they do not contribute to overpopulation. This seems to be a good compromise, and in fact it probably is for many human-animal families. The consideration is that animals were born intact and thus are meant to stay intact and therefore are generally healthier if left intact. There is a concern with this logic, however, though it probably is important to some animals and not others. Animals were indeed born intact, and by nature they are perhaps meant to be intact, but they were meant to be intact *and to breed*. There's the conundrum.

Many health problems we see in the reproductive system are in intact, nonbreeding animals. Additionally, the hormonal drives cannot be satisfied, and in some animals this creates mental stress. So, do we neuter or not? I think for most animals and people, neutering reduces stress and thus improves health, as most animals will not use their reproductive organs due to the concerns listed above. As I have said, this is a compromise position, consequential to a long pattern of domesticating and keeping animals. I think the pattern has flaws, but for now we have little option but to continue to keep them, and neutering, though morally questionable, seems to be a temporal necessity.

If we choose to neuter, when should we neuter? For years the standard has been at six months of age, after most of the reproductive system development has occurred but before the hormones "blossom." I prefer to wait longer, at least eight to nine months. This allows bone closure and other maturation as guided by sex hormones. This is especially important in male cats because the diameter of the urethra continues to grow as the system matures, and tomcats that are neutered too young are probably at greater risk of urethral obstruction. (Advocates of early-age neutering claim this is not a problem, but published studies have shown that early-age neutering results in smaller urethral diameter. See Chapter Eleven, "Urinary System," for more information about this disease.)

Today there is more and more impetus behind early-age neutering (four to eight *weeks*), especially at animal shelters. I am uncomfortable with this practice, although I understand its use in shelters as I served on the board of directors of a shelter for a few years. Once released from the shelter, most animals are not returned for neutering. These animals contribute to over-population, ultimately increasing the load on shelters that are already over-burdened. Despite this reasoning, I do not support early-age neutering in animal shelters, as I have seen many animals that became quite ill after neutering because the stress is simply too great; at six to eight weeks these animals are little more than newborns. I am adamantly opposed to early-age neutering in all other cases.

On the other side of the coin, many older veterinarians used to recommend allowing a female to go through a heat cycle before spaying her. While I used to dismiss this idea, I have come around to its wisdom. This plan allows development to full maturity before removing the organs. As the reproductive hormones affect other areas of development, such as skeletal growth, waiting may be a good idea. I recognize that the risk for some ailments such as mammary cancer are lessened by avoiding any heat cycles, but the risk in allowing one cycle is extremely minimal.

My recommendation is to wait at least until eight months for both females and males; wait a bit longer if you feel comfortable. For males, don't wait until much past ten months, as marking and territorial behavior can be rather persistent once it is ingrained. With female cats, waiting until they enter estrus is a bit tricky, as they do not ovulate until they copulate, so the un-bred female will go in and out of estrus, five to seven days on and off, for several cycles, which can tax the cat as well as her human guardians. If necessary, you can plan the ovariohysterectomy (spay) for two or three days after she comes out of a heat cycle. This will at least be during a quiescent period, which is better for the surgeon and the cat, as the uterus during heat is swollen and more difficult to remove, plus the sudden drop in hormones is hard on her body if she is spayed during estrus.

Breeding

As a veterinarian, I am certain I have biases, and this is one of those areas where they appear. On the one hand, certain breeds of dogs and cats have fascinated me or have captured my attention due to beauty or personality or both. But on the other hand, I have seen so many unhealthy animals who derived much of their weakness from inbreeding. In this case I am using the term *inbreeding* to denote purebred, as this is how a breed is created, and even though some genetic diversity occurs over time as the breed grows, the original stock was inbred. Purebred animals are, with very few exceptions, unhealthier on the whole than mutts.

I realize there is much argument about the truth of this statement, but I don't believe many veterinarians would disagree. Purebred animals have many more health problems than mixed-breed animals. Genetics may not be the entire answer; I doubt that it is. Most purebred animals receive far more vaccines and drugs than mixed breeds, and I am certain this contributes greatly to the demise of their health. But there is still an inherent weakness that probably makes the purebreds more susceptible to damage from these and other stressors.

If we go back to our questions above and ask whose needs we are serving, it is not the animal; I doubt that many dogs or cats care about appearance very much. (Of course they care about cleanliness and those aspects of appearance, but that is not my point here.) As to the second question, Do our actions harm or limit the animal?—I believe they do. The justification for breeding must therefore outweigh this concern. In many cases the health may not be severely impaired, so perhaps this is of little concern. In some cases, however, the health is quite impaired; I believe that breeding animals that fit this category is morally wrong. Of course, people have different opinions about where to draw the line, and certainly the middle area is not clear, but in many cases there is little doubt.

My experience working with an animal shelter further strengthened my bias. Not only did I serve on the board of directors, but I also spent some time at the shelter that included killing unwanted animals by lethal injection. (I could use the word *euthanasia,* but it does not change the situation.) This task is as horrible as you may imagine. I really struggle with the logic of breeding more animals by conscious choice when thousands are killed by the hour across this country for lack of homes. If we now return once more to our questions, I don't see much room for support for breeding. For every purebred animal born, another animal must die because there is no room at the inn.

I understand that this is a strong statement, and perhaps a bit unfair as so many people who breed are very responsible and have great love for animals in their hearts. And it is perhaps easy to point a finger at "puppy mills" that breed litter after litter for the money with no care for either the animal or the breed other than for the potential revenue it may bring. Surely these are the worst offenders. But we all must examine our actions and see if we can make a difference somewhere. As I suggest in Chapter Seventeen, "The Bigger Picture," our consumption has brought the earth to the brink of catastrophe, and our animals consume tremendous amounts of resources along with us. Any meaningful change in our world, any reduction in our impact, must take animal overpopulation into account along with human overpopulation. Further, we constantly destroy wild animal homes in order to expand our human and domestic animal populations. I think we are clueless to the value, to the intricate interconnectedness of these wild animals to our lives, to the fabric of our world. Unless we value these others and give them room to live alongside us, I suspect catastrophe to be unavoidable. Breeding more animals just for our fancy closes this door as surely as does cutting down rain forest and draining marshland to raise more cattle or put up subdivisions and shopping malls. The time of luxury is passing, and the decisions we make now involve survival.

For those who choose to breed, take steps to ensure the health of the animals you will bring into the world. Be as certain as possible that you are not creating lives of sickness. In essence, follow the Golden Rule in all actions. Remember also the question, just because we can do something, does this make it correct?

Chapter Content

This chapter will cover problems with males first as there is not too much information compared to that for females, and I did not want the section buried at the back of the chapter. I am also following homeopathic convention, sexist though it may be. I will then address problems of females, followed by a section on pregnancy and neonatal care. As you may have guessed by now, I do not encourage breeding, but I do encourage responsible breeding if you choose to breed. I do not address infertility or other breeding problems, as I generally believe these occur for a reason. In humans there is a much greater incidence of birth defects among children of parents that had difficulty becoming pregnant. Nature has her methods of reducing birth defects, and trouble may ensue if we attempt to override these measures.

The approach to disease in this chapter will be somewhat more oriented toward specific problems than other treatment chapters, but you should still follow homeopathic principles and try to pick a remedy that fits the entire animal rather than the one symptom alone.

MALE REPRODUCTIVE SYSTEM

Function

The reproductive system in the male serves two main functions. The first is production of testosterone, a steroid compound that initiates male behavior and male body development. The second function is production of sperm and seminal fluids to nourish sperm, the male's contribution to the formation of offspring. Sperm formation requires a temperature that is a few degrees lower than that of the body, so the testicles are housed in the scrotum. The exposed location provides the needed temperature. The testicles are formed in the body (next to the kidneys) and drop as the young animal matures. They should be fully in the scrotum by four to eight weeks of age. Although a testicle that is retained within the body will not normally produce sperm, hormone production is unaffected by the higher body temperature and continues normally. The increased temperature increases the likelihood of testicular cancer, however, so these animals should be neutered.

The penis is encased in the sheath, or prepuce, which is attached to the underside of the body in the dog and below the scrotum in the cat. Only when erect is the penis normally outside the sheath in the dog, while cats will extend the penis during urination.

The prostate gland is also considered part of the male reproductive system, as it straddles the urethra and encompasses the spermatic ducts as they enter the urethra. The prostate gland secretes fluid that constitutes the major part of the semen volume, essentially supporting and carrying the sperm along as ejaculation occurs.

Diseases of the male reproductive system involve inflammation for the most part, outside of infertility problems. Dogs will occasionally (though uncommonly) have difficulty either extruding or retracting the penis if the preputial opening is small. This is extremely rare in cats. Retained testicles occur occasionally in dogs; this is also rare in cats.

Discharge from the Sheath (Balanoposthitis, Sheath Inflammation)

This is rather common in dogs and for the most part it is not harmful. It may be difficult to eliminate in many cases. You will see a yellow to yellow-green thick discharge that may occasionally drip. The dog may lick the area frequently. Veterinarians sometimes call this a balanoposthitis.

Wash the prepuce out once or twice a day with a saline and *Calendula* or saline and *Hypericum* (St. John's wort) solution. Use one-fourth teaspoon of salt and ten to twenty drops of the herb per cup of boiled (but not hot) water (or one teaspoon of each per quart). This should soothe and disinfect the sheath.

Homeopathic Medicines for Discharge from the Sheath

Try *Thuja* first, and if this does not help, use one of the following remedies. Don't use *Mercurius* or *Silicea* after one another.

Cinnabaris

These dogs usually have an intense inflammation in addition to the discharge. The prepuce is quite painful and may be red. The dog may be very thirsty and may start easily from sleep.

Hepar sulphuris calcareum

Dogs needing *Hepar sulph* may be irritable, and the discharge is often very foul. The prepuce may also be quite painful though the inflammation will not be as great as with *Cinnabaris*. The dog may snap when you try to examine or clean the sheath.

Medorrhinum

This deep-acting nosode is best used under an experienced homeopath's guidance, but it can be useful for chronic balanoposthitis.

Mercurius (vivus, solubilis, or corrosivus)

Mercurius vivus and *Mercurius solubilis* are essentially the same remedy; *Mercurius corrosivus* is different, but the indications are very similar in many cases. The discharge tends to be more green than yellow. These dogs will often be irritable and especially hate to be corrected.

Nitric acid
When this remedy is needed, the dog may be quite vicious when examined because the pain is like a splinter and is simply overwhelming. These dogs are often very chilly. There may be pain while urinating, so the dog may whine or be reluctant to urinate. He may also lick the penis and prepuce immediately after urination.

Silicea (Silica)
Here the discharge is usually bland and yellow, and the inflammation is minimal. These dogs are usually easygoing. They may be on the thin side and leaning toward poor health.

Sulphur
Sulphur dogs are generally friendly and very easygoing. They often appear dirty and unkempt, as they have little care for their appearance. To them, life is too much fun for cleaning.

Phimosis and Paraphimosis

These related conditions occur as a result of a small opening in the prepuce. This makes passage of the penis through the preputial opening difficult to impossible. Phimosis is a condition whereby the penis cannot extrude through the opening, and paraphimosis is the condition when the extruded penis cannot retract back into the prepuce. Paraphimosis is much more serious as the tight preputial opening often compromises circulation to the penis, and there is a risk of gangrene.

The narrowing of the opening may be either congenital (occurring as a birth defect) or the result of swelling of the prepuce. The former condition requires surgery and is not amenable to remedies, while the latter situation may respond to homeopathic treatment.

Preputial inflammation is usually the result of a balanoposthitis (see above), although occasionally an injury will cause swelling.

General Care for Phimosis and Paraphimosis
See your veterinarian right away if your dog (or cat) has a paraphimosis (penis

extruded) and you cannot get the penis back in the sheath within fifteen to thirty minutes, especially if the color of the penis begins to darken. It should normally be bright red like the color of healthy gums, or a little brighter.

To assist him in retracting the penis, give one of the homeopathic medicines listed below if available, then apply cold, strong saline solution (one teaspoonful of salt per cup of water) for a few minutes. Next apply petroleum jelly, K-Y Jelly, or *Calendula* ointment to the penis and attempt to slide it back into the prepuce. If you are successful, rinse the sheath with the *Calendula*-saline or *Hypericum*-saline solutions (see above under "Discharge from the Sheath"). Treat the condition as a sheath inflammation/discharge.

If there is only a phimosis, you may not readily notice the condition unless he is a breeding animal and cannot extrude the penis. If you discover a phimosis, treat it as a sheath inflammation also. Have the animal examined by a veterinarian to see if surgery is indicated.

Homeopathic Medicines for Paraphimosis and Phimosis

If the swelling and paraphimosis or phimosis occurs following an injury, give *Arnica*; if this does not relieve it, give *Bellis perennis* or *Conium*.

If inflammation causes the condition, try one of the following remedies:

Apis mellifica
The prepuce will be swollen and may be whitish and cool to touch. The swelling is usually soft (edematous).

Cinnabaris
See above, under "Homeopathic Medicines for Discharge from the Sheath."

Colocynthis
The condition may occur following an episode of anger or irritability; these animals can be quite irritable. The pains are cramping and may cause the dog to jerk, twist about, or bend double in an attempt to relieve the pains.

Mercurius (vivus or solubilis), Mercurius corrosivus
See above, under "Homeopathic Medicines for Discharge from the Sheath."

Nitric acid
See above, under "Homeopathic Medicines for Discharge from the Sheath."

Rhus toxicodendron

As with the *Apis* state, the prepuce is swollen and soft (edematous), but it is more likely here to be red and irritated. These dogs are usually restless and may be thirsty.

Retained Testicle (Cryptorchidism)

As I mentioned above, the testicles usually descend into the scrotum by four to five weeks of age; if they have not descended by six to eight weeks, the puppy or kitten is said to be cryptorchid (or monorchid if only one has descended). Most of the time the retained testicle is in the abdominal cavity, although sometimes it can be felt somewhere beside the penis if it had moved partially down. We generally recommend castration, especially for those in the abdomen, because there is a higher incidence of testicular cancer in retained testicles. Cryptorchidism is much more common in dogs than in cats.

Occasionally a homeopathic remedy will cause the testicle to finish the descent if the remedy is given while the animal is still very young. These animals should not be bred, as the condition is often hereditary. A male with retained testicles cannot be shown (in dog shows), and it is possibly unethical to show one who had a retained testicle that came down after treatment. Some veterinarians will surgically bring a testicle down (if it was mostly down), but I understand these animals cannot ethically be entered in dog shows.

Homeopathic Medicines for Retained Testicle

Remember that if the testicle is not partially descended, it will not likely respond; response is not common in most cases but may be worth a try if you do not intend to neuter him.

Aurum

These animals are often low-spirited and may have a lot of other problems such as eye inflammation and chronic discharges from the nose. They may have a "heavy footed" walk. They often hate to be disciplined.

Calcarea carbonica

Calcarea animals are often big-boned, obese, and clumsy. They may be slow in learning to walk. Milk may cause diarrhea in these pups.

Calcarea phosphorica
These dogs are very similar to those needing *Calcarea carbonica* but are thin rather than heavy. They may appear rather delicate.

Clematis erecta
I have not used this remedy here, but Christina Chambreau, a colleague, reports good success in some cases of retained testicle with *Clematis*. The remedy has good affinity to testicular and genital issues, and there may be a concomitant preputial discharge.

Psorinum
This homeopathic remedy is usually a prescription item, but it may be useful for the pup that has a dirty, flaky, and sometimes oily coat.

Syphilinum, Thyroidinum, and *Tuberculinum*
These homeopathic remedies may also be helpful, but they are deep-acting and available by prescription only. While *Psorinum* is generally safe to use on your own (if you have access), these remedies should be used under the direction of an experienced practitioner.

Inflammation of the Testicles (Orchitis)

This condition is rather uncommon, but when it does occur, it is usually very painful. As with other genital diseases, cats are affected less often than dogs. The testicle(s) will become hot and swollen, often rather quickly. Sometimes the scrotum turns red and/or discharges a clear fluid (serum). In rare cases an abscess develops and the scrotum will rupture, discharging the accumulated pus.

If your dog develops orchitis, you should take him to a veterinarian for an examination and a test for canine brucellosis *(Brucella canis* infection). This organism is transmissible via sexual intercourse as well as occasionally by contact with urine or urethral discharges. Various *Brucella* species affect cattle, sheep, pigs, goats, and horses as well. The organism can also cause prostate infection, and in females it may be responsible for sterility and repeated abortions. The disease is also contagious to humans, and it is a serious illness. In humans it is called undulant fever or Malta fever.

Most cases of orchitis leave the dog infertile due to residual damage to the testicle. The conventional treatment is castration plus intensive antibiotic therapy. If brucellosis is present, some veterinarians recommend euthanasia because of the possibility of transmission to humans.

If brucellosis is not present, you may try one of the following homeopathic medicines. If you do not see a quick response, consider antibiotic treatment plus castration, as this condition can be very painful and it is unfair to wait too long.

Homeopathic Medicines for Inflammation of the Testicles (Orchitis)

Arnica montana
Trauma is *Arnica*'s sphere; if your dog develops orchitis after trauma, try this remedy first. The pain will usually be so intense that he will be fearful of approach or touch.

Baptisia
When this remedy is needed, the animal is often *very* ill and listless. He typically looks and acts as if he feels terrible (which he does). His gums may be deep red, and if you press on them the color returns slowly (two or three seconds instead of immediately). Nausea and diarrhea may accompany the orchitis.

Belladonna
Belladonna conditions are often sudden and intense. The testicles will usually be hot, sometimes red, and very painful. The patient is typically restless, hot, and thirsty, and he may be irritable and aggressive.

Clematis erecta
This remedy is a good one to consider for orchitis, especially if only the right testicle is affected. The affected testicle becomes very painful and very hard, even stony hard. The urination may be difficult at first, with interruptions of the stream until he finally gets a good flow going. He may be worse at night and better in open air.

Conium maculatum
Here the inflammation may occur after either excessive sexual activity or because of suppressed activity. It may also follow injury. When *Conium* is needed the testicles may become stony hard like the *Clematis* state, but the

pain is not so intense. The dog may have a history of easily becoming sexually excited.

Hamamelis
Like *Arnica,* this remedy may be useful for orchitis following an injury, though not all *Hamamelis* cases start with injuries. The testicles will be swollen, hot, and very painful. Any motion or jarring is very painful, and he prefers to lie quietly, usually inside, as open air may worsen the condition as well.

Mercurius (vivus or solubilis)
When *Mercurius* is needed there is often a discharge from the penis and prepuce; the discharge is usually greenish and may include some blood. Think of this remedy if you see ulcerated skin over the testicles as well as the swelling. These dogs may also have poor teeth and gums.

Pulsatilla
Like *Clematis,* this remedy is good for right-sided orchitis (occasionally left). In this case, there may be a yellow discharge from the prepuce as well. The affected testicle will be very painful but will not be hard. There may be a prostate inflammation as well. These animals tend to be thirstless and intolerant of stuffy rooms, and they are usually mild-mannered and very desirous of attention.

Rhododendron
When this remedy is needed, the condition usually develops or worsens at the approach of stormy weather (rainy and windy, also thunder). He will improve as the storm breaks. Cold damp weather may also incite illness, and sitting on cold stones may initiate an orchitis. The testicles are intensely painful. The right side is more commonly affected, though the left may be the site of inflammation as well.

Rhus toxicodendron
The scrotum is often swollen and soft (edematous) along with the testicular inflammation when *Rhus tox* is needed. There may be moist skin inflammation on the scrotum and between the scrotum and the thighs. He may also have a persistent or recurrent erection.

Injuries to the Testicles

For blunt trauma and bruising, *Bellis perennis* and *Arnica* are the first remedies to consider. If the condition does not resolve and the testicles become swollen, try *Conium*.

For lacerations, give *Staphysagria* first, and use *Calendula* solution topically (one-fourth teaspoon of salt and ten to twenty drops of *Calendula* tincture per cup of boiled but cool water). If there is no improvement, give *Calendula* in oral potentized form (i.e. 30C, 6C, etc.). You may also substitute *Hypericum* (St. John's wort) tincture for the *Calendula* tincture.

For puncture wounds, first try *Hypericum*, and if there is no response, give *Ledum* (use *Ledum* first if the wound is cold to touch). Clean the wound with either solution as described above for lacerations.

Prostate Affections

Many intact dogs develop prostate diseases as they age, especially if they are not actively breeding. Tomcats very rarely have prostate troubles. Just as is well recorded in humans, the canine prostate functions best if it is regularly activated by sexual intercourse; this is one of the problems with keeping an intact but sexually inactive animal. Problems may occur as early as one to two years, though around six years is more common. The prostate will begin to enlarge; this will sometimes create difficulty with urination and/or defecation. The underlying condition may be either inflammatory or noninflammatory. The latter condition is called prostate hypertrophy, indicating that the prostate is larger than normal. This condition is not cancerous, but a large percentage of hypertrophied prostate glands progress to cancer if untreated.

Inflammation may be associated with a bacterial infection, though as in other areas the inflammation and susceptibility to infection must occur to allow the bacteria to grow; the bacteria are not the cause. When inflammation is present the dog may have blood in the urine; the blood will come at the end of urination rather than throughout urination. This is virtually diagnostic of prostate inflammation.

General Care for Prostate Affections

If your intact male dog develops problems urinating or defecating, or if he has blood in his urine, have a veterinarian examine him right away (though it is not usually an emergency unless he *cannot* urinate or defecate) to determine the cause. You may then opt for homeopathic treatment, but your veterinarian can help you monitor his condition as well as provide treatment if necessary.

Conventional treatment for an inflamed prostate includes antibiotics with the assumption that it is infectious. Most veterinarians recommend castration for any prostate disease because of the tendency to progress toward cancer, as prostate cancer is highly fatal and difficult to treat. I generally agree with this recommendation. The risk is too great, and castration is very effective as part of the treatment.

Castration plus homeopathic medicines can be an effective combination. Sometimes homeopathic remedies alone can reverse the prostate condition, so if your desire is to avoid castration, you may try homeopathic treatment first. If you do not see a response within a couple of weeks for an inflammatory condition or within a couple of months for prostate hypertrophy, consider castration. You will need a cooperative veterinarian to help you assess the progress as this necessitates a rectal examination.

Supplements that promote prostate health include zinc, essential fatty acids, antioxidants, kelp, and lecithin. Zinc is particularly important; give small dogs (up to thirty pounds) 12.5 mg per day, medium to large dogs 25 mg per day, and very large dogs (over eighty pounds) 50 mg per day. Essential fatty acids include omega-3 fatty acids and gamma-linolenic acid (GLA). Omega-3 fatty acids can be obtained from flax seed oil; give one-fourth teaspoon per ten pounds daily. GLA is especially important and is available in borage or evening primrose oils. Give small dogs 125–250 mg per day, medium to large dogs 500–1,000 mg/day, and very large dogs 1,000–1,500 mg/day. Vitamin E is a good antioxidant for the prostate; give 5–10 mg per pound daily; use mixed tocopherols for best effect. Vitamin C may help as well; give 5–10 mg per pound two to three times a day, using natural vitamin C if available. For kelp, give one to three tablets per day (or one-fourth to one teaspoon), and for lecithin give one-half teaspoon to one tablespoon per day. Give the lecithin before meals if possible. Finally, a pinch of royal jelly in the food may also be beneficial.

Homeopathic Medicines for Prostate Affections

These remedies may help for either inflammatory or hypertrophied enlargement, though as indicated, some are better in one sphere than the other.

Chimaphila umbellata

This remedy is especially good for inflammation with impeded urination. The dog must strain to start the stream of urine, and there is often mucus in the urine. He may stand with his rear legs wide apart to urinate. Urination is often painful, and walking relieves the pain. Cold, damp weather often initiates a *Chimaphila* state.

Conium maculatum

This is one of the main remedies for prostate hypertrophy in older men; it has a similar affinity in the dog. Urination is difficult to start, and it may start and stop several times. The dog may also dribble urine. He may have a weakness in the rear legs as well. The prostate may be extremely hard upon palpation.

Eupatorium purpureum

Here the prostate is affected along with the kidneys and bladder. The back is usually painful, indicative of kidney involvement, near the area where the last ribs meet the spine. There may be symptoms of bladder inflammation, like straining and protein in the urine.

Ferrum picricum

This remedy is also useful for senile hypertrophy of the prostate with urinary difficulty. In this case the dog will get up to urinate several times at night. He may have warts as well.

Picric acid

These dogs will usually be very exhausted and weak and may have very weak rear limbs. This is similar to *Conium* but more intense and progresses more rapidly. The prostate is usually hypertrophied, but this remedy works best when the hypertrophy is not too advanced. Accompanying the prostate troubles is a tendency to experience persistent, even painful erections. The erections often begin as soon as the dog goes to sleep.

Pulsatilla

Pulsatilla is another important remedy for the prostate. It is best for acute inflammation of the prostate rather than hypertrophy. The prostate is usually painful and there is often a thick yellow discharge, sometimes with blood. These dogs are usually thirstless and intolerant of stuffy rooms, preferring to be out in the open air. They love sympathy and attention.

Sabal serrulata

This remedy is made from the saw palmetto, which is useful as an herb for prostate affections. The homeopathic preparation is also very good for an enlarged prostate. There is usually a discharge of prostatic fluid, and the testicles may be atrophied (shrunken). These dogs dislike sympathy and may become irritable if consoled.

Selenium

This mineral remedy is good for dogs that are weak and debilitated and are worse from heat. The prostate is hypertrophied (enlarged), and urine dribbles when the dog walks around. Prostatic fluid also drips almost constantly. Hot days are intolerable, and these patients improve as the sun goes down and the temperature drops.

Staphysagria

Like *Pulsatilla*, this remedy is best for acute inflammatory prostate enlargement. The urethra burns when the dog is not urinating, so he may urinate frequently, and he will often lick his genitals constantly due to the pain. He may strain to urinate for long periods.

Thuja occidentalis

If none of the above remedies seems appropriate, or if they do not have the desired effect, try this remedy. Vaccinations often cause genitourinary troubles, and this remedy is especially useful when this is the case.

Hypersexual Behavior

Though most cases of hypersexual behavior (especially masturbation in neutered animals) are evidence of chronic disease and thus require constitutional treatment, there is an occasional exception. Some male dogs, more commonly smaller breeds, mount other animals and humans (usually the legs) constantly. This behavior will sometimes respond to the homeopathic medicine *Yohimbinum*. Don't give the herb yohimbine, as this may increase the sex drive in males. *Medorrhinum* may also help, but should be prescribed by an experienced homeopath.

Scrotal Swelling following Neutering

Sometimes the scrotum fills with blood after neutering. While not harmful, this can be painful. *Bellis perennis* is usually the best remedy, but you can also consider *Arnica, Phosphorus, Hamamelis,* and *Millefolium.*

FEMALE REPRODUCTIVE SYSTEM

Function

The female reproductive system has three main functions: first, the ovaries produce the female hormones, estrogen and progesterone, which stimulate development of an animal's female body and guide her reproductive cycles, including pregnancy and milk production. Secondly, the ovaries produce eggs that, when fertilized by sperm, begin the development of embryos; these become fetuses as they develop into a new individual of the species. The third function is provided by the uterus as it provides a home for the developing individuals until they can live outside the mother's body.

The ovaries arise in the abdomen near the kidneys, similarly to the testes in the male, but the ovaries stay in that location. When eggs are produced, they travel through a small tube called the oviduct, which essentially deposits them into the upper end of the uterus. Fertilization normally occurs in the uterus, and the fertilized egg attaches to the inner surface of the uterus, where it develops into a baby. The terminal end of the uterus is the cervix; this is normally closed to a narrow diameter until delivery. Continuing toward the body opening, the next chamber is the vagina; the cervix joins the vagina and the uterus. The vagina is the canal that accepts the penis during copulation. The terminus of the vagina—the opening to the outside—is the vulva.

The breasts are often considered part of the reproductive system, although they are technically separate. If we add them, however, we add a fourth function, milk production. I will cover some mammary problems in this chapter under the "Pregnancy and Neonatal Care" section.

Female cats and dogs (queens and bitches) have reproductive cycles that are triggered by light levels. Bitches normally cycle every six months, usually spring and fall, though there is a lot of variation, possibly due to separation from the natural environment and natural lighting. The estrous cycle (heat cycle) usually lasts about twenty-one days; the onset is announced with bleeding from the uterus that discharges through the vulva. Ovulation occurs mid-cycle; the bitch won't usually "stand" for breeding before ovulation, although males are attracted from the outset. If she is not bred, she may experience a false pregnancy that lasts approximately the same duration as a real gestation (gestation is fifty-eight to seventy days, average sixty-three to sixty-five days). She may begin nesting behavior and even develop milk in some cases. This is within the realm of normal responses, possibly a remnant of pack behavior as a way to prepare nonalpha females for assisting the alpha female in mothering. The cycle can vary tremendously among different bitches, so this is only a guideline. Veterinarians can test hormone levels to determine a more exact picture of an individual bitch's cycle.

The queen is rather different than the bitch in her cycles. She cycles spring and early fall as triggered by light, but she does not ovulate until she has bred with a male. Her heat lasts about a week; if she has not bred and ovulated, she will go out of heat for a few days and then resume heat for another week. This may repeat three to four times until she either ovulates or eventually stops cycling until the next fall or spring, though in some cases it continues even longer. Queens typically do not bleed during the estrous cycle. They will develop some vulvar swelling and perhaps a clear discharge (minimal). Their behavior gives it away, however, as they roll around, howl mournfully (lustily?), rise up on their back legs, and generally draw attention to themselves. They often become very affectionate with humans, though sometimes they become irritable. When I worked at an emergency clinic, people frequently called about cats in heat—and sometimes brought them in for an examination—because they were sure the cat was in some distress. This was always a nice relief from the other cases that were often such sad occasions.

The gestation time is virtually the same for cats as for dogs (fifty-eight to seventy days; average sixty-three to sixty-five days). In contrast to bitches, queens rarely go through a false pregnancy if they do not conceive.

The primary symptom encountered in the female reproductive tract that is not associated with pregnancy is inflammatory or infectious discharges from the vulva. Some females (mostly bitches, as queens have very few reproductive-system difficulties) have problems with erratic cycling or cystic ovaries. These are generally deep-seated problems and usually require constitutional treatment by an experienced practitioner. I will address discharges in this section, followed by a section on pregnancy and neonatal care. The latter will include problems with milk production and mastitis (inflammation of the mammary gland).

Discharges from the Vulva

Discharges of pus from the female reproductive tract can have vastly different implications, especially if she is intact (unspayed). Occasionally a female (primarily bitches, rarely queens) will develop a condition called pyometra (pus in the uterus). This is essentially an abscess within the uterus, and it occurs around a month after the end of a heat cycle. It is most common in middle-aged dogs (five to ten years old), though it can occur at other ages. Progesterone helps condition the uterus for pregnancy, and part of this involves minimizing the immune response so the fetuses are not rejected, but this increases the susceptibility to infection. Pyometra also occurs very commonly after a "mis-mate shot." This is an injection of an estrogen compound to incite an abortion within a few days of an accidental (to the guardian, anyway) breeding. The added estrogen increases the effect of progesterone on limiting immunity. I do not recommend these injections for this reason.

Pyometra is a serious condition and potentially life-threatening; I don't recommend attempting treatment at home. In fact, I recommend surgery (spay) in most cases, as these are difficult to treat. Typically, the bitch is thirsty and urinates a lot (larger volumes, not just more frequently) in addition to the discharge; she may be quite listless, and her gum color may be poor if she is toxic from the infection. If you press on her gums and release, the color may return slowly. Normally it returns immediately, but when an animal is toxic it may take two to three seconds or longer. This is not a good sign and you should take her in to a veterinarian immediately if you see this condition.

In some cases of pyometra the cervix is closed and there is no visible discharge, but the other symptoms (thirst and urination as well as listlessness four to eight weeks postheat, poor gum color) may clue you in to the illness. These animals are usually much sicker and need more immediate attention. As with any listless animal, take her in to a veterinarian to determine the illness and then decide if it should be treated at home. In the case of pyometra, and especially closed pyometra, I don't generally recommend home treatment.

If your female is spayed or if you have had her examined and she does not have pyometra but only a vaginal inflammation, home treatment is appropriate. In rare cases, a spayed female may develop a pyometra if the spay was not properly executed, so if your spayed animal develops pyometra symptoms, have her examined right away. Discharges may also develop after delivery. In this case there is either a retained placenta or a uterine infection, but the infection is not so serious as the uterus is better able to handle the infection (progesterone levels are not so high). See the section on pregnancy and neonatal care for treatment of retained placenta and post-partum infections.

An infection or discharge that is not from the uterus is a vaginal inflammation (vaginitis). This is rarely serious, although it may be persistent and difficult to treat. Typically, you will see a discharge that varies from clear to mucus or pus; white to yellow or yellow-green. There may be a foul odor (uncommonly) and the discharge may be irritating to the skin around the vulva. The odor may smell like a female in season to a male dog, and you may see males who are interested in her even though she is not in season. This may be your first clue that there is a problem. This sometimes occurs with bladder infections as well. Another similarity to bladder infections is that some females with vaginitis will urinate frequently, but in small amounts rather than the increased volume we see with pyometra.

General Care for Discharges from the Vulva

If you see a discharge from your companion's vulva, you must assess the severity of her condition:

- Is she spayed?
- If she is intact, when was her last heat cycle?
- Is she listless?
- Are her gums nice and pink (like yours, or like under your nails)?
- Do the gums refill with blood within one-half second when you press gently and release, or does it take longer?
- Is she excessively thirsty or urinating more than usual?
- Does the discharge irritate the skin around the vulva?

See your veterinarian immediately:
- if she shows possible symptoms of pyometra (see above): four to eight weeks postheat, listless, increased thirst and urination, discharge (sometimes absent), or poor gum color or refill time;
- if she is listless, regardless of other symptoms.

Have an examination soon:
- if the discharge is irritating to the skin;
- if the discharge does not clear within a few days to a couple of weeks.

Next, assess the nature of her symptoms:
- What color is the discharge?
- Does it irritate the skin around the vulva?
- Does she lick the area constantly or scoot on the ground?
- Does she urinate frequently but not in large volume?
- Are there accompanying symptoms, or changes in her mental state?

Give her vitamin C (5–10 mg/pound, two to three times a day) to help her resist the infection. Nettle tea and cleavers support the urogenital system and cleanse the body. Immune-building herbs such as echinacea, cat's claw, astragalus, and goldenseal may help as well. Use one or two of these at a time. The best method is to make a tea by pouring boiling water over the herb (about one teaspoon of dry herb per cup of water) and allowing it to cool. Give one-fourth teaspoon of the liquid per ten to twenty pounds, two to three times a day. Goldenseal is very strong, so use it for only about a week at a time. If you cannot get the fresh herb, use the tincture and give five to ten drops per ten to twenty pounds, two to three times a day. If possible, get a glycerin tincture rather than an alcohol tincture. If you have the alcohol tincture, place the dose in a spoon and allow it to sit for a few minutes (you may warm it slightly) to allow the alcohol to evaporate before administration. This is especially important for cats.

Topically, use a douche of *Calendula* (prepare the tea as above or use the tincture and add ten to twenty drops per cup of water) or vinegar and water (use one or two tablespoons vinegar to a cup of water). *Hypericum* (St. John's wort) may be used instead of the *Calendula*. Use an ear bulb syringe and gently insert it into the vulva about one-quarter to one-half inch, then gently flush. For cats and small dogs you may need to use a small plastic dropper or a hypodermic syringe (without a needle).

Try one of the following homeopathic remedies. If you see no improvement after a few days, try a different one, and if you still see no improvement, consult a homeopathic veterinarian for assistance. Be sure to have her examined at once if any signs of pyometra appear (see above). I have listed some remedies that may assist treatment of pyometra, but as I stated above, I recommend surgical treatment unless you feel it is important to keep her intact. Even in this case you should work closely with a veterinarian (homeopathic if possible), as the condition is dangerous.

Homeopathic Medicines for Discharge from the Vulva

Aletris farinosa

When *Aletris* is needed the patient is generally weak and anemic, and she moves as if she is weighed down. The discharge is usually white and stringy. She may be nauseated upon eating the smallest quantity of food. These animals may have a history of repeated spontaneous abortions due to weakness.

Alumina

These patients are also rather weak and are made worse by any exertion. They tend to be thin, dry, and constipated. The discharge is clear, sometimes ropy, and profuse, even dripping down the legs. It burns the skin around the vulva. There may be difficulty walking due to numbness of the rear legs.

Calcarea carbonica

These patients tend to be chilly, heavy, awkward, and slow moving. The discharge tends to be thick and milky or yellow and may occur in young animals.

Caulophyllum

This remedy is made from the herb blue cohosh, a favorite of midwives for many years as it stimulates and tonifies the uterus. It is most useful during and after pregnancy, but occasionally is indicated for discharges, especially in young animals. The discharge is usually profuse and irritating. This remedy may assist with open pyometra, as it stimulates uterine contractions and helps clear the pus.

Copaiva

Here the discharge is usually bloody and quite foul. This remedy may be useful in pyometra. The vulva and the anus are typically itchy and irritated, so you may see her lick or scoot frequently. She may have mucus-covered stools and/or hives as an accompaniment to the discharge.

Echinacea
This herb is also useful as the homeopathic medicine for severe infections (sepsis) where she is deeply impacted. She will usually be rather ill, and her gum color may be muddy or dark instead of bright pink. This is a good remedy for pyometra when she is quite ill. Use it to boost her immunity before surgery, or if you wish to avoid surgery it may turn her around, but you should work with a veterinarian. The discharge is usually foul and irritating.

Graphites
These animals often have terrible skin troubles as well as the vulvar discharge. The skin tends to be cracked and raw and may have honey-colored discharges. The vulvar discharge will usually be white, profuse, and irritating. In this case, the illness is deep-seated and you should work with a homeopathic veterinarian.

Hydrastis
When this remedy is needed, the discharge is often thick, rubbery, and burns the skin around the vulva. It tends to be yellow and may form into ropy strands. A similar discharge may occur elsewhere. The vulva is very itchy and burning, so she will lick and scoot frequently. This remedy is especially useful in older, weak, depressed, and emaciated animals.

Kali bichromicum
The discharges in this case are quite similar to those when *Hydrastis* is needed—yellow, ropy, and irritating, producing itching and burning in the vulva. A differentiation is that animals needing *Kali bichromicum* are more indifferent or irritable and they avoid company, and those needing *Hydrastis* may be older and very depressed.

Kreosotum
This is another remedy with acrid, burning discharges that cause the animal to lick and scoot constantly due to the pain. The discharge is foul and may be bloody or yellow, and it may occur during pregnancy. She may have severe inflammation of the mouth as well, with spongy, bleeding gums and loose teeth. Weakness in the rear legs and urinary problems may accompany other symptoms. These animals tend to be very irritable.

Lilium tigrinum

When this remedy is needed, the patient is generally depressed, anxious, and snappish, and she may exhibit sexual behavior such as masturbation or humping. The discharge is thin, brown, and irritating. She will lick the vulva constantly due to the irritation and the sexual sensations.

Mercurius (vivus or solubilis)

Mercurius is similar to Kreosotum in its affinity to mucous membranes of the mouth and the vagina. The gums are often inflamed and sore. The discharge from the vulva may be white and thick, or it may be greenish, foul, and even bloody. In either case, it is irritating. Diarrhea with straining is common when Mercurius is needed and may accompany the vaginal inflammation. These animals dislike discipline and may snap if corrected.

Nitric acid

These animals have an acrid, burning discharge that is brown to yellow and thin. The hair around the vulva may be missing because of the irritation. There may even be ulcers on the vaginal mucous membrane. The inflammation is generally quite painful, and the patient is violently irritable, thus she may snap aggressively at any attempt to examine or clean the area. She is usually very chilly.

Pulsatilla

These animals are usually friendly and sweet, sometimes to the point of neediness. The vulvar discharge is thick and creamy, and it may be mildly irritating. The color is usually white to yellow but may be greenish. Young animals that develop a discharge before their first heat may need Pulsatilla. This remedy may be helpful in pyometra, as it is a major uterine remedy. These patients tend to dislike stuffy rooms and prefer open air; they tend to drink little (unusual for pyometra).

Pyrogenium

Like Echinacea, this remedy is excellent for septic states. The animal is usually quite sick, with foul-smelling discharges. She often has aching pains that force her to move about constantly. This remedy is useful in pyometra when she is quite ill and may be helpful to build her strength even if you opt for surgery. If your companion is this sick, you should work with a veterinarian.

Sabina

When *Sabina* is needed, the discharge is thick, yellow, foul, and irritating. The patient may exhibit sexual behavior, though not as strongly as those needing *Lilium tigrinum*. *Sabina* animals are usually very sensitive to noise and may startle easily at sudden noises. They may have accompanying urinary difficulty, and they may have begun their heat cycles at a very young age. Consider this remedy for pyometra.

Secale cornutum

Like *Caulophyllum*, this remedy tonifies the uterus and stimulates uterine contractions. It is most useful after birth but may be indicated for pyometra or vaginitis with discharge. The discharge is brown and very offensive. There may be a bloody watery discharge as well.

Sepia

Last but not least, *Sepia* is a remedy with great affinity to the uterus. These animals are often indifferent to their family including offspring. They are very chilly even when they are in warm rooms. The discharge is yellow to green and itches the vulva. There may be a discharge in young animals (before their first heat) that is lumpy and milky.

PREGNANCY AND NEONATAL CARE

As I stated above in the overview for this chapter, I believe we should give careful consideration to any decision involving breeding animals because of existing problems with overpopulation. Such reasons as breeding for money or status do not carry sufficient weight. And as beautiful as the birth process is, I do not think breeding an animal so that children can experience this beauty is justifiable in today's world.

It is thus with some hesitation that I provide this section, but I hope that those of you who have carefully proceeded to a decision to breed will do so with the utmost care. Read other books on nutrition and pregnancy, as this is not complete. I am not an expert in this area to the degree I am in others. Please read carefully the chapter on vaccinations (Chapter Sixteen, "Vaccination") as these are especially damaging in young animals, and most vaccines are unnecessary. And if you have not read the chapter overview (above), please do so as well, and read Chapter Seventeen, "The Bigger Picture," and reconsider your decision.

Some of the suggestions here are rather rote, such as those for pregnancy maintenance, while others are more individualized. This is partly because certain conditions are common and thus individual prescribing is difficult, and partly because not many remedies are known for the conditions.

Pregnancy

For pregnancy maintenance and optimal function of the uterus during pregnancy you can give homeopathic remedies during the last two weeks of gestation. Give *Caulophyllum* 6C, 12C, or 30X every other day. On the alternate day give *Calcarea phosphorica* 6X or 6C. These remedies tonify the uterus, and the *Calcarea phosphorica* also promotes calcium uptake and utilization so the mother can provide calcium for bone and milk formation. It is important to provide extra calcium in the diet as well during the last three weeks of gestation and during nursing. Bone meal is best, as it provides calcium and phosphorus, and you avoid the problem of upsetting the balance between these two elements. You do not need to give much; about one-fourth to one-half teaspoon per ten pounds daily is enough. Better yet, if you offer her fresh raw bones (not cooked—they splinter), she will probably eat these and obtain the extra calcium and phosphorus that way.

Raspberry leaf is also beneficial for pregnant mothers. Make a tea with one tablespoonful of dry leaves per quart of boiled water. Pour the water over the leaves and allow it to steep until cool. Give one dropperful per ten to twenty pounds, one or two times a day.

Labor

As labor approaches, she will become restless and will search for a place to deliver her babies. Usually this is someplace dark and secluded. She may carry clothing or other soft items to her chosen area to make a nest. This usually occurs a few days prior to delivery. On the day of delivery, the restlessness increases. She usually stops eating a day or two before delivery as well. She may also simply disappear and go to her nest. Begin giving *Arnica* every six to twelve hours the last day before delivery (as best as you can guess this) to prepare her for the pain of delivery. If she is having mild contractions but not delivering in good time, give *Caulophyllum* 30C once every one-half to one hour for three to four doses. If there is no response, try *Secale cornutum* in the same manner. If she seems to have no uterine tone or contractions, give some extra calcium as this is needed for uterine muscle contraction. Give the remedy *Plumbum metallicum* if *Secale* has not helped and she is generally weak. If available, the remedy *Opium* is also helpful, especially if her weakness is combined with sleepiness. (Even though there is no detectable drug present in the homeopathic form of *Opium*, the FDA considers it a Schedule I narcotic, so it is not available in the United States.)

For anxiety before delivery, try Rescue Remedy (the Bach flower preparation) or its equivalent. You may also give the homeopathic medicine *Gelsemium*.

For pain during delivery, *Arnica* is usually effective. Other remedies for labor pains include *Secale*, *Nux vomica*, and *Coffea*.

Postpartum Conditions (after Delivery)

Pain

Following delivery, use *Arnica* as needed to control the pains. If this is not helpful, try *Hypericum*, *Ruta graveolens*, or *Bellis perennis*. Use any strength up to 30C every few hours.

Hemorrhage

Bleeding is normal following delivery, but it should significantly abate within one to four hours. Minimal bleeding may occur for a day or so, but this should be no more than a trickle. If she bleeds more than this, give the homeopathic medicine *Ipecac* every fifteen minutes to every hour or two as needed. If this does not stem the bleeding, try *Phosphorus* or *Millefolium*, or if the blood is dark, try *Lachesis*. If she has a retained placenta (see below) and bleeds excessively, try *Pulsatilla*.

Retained Placenta

Occasionally, the placenta is not completely cleared after delivery. Delivery of the placenta (afterbirth) normally occurs within a few hours to a day after delivery. If the placenta is retained, you may see continued bleeding or discharging fluids that become foul-smelling. If you believe the mother did not clear everything, give her *Caulophyllum* or *Secale* in the highest potency you have. You may need to repeat the dose every few hours. If bleeding occurs due to a retained placenta, give *Pulsatilla*.

Postpartum Infections

If infection develops after delivery, it may be due to a retained placenta or to trauma and contamination during the birth process. See a veterinarian for assistance with these conditions. The conventional treatment is antibiotics, but since the puppies or kittens will also get the antibiotics via the milk, you may try one of the following homeopathic medicines instead, unless she is very ill.

Start with *Caulophyllum* or *Secale* (as above, under "Retained Placenta") to encourage uterine contractions and cleansing of all afterbirth. Additionally, give her echinacea and goldenseal (herbal) to assist her immune system. Prepare a tea by steeping one tablespoonful of each in a pint of water; give one dropperful per ten pounds, two to three times a day. Give vitamin C as well (5–10 mg/pound, two to three times a day). Then choose one of the remedies described above in the section on "Discharges from the Vulva" to stimulate the healing process. Especially consider *Echinacea, Pyrogenium, Sabina,* and *Sepia*—although you should use the remedy that fits her symptoms the best; it may be one of the other remedies.

Consider also these remedies:

Arnica montana
Use *Arnica* if the birth was especially traumatic and she is painful and afraid of touch.

Arsenicum album
This remedy may be needed if she is chilly, thirsty, and restless. She may also be weak and vomiting, and may have a black, bloody discharge.

Rhus toxicodendron
This remedy picture is similar to that of *Arsenicum* but is not so severe. There is often red swelling of the eyelids or the vulva.

Eclampsia

Occasionally, the calcium requirements of late gestation and nursing deplete the blood and body calcium of the mother. This is primarily (probably only) a problem in the bitch rather than the queen. When the calcium level falls, this affects nerve and muscle function and results in a state of continued muscle contraction. This includes the heart muscle. The result is a dog that is in a constant spasm and who is panting, hyperexcitable, and overheated. The muscles twitch and jerk constantly and incessantly. She looks like you might imagine if she were plugged into electric current. *This condition is potentially fatal and should be treated by a veterinarian immediately.* Intravenous calcium will rapidly stop the condition. Do not avoid treatment, but you may try one of the following remedies along with oral calcium while you are on the way to the veterinary clinic. Use caution as you give anything orally, as her muscle spasms may cause her to bite you inadvertently.

Homeopathic Medicines for Eclampsia

Use whatever one you have at hand—don't take time to go to a store or a friend's to get one. Just get her to a veterinary clinic. If you have a choice, give the highest potency available.

Belladonna
She will have dilated pupils and will be very hot. She may be aggressive.

Cicuta virosa
Here the pupils may be dilated, crossed, or turned outward. Her head may be twisted to one side. The spine or neck may be bent backward, and she may have facial contortions. There may be bloody foam coming from her mouth.

Hyoscyamus
In this case, there may be some weakness along with the trembling and spasms. The pupils may be dilated. In the early stage the tremors may alternate with sleepiness.

Magnesia phosphorica
Mag phos is great for cramping anywhere, and can be helpful here to minimize the discomfort. Use the tissue salt, in a 6X, and give one to four tablets every five minutes or so. You may also dissolve four to six tablets in an ounce of water and give this by dropperful, repeating as needed. Most health food stores have this remedy.

Nux vomica

These animals may be irritable along with the muscle spasms. This remedy is common and may be more available. Noise often incites more spasms.

Stramonium

The spasms may occur in one leg or another, or one part of the body or another. She may also stumble as if she were drunk. Bright lights often trigger the spasms. Her pupils may be dilated.

Strychninum

Strychnine poisoning is very similar to eclampsia tetany. The muscles twitch and jerk violently, and any touch or noise incites a great spasm. This remedy is made from strychnine, and it is a good choice if available.

Finally, if none of these are available, try *Calcarea carbonica* or *Calcarea phosphorica* to encourage calcium utilization by the body.

Neonatal Care

Rejection of Puppies or Kittens

Most mothers take to their babies immediately after delivery is complete. At this time the mother cleans the infants and begins to nurse them. Occasionally a mother will not be so enthusiastic. Some will ignore the babies and want attention themselves; some will even be aggressive toward the infants; and some will simply ignore their young. Consider *Sepia* first, especially for mothers who show no interest in the babies. If the mother is aggressive toward her young, *Secale cornutum* may change her attitude. And for the mother who wants attention herself and thus places the infants behind her needs, try *Pulsatilla*. These "*Pulsatilla* mothers" may find nursing painful or they may have scanty milk, so they may cry out when the puppies or kittens try to nurse (see the section on mammary problems).

Weak Kittens or Puppies

For newborns that seem weak and listless, first give *Arnica* for the shock and trauma of birth. Also give Rescue Remedy (the Bach flower remedy) or its equivalent. If this does not revive them, give *Thuja*, or if they are weak and especially cold, give *Carbo vegetabilis*. If they cry constantly, *Thuja* or *Pulsatilla* may be beneficial.

For those kittens or puppies that still do not respond or that simply do not thrive despite a good mother and a lack of obvious problems, try either *Baryta carbonica, Calcarea carbonica, Magnesia carbonica,* or *Calcarea phosphorica.* Those needing *Calc carb* tend to be bulky and clumsy. *Mag carb* newborns are often very anxious and nervous. If *Baryta carb* is needed, the puppy or kitten is very dull and may hide constantly. *Calc phos* newborns will usually be thin and more frail than heavy. Always have a puppy or kitten that is especially weak examined by a veterinarian, as there may be a birth defect.

Runts, Dwarfishness

Runts are in the same category as those above, although the condition leads to permanent changes in the body. I recommend consulting a homeopathic practitioner, as some of the best remedies are very deep-acting ones that are available by prescription only. Otherwise the remedies listed above *(Baryta carb, Calc carb, Calc phos,* and *Mag carb)* may be useful. Also consider *Lycopodium clavatum* for puppies that are "momma's boys" (they are mostly male), and *Sulphur* if the animal is scruffy, thin, and dirty.

Mammary Problems

Inadequate Milk Flow

Sometimes the mother does not begin producing milk right away, or she just does not produce enough milk for her offspring. Be sure not to feed her any parsley, as this may diminish the flow. In some cases homeopathic remedies may improve this condition. Try one of the following, according to her condition:

Asafoetida
In these mothers, the milk appears late and then diminishes too soon. They may be rather sensitive individuals.

Calcarea carbonica
Heavy mothers who have large or swollen breasts but little milk.

Calcarea phosphorica
Thin mothers who look undernourished even though they are well fed. There may be a calcium deficiency in these animals. Use this remedy along with extra calcium.

Lac caninum

The milk flow starts out fine but then diminishes too soon and too rapidly.

Lactuca virosa

Lactuca is "a true galactogogue" in that it improves milk flow. It is good for negative thinking in general, so perhaps for mothers who are reticent about caring for their young; the lack of nourishment they provide is physical as well as emotional. Use in low potency (3X, 6X, 6C).

Medusa

This is the jellyfish, and concomitant symptoms can include a puffy, edematous face. It can restore lactation in mothers with a history of inadequate flow.

Pulsatilla

Use this remedy for mothers that prefer getting attention from their guardians to giving attention to their babies. The milk flow is often scanty and the breasts swollen and painful when nursing, so she cries out when the newborns try to nurse.

If none of the above remedies seems appropriate, try one of the following (listed in order of usage frequency):

Urtica urens in 30C and higher potency (low potencies may diminish flow.)
Ricinus communis in low potency—3X, 6X, 6C
Spiranthes in low potency

Herbs that can promote milk flow in humans include alfalfa, blessed thistle, fennel, fenugreek, chaste berry, goats rue, and vervain.

To Dry Up Milk Following Weaning

Give *Urtica urens* in low potency—3X, 6X, 6C—every few hours. *Lac caninum, Pulsatilla,* or *Spiranthes* may help if *Urtica* does not; give 30C one or two times. Parsley water or parsley tea will often reduce milk production. Warm compresses may alleviate the mother's discomfort. Other herbs to diminish flow include lemon balm, sage, peppermint, spearmint, bugleweed, sorrel, and periwinkle.

Bad Milk

Occasionally the milk becomes mildly infected, and the puppies or kittens may also become ill, or they may refuse to nurse. If you lightly squeeze on the nipple to get some milk, it will appear yellowish or even bloody (pinkish) instead of white. Feed the babies with a bottle until the milk clears if the mother is experiencing pain or the milk seems very foul. If it is only mildly discolored and the newborns continue to nurse, this can be helpful to clear the infection.

Herbs that can be helpful include raspberry leaf, dandelion, nettles, echinacea, and goldenseal. Make a tea of one to three of these by using up to a tablespoonful of dry herb per pint of boiling water. Pour the water over the herb and allow to steep until cool, then give one dropperful per ten to twenty pounds, two to three times a day. Don't use goldenseal for more than a week or two (only a week in cats) without stopping for a week, as it is a strong herb. If you can get her to take a dropperful or two of diluted apple cider vinegar (one tablespoonful of vinegar per cup of water) two or three times a day, this may also help. Acidophilus is helpful in all infections as well.

Try one of the following homeopathic remedies; see your veterinarian if the milk does not clear within a few days.

Borax

The milk tends to be thick and it has a bad taste, so the kittens or puppies often refuse to nurse. The newborns or the mother may have mouth ulcers, and either may be extremely frightened of downward motion such as when you put them down or they (or you, carrying them) are going down steps.

Calcarea carbonica

When *Calc carb* is needed, the milk is thin and has a poor taste. The mother's breasts may be swollen with poor milk flow, and her nipples may be cracked and painful. She may be heavy and big-boned.

Chamomilla

Here the milk is also bad, and the puppies or kittens refuse to nurse. The mother or the babies may be whiny and restless but difficult to console by petting or holding them. Sometimes carrying them around will help. The nipples and breasts may be quite painful.

Mercurius (vivus or *solubilis)*
These mothers are often irritable, and they may have a putrid discharge from the vulva in addition to the discolored milk. Diarrhea may also accompany these symptoms.

Silicea (Silica)
Mothers needing this remedy tend to tire easily. They often appear delicate. The milk is yellowish, and the nipples may be sore and cracked. There may be a bloody discharge from the vulva when the babies nurse.

Mastitis

If the breasts become hot, swollen, and painful, the inflammation has progressed beyond a mild condition. There may be an intense infection or possibly only a plugged milk duct. Have the mother examined by a veterinarian to determine the extent of the inflammation. Conventional care is usually antibiotics. If the condition is not too bad, you may wish to try home treatment at first; you may also use these recommendations along with conventional treatment if you feel the latter is necessary. Nursing can help if the milk ducts become plugged. Try warm compresses and massage (if she will allow it) to release the milk, then place a puppy or kitten on the affected teat. Additionally, use the herbs as suggested above under "Bad Milk."

Use one of the following homeopathic remedies as indicated:

Apis mellifica
The mammae will generally be bright red, shiny, and swollen but fluid-filled (edematous). They are usually painful. The mother is usually thirstless and prefers cool, open air.

Arnica montana
Use this remedy first if the mastitis occurred after an injury. See also *Bellis perennis.*

Belladonna
In these cases the breasts are very red and hot, and the mother is often very agitated and restless. Her pupils may dilate with the pain, and she may become irritable.

Bellis perennis
This remedy is very useful for mastitis after injury, especially for blunt trauma. It is similar to *Arnica*, and possibly more useful for breast injuries.

Bryonia alba
When *Bryonia* is needed, the breasts are also hot, very hard, and painful. Any motion increases the pain, so the mother stays still. She is usually thirsty and may be irritable.

Conium maculatum
Conium is often needed for mammary complaints when the breast is stony hard or has stony hard nodules. This remedy may also be useful in mastitis after an injury if hard knots occur as a result. It is often useful in older animals and those who are weak.

Hepar sulphuris calcareum
Hepar sulph is a good remedy for abscesses and may be useful for mastitis that forms an abscess. The affected breast will be extremely sensitive to touch, and the discharge or the milk will be very foul-smelling. These animals are usually chilly, and they can be very irritable.

Lac caninum
The symptoms are similar to those of *Bryonia* in that any jarring, such as walking up or down stairs, intensifies the pain. When this remedy is needed, the condition often alternates sides of the body. Thus the inflammation may start on one side but move to the other and then back to the original side; this can occur surprisingly quickly.

Phytolacca
This is a remedy with strong affinity to the mammary glands. When it is needed for mastitis, the glands are usually very hard, quite painful to touch, and may be purplish. The milk is often thick, coagulated, and stringy. These inflammations heal very slowly. The pains are so severe that she may moan. *Phytolacca* inflammations often occur after the patient has become chilled.

Urtica urens

This remedy may be needed for mastitis if the breasts are edematous (soft, fluid swelling) and have a rash or reddish blotchy appearance. Remember that low potencies of *Urtica* diminish milk flow and higher potencies (above 30C) encourage flow. Milk flow is usually helpful for mastitis, so use 30C if available.

Injury to the Breast

In the initial stage try *Arnica* or *Bellis perennis;* if further inflammation develops, consider *Conium* or *Phytolacca.* See above for descriptions.

Chapter Fifteen
THERAPEUTIC INDICATIONS BY CONDITION

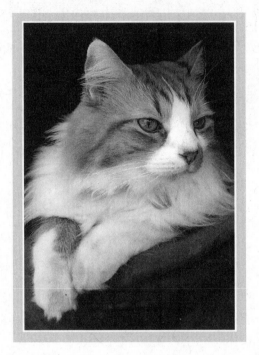

Overview

Abscesses

Allergic Reactions

Bites of Cats and Dogs

Bites of Snakes

Cuts and Lacerations

Diabetes Mellitus

Drug Reactions

Euthanasia

Fear

Fear of Noises

Fever and Infections

Fleas

Food and Garbage Poisoning

Grief

Heart Disease

Heartworm

Hemorrhage

Hyperactivity

Liver Disorders

New Puppy or Kitten

Overheating (Heatstroke, Sunstroke)

Surgery

Thyroid Disease

Vaccine Reactions

Worms (Intestinal)

Overview

In this chapter I will cover various conditions that do not fit into other chapters in the book. Some are specific situations such as injuries or what to do if your companion needs surgery. Others are more serious conditions, like thyroid disease, which should be treated by an experienced homeopathic veterinarian rather than at home. For the latter situations, I will give suggestions for supportive care but not for primary care. They are often treatable with homeopathy but are too complex for unskilled prescribers to treat.

Even though many of the following conditions are addressed somewhat specifically rather than from a classical homeopathic perspective, the classical approach is still important. The remedy you choose must fit your companion's overall state. Thus if your dog sprains his leg, you might immediately reach for *Arnica*, but perhaps he is not afraid of touch or the leg is not really painful. Instead, he limps badly when he first rises from lying down but quickly improves. *Rhus tox* might be a better choice and may help him, whereas the *Arnica* does not. This is the crux of homeopathy—seeing him as an individual who responds in his own way to a stress, and treating his response rather than just the common stress. See the introductory chapters on homeopathic principles for more information if you have not already read them. Or read them again; this information is difficult to grasp on one pass. And don't forget to read about the remedies in the *materia medica* to confirm your choices.

Abscesses

The first sign of an abscess is usually a soft swelling under the skin. It may be painful, although many times there is little or no pain. Often you will recall that your cat was in a fight a day or so prior to the appearance of the swelling. Abscesses occur much more frequently in cats than dogs, and cats generally handle them better than dogs. When a dog has an abscess, it is more likely to cause generalized illness, and it is more serious, though most can still be handled at home.

An abscess occurs when an infection develops in a part of the body that is capable of opening into a pocket. Most commonly this happens under the skin as a result of a puncture wound. Bites and scratches from fighting are the primary cause. Sometimes an abscess will develop elsewhere if there is a space that can become a pocket. The area around a tooth root is a good example of this. These pockets fill with pus, which is an accumulation of dead bacteria and dead inflammatory cells (primarily white blood cells) that have moved into the area to attempt to eliminate the bacterial overgrowth. Pocketing is also the result of the body's walling off the infection to spare the rest of the body; in this way an abscess is good management of infections.

Eventually, if the inflammatory cells cannot clean up the infection on their own, the pus accumulates to the point that the abscess must rupture. The rupture occurs because the increased pressure from the pus interferes with circulation on the surface and weakens it, allowing the pus to exit. Usually, this creates an opening through the skin to the outside of the body and facilitates elimination of the infection. In rare circumstances with internal abscesses, the rupture may drain into a body cavity (such as the abdomen or chest). This is serious. In this section, I am only addressing abscesses that can rupture to the outside—usually those under the skin.

After rupturing to the outside, in most cases the body finishes the cleanup on its own. In a few cases, the wound will close over and the abscess will recur; this sometimes happens numerous times. The resultant wound from a big rupture can look quite nasty, but these usually heal fairly well and much more rapidly than you might expect.

Although conventional veterinarians usually prescribe antibiotics for abscesses, these are rarely needed. Most animals can heal an abscess with the support of homeopathic treatment.

General Care for Abscesses

The main conditions that require the assistance of a veterinarian are listlessness (any listless animal should be examined right away) and abscesses that do not heal within a few days to a week. If the abscess does not rupture or diminish within a couple of days and your companion seems to worsen, take him in right away. If his energy remains strong, you may work with him a bit longer.

If the abscess is immediately adjacent to the eye, the anus, or the genitals, you should also have an examination to be sure there is no risk to these organs. Additionally, if there is a draining opening on the feet it may indicate a foreign body, especially if you live in the western United States where foxtails (grass seed heads) are common. For foreign bodies, see the section "Foxtails and Foreign Bodies" in the ear portion of Chapter Six, "Skin and Ears."

As with any infection, immune-building vitamins and herbs can help. Vitamin C (5–10 mg/pound, two to three times a day, with natural C if available), vitamin E (5–10 mg/pound, once a day, mixed tocopherols) and vitamin A (75–100 IU daily) are helpful. Echinacea and goldenseal can also boost the immune system, although I recommend limiting goldenseal administration to a week. The best method for administering herbs is a tea (infusion). Use the dry herbs (one teaspoonful dry herb to one cup water) and pour boiling water over them. Allow it to cool, and strain off the herb. Give one-half to one dropperful per ten pounds, two to three times a day. If you have a commercially prepared tincture, give about five drops per ten pounds, two to three times a day, as these are generally stronger than a tea.

Before the abscess has ruptured, you will see the swelling, and you may see evidence of a fight or other wound. In most cases it is best to encourage the abscess to rupture to facilitate removal of pus. Warm compresses stimulate development of the abscess (bringing it to a head). These should be applied three to four times a day. Simply run warm water onto a cloth until it is saturated and then hold this over the abscess for about five minutes. Longer may be more helpful. Some animals will not tolerate the pressure, as the abscess is painful. This helps to differentiate the indicated homeopathic medicine. The correct remedy will usually hasten rupture and thus healing. In some cases with small abscesses, the remedy may initiate reabsorption of pus and healing without rupture. When this happens, the swelling will simply diminish *as the animal improves overall.*

If the abscess does not rupture and does not reduce in size within a day or two, the abscess may need to be lanced. This may be needed about 10 to 15 percent of the time. Ask your veterinarian if she can simply lance the abscess without using anesthesia, since this is usually unnecessary. A quick lancing is relatively painless and much less traumatic than hospitalization and anesthesia. The argument for anesthesia is that the abscess can be cleaned better, which is true, but it is mostly unnecessary.

Once the abscess has opened, it is important to keep the resulting wound clean and open so any pus that forms can continue to discharge. This is accomplished by continuing the warm compresses as well as flushing the wound with a solution of *Calendula* and *Hypericum* (St. John's wort) in saline. You may also use *Aristolochia clematitis* (if available), a very good wound cleanser—possibly better than *Calendula*—or goldenseal. Use one-fourth teaspoon of table salt and ten drops of each herbal tincture per cup of water. If you boil the water first, it will sterilize it; as it cools, add the salt and the herbs. Allow it to cool to body temperature before using the rinse. Use a basting syringe or an ear syringe to gently rinse out the abscess. Do this three to four times a day until the wound is clearly healing on its own. *Calendula* stimulates healing and will improve the rate of closure. In some cases of deep abscesses, it will close the wound before the infection is cleared. In abscesses that are especially large or deep, you might use *Hypericum* alone for the first few days and add the *Calendula* later. In this case, use fifteen to twenty drops of *Hypericum* per cup of water and salt.

After the infection has cleared and the wound is clean but not healed, you may use a *Calendula* ointment (so it stays on the wound longer) to stimulate closure.

Homeopathic Medicines for Abscesses

Most abscesses will respond to one of a very few remedies, though there are over a hundred remedies that may be indicated. I usually start with either *Silicea, Hepar sulph,* or *Gunpowder,* as these are effective in many cases. Since I wrote the first edition, I became acquainted with *Gunpowder* as a homeopathic remedy, and it is a marvelous remedy for abscesses and bite wounds. I now consider it as one of the top choices. If you do not get a response or if another choice seems indicated, however, try another remedy or call for assistance. I remember a case that was not responding to either remedy. The guardian had told me a couple of times that her cat was very easily startled, but I had not paid sufficient attention to that detail, as I thought *Silicea* would heal the abscess. Finally, I took the statement more seriously and prescribed *Phosphorus,* a remedy that is well known for this noise sensitivity and tendency to startle. The abscess healed quickly and nicely from that point on. We must individualize our cases if we desire success, and we all forget this at times.

Arnica montana

We know *Arnica* best for trauma, and it can prevent formation of abscesses if given at the time of an injury. I usually use it right away after a bite wound to try to avoid an abscess. It may be useful for abscesses that have formed if they have the *Arnica* characteristic of great pain and fear of touch. *Hepar sulph* is similar, but the animal is aggressive and may scratch or bite, whereas the *Arnica* patient mostly tries to get away.

Calcarea sulphurica

This remedy is useful once the abscess has ruptured and the pus is discharging, as it speeds further healing. If your first remedy gets the abscess draining but cannot complete the healing, consider this one (also *Sulphur*). The pus is usually yellow.

Calendula officinalis

Calendula may be used in potency in addition to topical use to stimulate wound healing. Remember that in deep wounds it may close the surface too quickly, so use it only with wounds that are well closed under the skin (see above).

Guiacum

For stubborn abscesses that do not open up and drain, consider *Guiacum*, as it has a reputation for promoting suppuration of abscesses. It just may get the abscess to rupture open, which in many cases is critical to healing.

Gunpowder

Yes, this is actually gunpowder, and it is a great remedy for bites and abscesses. It has become one of my favorite remedies in these circumstances. It is especially helpful when the infection involves bone, but is useful in many abscessed/infected wounds.

Hepar sulphuris calcareum

This is one of the three big abscess remedies. The state that calls for *Hepar sulph* is a condition in which the pus is especially foul-smelling (yes, some are worse than others) and the wound is particularly painful. These animals often scratch or bite when you try to examine or treat the wound. Even if they don't bite, they will often growl fiercely enough to make you nervous.

Lachesis

This remedy is made from the venom of the bushmaster snake. Imagine a snake bite wound, and you have a picture of what the remedy can treat. These abscesses are severe, and there is a lot of damage to tissues around the area. The pus or wound edges may be bluish to blackish; there may also be dark blood coming from the wound. These animals may also bite or scratch, though they will tolerate a moderate amount of handling before they reach the breaking point. (Despite their undeserved reputation for aggression, most snakes prefer not to bite and only do so as a defense except when seeking food. To do otherwise simply wastes venom.)

Mercurius (vivus or solubilis)

This remedy is also indicated for more serious abscesses. Here the pus tends to be greenish-yellow, and it may irritate the skin around the opening. The lymph nodes ("glands") may be swollen near the area. These patients are similar to those needing *Hepar sulph*. They may have diarrhea as an accompaniment. Often these animals are ill and somewhat listless from the abscess.

Myristica sebifera

The primary indication for this remedy is removal of foreign bodies. I list it here because many apparent abscesses turn out to be discharging pus in an attempt to remove a foreign body. This remedy is excellent in these cases.

Nitric acid

These animals are at least as angry and vicious as those needing *Hepar sulph*. The wound is very painful, and these animals may viciously attack anyone who tries to attend to the abscess. The pus is quite foul. The abscess may be near a body opening (anus, prepuce, vulva, mouth, nose) where the skin and the mucous membrane meet.

Phosphorus

The startling reaction (see above in the introduction to this section) is most characteristic. There may also be bright red blood along with the pus.

Pyrogenium

When the abscess is foul and the animal is very ill, this remedy may be needed. The patient is generally restless, as he is achy due to the generalized infection and cannot find a comfortable position. The wound and the pus will typically be quite foul, though it may not discharge much because his reaction is very low. This remedy is often needed when the abscess has opened several times and the patient continues to deteriorate (compare with *Silicea* and *Sulphur*).

Silicea (Silica)

This is one of the most useful remedies for abscesses. In these cases the pus is bland and yellowish to brown. While all pus has a bad odor, the pus here may be less foul than in other cases. The cat may be sluggish and somewhat weak but not so severely debilitated as those needing *Pyrogenium* or *Mercurius*. Another indication is that the abscess may drain constantly while the animal remains generally healthy (see *Sulphur*). The key is that these animals have difficulty mounting a strong enough response to heal the wound. This remedy often will initiate rupture of abscesses that are slow to come to a head.

Sulphur

I find this remedy helpful for those abscesses that continue to rupture and close a number of times, though the animal stays relatively healthy. Often these patients are dirty and do not bother to attempt to clean themselves, or give a half-hearted effort—rare in a cat. Whereas *Sulphur* patients are typically warm, when they have abscesses they may be chilly. Like those needing *Silicea*, these animals cannot mount a strong inflammatory response.

Tarentula cubensis

If the abscess is purplish and painful, this remedy may alleviate the condition. Often the animal is quite restless and painful when *Tarentula cubensis* is needed. Severe inflammation and malignant suppuration call for this remedy—meaning conditions wherein the infection is rather intense and aggressive compared to the typical abscess.

Allergic Reactions

In this segment, I refer to immediate short-term reactions rather than chronic allergies such as those that underlie many skin illnesses. The most common allergic reactions are to stinging insects; these are covered in Chapter Six, "Skin and Ears."

Vaccines are another frequent culprit, and these are covered later in this chapter. Often, however, you simply do not know the inciting event. In these cases one of the remedies below may be helpful.

The most common allergic reactions are swelling, redness, and hives. Often itching accompanies the visible response. Sometimes when swelling occurs, the patient develops breathing difficulty as well, and this can be dangerous. Breathing troubles usually show up within fifteen minutes to an hour after the other symptoms.

Most allergic reactions are manifested by histamine and related compounds. Histamine does not cause the allergy; rather it is released in response to the allergen and creates the above reactions either locally or systemically.

Antihistamines are drugs that block the effect of histamine. For this reason, they can be helpful in allergic reactions. I do not usually recommend drugs, and for most allergic reactions I would not use antihistamines, but if swelling occurs and/or there is any hint of breathing troubles, an antihistamine could be a lifesaver. These drugs must be given quickly, however, as they do not reverse the histamine effect, they only block further impact. If your companion has a history of respiratory difficulty due to an allergic reaction, giving an antihistamine immediately is probably a good idea. If the response is mostly skin irritation, I would not recommend antihistamines unless the response is very intense and homeopathic medicines prove ineffective.

General Care for Allergic Reactions

See a veterinarian immediately:
- if she develops any breathing difficulty;
- if swelling around the face is severe, because breathing problems may follow shortly. In these cases, it is often best to head for a clinic in case respiratory troubles start.

See your veterinarian soon:
- if you see no response to treatment within a few hours (facial swelling) to a day or so (hives);
- if the condition worsens.

Vitamin C (5–10 mg/pound, two to three times a day, using natural C if available) and vitamin E (5–10 mg/pound, once a day, mixed tocopherols) may be helpful in preventing allergic attacks in sensitive animals. The B vitamins (about 1 mg–mcg—as appropriate for each B vitamin—per pound) may help minimize the reaction. Coenzyme Q_{10} may also minimize the reaction.

If you must use antihistamines, Benadryl (diphenhydramine) and chlorpheniramine are fairly commonly available. Use the former at 1–2 mg/pound and the latter at the dose of 2 mg per ten to twenty pounds—up to 8 mg total (chlorpheniramine) in a big dog. Diphenhydramine may be given every eight hours and chlorpheniramine every twelve hours if needed. Often only one or two doses are needed.

The other drugs that help with allergic reactions are corticosteroids ("cortisone"). These will reverse an allergic reaction. Use these in an emergency only (i.e. for breathing difficulty) as directed by your veterinarian. However, if you take your companion in for an allergic reaction but he does not develop breathing troubles, I suggest avoiding corticosteroids. Allow the body to handle the reaction, or use antihistamines if necessary. The other symptoms are not a problem.

Homeopathic Medicines for Allergic Reactions

Apis mellifica

This is the primary remedy for swelling and for respiratory difficulty. If you see facial swelling, give *Apis* right away. It may prevent respiratory problems, but if you see respiratory impairment, give the remedy and take your companion directly to a veterinary clinic.

Arsenicum album

This remedy may help if the animal is restless and weak. The skin may itch intensely and may have hives, or there may be no physical change. *Arsenicum* may be helpful when breathing is impaired without facial swelling.

Histaminum

This is histamine, the primary chemical messenger that carries out the allergic response. It can sometimes provide acute help with any allergic reaction. Itchy skin and itchy, watery eyes are common indications.

Medusa

Medusa is made from a jellyfish, so you can imagine the swelling that may occur when this remedy is needed. The *Medusa* state is like the *Apis* state but much more intense, with puffy swelling of the entire face, eyes, nose, ears, and lips. Affected areas may burn and sting, so the patient will rub the face or wherever the swelling is located. There may be blisters or other signs of an eruption on the face as well. This is an uncommon remedy, so you won't find it locally, but if your dog or cat suffers from allergies with facial swelling, consider ordering this remedy to have "just in case."

Rhus toxicodendron
This remedy, made from poison ivy, can help with hives that are accompanied by great itching and restlessness. The itching is improved by hot applications or hot bathing. There may be swelling around the eyes.

Urtica urens
Urtica is made from the stinging nettle. This is perhaps the best remedy for most allergic hives. The hives itch and sting intensely. Often there are red patches of skin as well. Increased frequency of urination may accompany the hives.

See also Chapter Six, "Skin and Ears," especially the section on "Insect Bites and Stings."

Bites of Cats and Dogs

Unless a bite wound is clearly superficial, I recommend that you have a veterinarian examine your companion if he has been bitten. This is especially true of dog bites, as there is more force behind the bite. If the wound is over an area that has internal organs underneath, an examination is even more important. On the other hand, if you are sure that there is only muscle underneath, you may not need an exam, though it never hurts to be certain there is not deep trauma.

One of the strangest things I have seen in practice—and I've seen it twice—was the result of a dog biting a cat. In both cases, the guardians knew that their cats had been attacked by a dog. When I examined the cats, there was no trace of a puncture wound on the skin, but upon examination I found that the underlying abdominal wall was torn. This in itself is actually rather common, as the skin is elastic while the abdominal wall is not. It is common to find more damage under a bite than one might expect based upon the skin damage, especially in cats, with their loose skin. What is so odd in these two cases is that not only was the abdominal wall torn, but a loop of intestine was lacerated as well. In both cats I examined the skin thoroughly, especially after discovering the intestinal wounds during surgery. I still find it puzzling. Usually there is a puncture wound in the skin and extensive damage below, and this is understandable. You never can be sure just what the extent of the damage is in these cases, so an examination is generally useful.

You can also use these remedies if you are unfortunate enough to be bitten by an animal, though you may need to seek medical care. I have assisted two clients with cat bite wounds on themselves, and the remedy *Gunpowder* was the next thing to a miracle, so I would start there if you are bitten, especially if by a cat. Of course, if you are bitten by an animal in a situation that did not make sense (an unprovoked attack), be sure to seek medical help. Tetanus is a possibility also, though not too common with bites.

Once you determine that the wound is relatively minor, home treatment is fine. Antibiotics are usually unnecessary, though they are commonly prescribed. Wound cleanliness is important, as is management of the trauma. See above in the section "General Care for Abscesses" for helpful supplements and an herbal wash for wounds. Use the wash three to four times a day to cleanse the area. See your veterinarian if the wound begins to smell badly or is not healing. One of the following homeopathic remedies may help speed the healing process. Consider also any of the remedies listed above, under "Abscesses."

Homeopathic Medicines for Cat and Dog Bites

Acetic acid
If your companion is extremely listless following a bite wound, this remedy may help him regain his strength. This is especially true if the wound does not seem severe enough to warrant the prostration.

Arnica montana
I generally use *Arnica* first as it is so useful for trauma of almost any sort. It can prevent abscesses and minimize tissue trauma. Reduced tissue damage means better and faster healing. It is especially useful for the animal who is afraid of touch because of the pain.

Gunpowder
Now my first choice for cat bites, this remedy is unexcelled in averting trouble from bite wounds and potential abscesses. It is a marvelous remedy here.

Hypericum perforatum
This remedy is great for wounds that involve areas with a lot of nerves, such

as the toes, tongue, and tail. It relieves pain in the nerves better than *Arnica*. If your companion is bitten in one of these areas and *Arnica* does not relieve the pain, especially if the pain is intense, try *Hypericum*. I was bitten on the finger by a cat once and took this remedy; I was pleasantly surprised at how rapidly the pain diminished—within a minute or two.

Lachesis

Lachesis is needed for bite wounds that turn dark blue to black. This is usually due to the especially traumatic nature of the bite. Often, this occurs from an aggressive fight when the bite was vicious. These wounds tend to become infected because the circulation to the wound is compromised.

Ledum palustre

As the best-known remedy for puncture wounds, *Ledum* is another good choice for bite wounds, especially if they are primarily punctures rather than lacerations. The wound may twitch and the area around the wound may be cold to the touch. *Ledum* is said to be a preventive against tetanus. It is usually the first remedy to give when the puncture is from a rusty nail or similar object.

Lyssin

This is the homeopathic nosode for rabies. It should be administered by a homeopathic veterinarian, but in cases where your companion was viciously attacked, it may be of use to prevent transmission of the aggressive tendency. See "Aggression and the Rabies Miasm" in Chapter Thirteen, "Nervous System."

Myristica sebifera

Myristica is "a remedy of great antiseptic powers," and may be useful with bites when the wound ulcerates. Inflammation is rather intense, with damage to skin around the wound. It is especially helpful in encouraging suppuration and discharging of foreign material, including infection.

Vespa crabro

This is the European hornet, and so when needed, bite wounds will be hot and painful, like a hornet sting. The patient may be dizzy or may lose consciousness. The eyes may be red, painful, and swollen.

Bites of Snakes

In the United States there are four groups of poisonous snakes that include over twenty species. The most common type is the rattlesnake family *(Crotalus* spp. and *Sistrurus* spp.). Next are the copperheads *(Agkistrodon contortrix* spp.) and the cottonmouths, or water moccasins *(Agkistrodon piscivorus* spp.). Finally, the rarest but most poisonous are the coral snakes *(Micrurus* spp.); these are related to cobras and mambas. Fortunately, coral snakes have small mouths, so they cannot easily bite humans except on the fingers, and even with most dogs this is a limitation. Coral snakes, copperheads, and water moccasins inhabit the southeastern United States only, while various rattlesnake species call much of the country home.

Despite their reputation for aggressiveness, in my experience most snakes are quite happy to leave humans alone unless they are threatened. With some species this requires quite a threat. Most of my experience with snakes (both growing up and as a practicing veterinarian) stems from my time in North Carolina. Copperheads and rattlesnakes (primarily the timber rattlesnake, *Crotalus horridus horridus)* were my primary teachers, although I saw a couple of water moccasins while I was growing up. As a veterinarian, well over 95 percent of the bites I saw were copperhead bites (and all of the bitten animals I saw were dogs—cats are generally too quick to be bitten and often catch snakes, including poisonous snakes). From this experience as well as talking with experienced woodsmen, I found that copperheads are rather aggressive and will often bite quickly. Apparently, their tolerance for intrusion is relatively low and the perceived threat is high.

In contrast, rattlesnakes—at least the timber rattlesnake—are fairly passive and tolerant. One time I was walking in the woods and came upon a dead chipmunk. I thought at the time that something was odd, but I did not recognize just what it was until later (the body was vividly marked, unlike what one would see in a long-dead animal). I reached down and touched the chipmunk, only to discover that the body was warm—quite a surprise. I looked about a foot away and immediately understood the situation, as I saw a rattlesnake patiently waiting for the chipmunk to die. I slowly stood up (believe it or not) and walked away. The snake had not moved the entire time, not even to rattle. I have heard similar stories about other people's encounters with timber rattlers. These snakes are not generally aggressive; indeed, they are passive. I have heard that some of the Western rattlesnake species are not so calm, but I do not know how true this is, or if it comes from our cultural snake phobia.

The cottonmouths apparently hold their ground rather than fleeing, though I do not know if they bite so readily as their copperhead relatives. I have no direct knowledge of coral snakes, but my understanding is that they are relatively peaceful. In addition, their mouths are quite small, and it is difficult for them to bite anything much larger than a finger or toe, though their venom is extremely poisonous.

Fortunately, the venom of the copperheads is relatively benign. I have never seen a dog die from a bite. The wounds swell tremendously and appear fairly painful, but they heal without incident in the vast majority of cases. Rattlesnake venom is much more deadly and causes great damage to the local area. Some dogs will die (though most survive), and the survivors are left with quite a wound because a large area of tissue dies and sloughs off. Cottonmouth venom is similar to that of copperheads, perhaps slightly stronger. Coral snake venom is toxic to the nervous system and is highly fatal, though it causes minimal damage to the bite area.

The best way to deal with snake bites is to avoid them. Use caution while walking in the woods or in open country where snakes live. It is impossible to deliver this message to your dog, but staying on well-used trails will minimize exposure. Please don't kill a snake just because you see it, however. Generally, if we leave them alone, they will respect us as well.

There is a vaccine made from western diamondback rattlesnake venom, but I do not recommend its use. I have seen some problems in animals following this vaccine, and its efficacy is questionable. The vaccine may not still be available, due to these issues, though to my knowledge it is still available as of this writing, at least in some states.

General Care for Snake Bites

If your dog is bitten by a snake, you should take him to your veterinarian. If you know it was a rattlesnake, I suggest you use the injectable antivenin if available and if the bite is recent—within a couple of hours. I do not recommend antivenin for copperhead bites, as the risk from the antivenin is greater than that from the copperhead venom. I have no experience with cottonmouth bites, but I would treat these as with copperhead bites unless your veterinarian believes the risk is as great as with a rattlesnake. Coral snake bites require antivenin, though I doubt the survival rate is good in many cases. As I mentioned, I have no direct experience with coral snakes, so ask a veterinarian in your area about the risk. (Coral snakes primarily live in the extreme Southeast and Texas, so fortunately they are not a concern for most of us.)

The wound can be treated like any bite wound with the flush solution given above in the section on abscesses. Additionally, *Echinacea, Cedron,* and the Western herb golondrina may help detoxify the venom if applied topically. Use one of the following homeopathic remedies, but seek assistance from your veterinarian.

Homeopathic Treatment for Snake Bite

Your remedy choice here is often hindered by what you have available. For any given remedy, use the highest potency you have on hand. Use in addition to veterinary care, not in lieu of care.

Immediately upon discovering the bite, give either *Ledum, Lachesis, Crotalus horridus,* or *Belladonna.* See the indications under dog and cat bites, above. If the dog is frantic, restless, and his pupils dilate easily, choose *Belladonna. Crotalus horridus* is the timber rattlesnake, so this remedy can be used as a sort of direct antidote; I had one cat patient who was bitten by a western diamondback rattlesnake, and *Crot-h* got him through. Apply any of the above herbs if available. *Cedron* or *Senega* may be given in low potency, like 6X, along with other remedies if you have them available. These are herbal remedies handed down from Native Americans, and they may offer supportive help. If the wound changes and begins to look worse, give *Arsenicum album, Lachesis, Cedron,* or *Vipera.* Consider also any remedy listed above for cat and dog bites or abscesses. If the patient collapses, give *Arsenicum* or, if he is extremely cold, *Camphora.* Give *Echinacea* or *Cedron* if he develops a generalized infection subsequent to the bite; this usually happens twelve to forty-eight hours after a rattlesnake bite and rarely after bites from other snakes. Consider also *Acetic acid* or *Carbo veg* for weak animals and *Pyrogenium* or *Carbolic acid* for infections.

For chronic ailments after snake bites, use *Mercurius* or *Phosphoric acid* according to symptoms, unless the symptoms indicate another remedy. It is also important to support the liver with snake bites, as the liver will be secondarily affected in most cases; see the section below on "Liver Disorders." I recommend consulting a homeopathic practitioner if your dog does not recover readily.

Cuts and Lacerations

Use the flushing solution described above, under "General Care for Abscesses," but see the note under *Calendula* below. *Aristolochia clematitis* or goldenseal may be better choices for deep or punctured wounds. Clean the wound three to four times a day. If the wound is longer than one-half to one inch, it may require suturing. See your veterinarian if you have any questions. Use one of the following homeopathic remedies to speed wound healing:

Arnica montana
We generally use *Arnica* for blunt trauma, and it may be helpful in cuts if the cut was from blunt trauma rather than a sharp object. It may reduce the pain in especially traumatic lacerations.

Calendula officinalis
As one of the primary remedies for lacerations, *Calendula* greatly speeds the body's healing of wounds. It has a reputation for occasionally healing the skin before deeper tissues clean and heal themselves, resulting in an abscess since inflammatory debris (pus) cannot escape. Use it for shallow wounds, or use it later in wound healing, after the deeper tissue has healed and only skin healing remains. This is true for topical use as well.

Carbolic acid
This remedy is useful in wounds that are seriously infected and slow to heal.

Hypericum perforatum
Both topically and in potency, *Hypericum* is helpful for wound healing. It often reduces the pain of wounds, especially in areas with a lot of nerves such as the toes, tongue, and tail. If the wound is especially painful, consider *Hypericum*.

Staphysagria
This remedy is also very helpful for alleviating pain, especially in lacerations from very sharp objects—including surgical wounds.

Diabetes Mellitus

Diabetes is a very serious condition, and treatment should always be under the direction of a veterinarian. Homeopathy can help, though cures are rare. A certain percentage of cats have a transient experience with diabetes, so if your cat develops diabetes, watch him closely to see if he recovers on his own.

All diabetic patients should be on the element chromium. It usually comes as either the compound chromium picolinate or as GTF chromium. Either is fine. Give fifty micrograms twice daily to cats, and give dogs fifty micrograms per fifteen to twenty-five pounds twice a day. You may also decrease the dose and give it three to four times a day. Chromium is necessary for proper insulin function, and it will usually reduce the insulin dosage requirement, so observe your companion closely when you begin supplementing with chromium if you are giving insulin by injection.

We now know that high carbohydrate foods, like grains, are a big factor, especially in cats. Not all cats or dogs have problems with some grains in the food, and these can be helpful for fiber content, which helps avoid constipation in domestic cats and dogs. Wild cats and dogs eat the hair and feathers along with the rest of the body, which helps move the high meat–low residue food through the gut. With homemade or commercial foods, we must use something for fiber, and grains and vegetables can provide this. Also, as meat production is so environmentally costly, I think we should limit the amount of meat when we can. So I usually use some vegetables and grains for those animals who can tolerate them. Dogs tolerate more grains and starchy vegetables than cats do, as dogs are opportunistic carnivores—they will eat other foods when the opportunity arises. Diabetic animals, however, should have no high carb foods, so use fiber like bran or psyllium and low-starch vegetables like greens, broccoli, and green beans.

Many other foods and herbs have activity that reduces blood glucose. Dandelion, blueberry, and ginseng are helpful herbs. Green beans and mesquite pods are helpful foods. Niacinamide is occasionally helpful for humans with juvenile onset diabetes. Response to most of these is individual, and they are all safe, so you need to try different ones to see if any prove helpful for your companion. Garlic is also helpful, but long-term garlic use may incite anemia, particularly in cats, so I would not give this regularly. *Cephalandra* in tincture or in low potency can sometimes be helpful, as can Gymnema or gymnosperma. Insulin in potency (6X–12X or 6C) can help also in some cases. Usually these would be used in addition to treatment with an experienced homeopath.

Drug Reactions

I am referring here to immediate acute reactions to drugs rather than chronic illnesses such as liver disorders. The latter should be treated by an experienced homeopath.

The most common drug reaction is diarrhea and/or vomiting; usually this occurs after antibiotic therapy due to suppression of normal intestinal bacteria as well as (sometimes) acute liver or kidney inflammation. If possible, the first measure is to stop the offending drug. Consult with a veterinarian about stopping the drug. If your companion has diarrhea and it continues, give acidophilus either by capsule or in yogurt. Slippery elm bark or activated charcoal may also help. Try one of the following homeopathic remedies as well:

Arsenicum album
These patients will vomit as well as develop diarrhea. The vomiting is often triggered upon eating or drinking even small amounts. Vomiting and diarrhea may occur at the same time.

China (pronounced "keena")
This remedy is useful for diarrhea, particularly if the patient begins to weaken as the diarrhea continues.

Lycopodium clavatum
Lycopodium is needed in animals that are very sensitive to drugs and develop diarrhea with a lot of gas. These animals may easily develop diarrhea from changes of food.

Nux vomica
Nux is perhaps the primary remedy for drug reactions. These animals develop diarrhea, and they usually strain during the stool. They may also strain before or after the stool. The sensation is that they never quite finish emptying their bowel. They may be irritable, and they occasionally develop urinary difficulty as well.

Pulsatilla

These patients may develop diarrhea or constipation after antibiotic therapy. They tend to be clingy and need a lot of attention. They are usually thirstless despite the diarrhea.

Thuja occidentalis

Thuja is also useful for drug reactions, though unlike most animals, those needing this remedy tend to develop urinary troubles as a result of the drug.

Euthanasia

I used to be clear about euthanasia being a blessing among our options as veterinarians. When faced with a terminally ill animal who is suffering, it seems wonderful to be able to shorten the time she suffers. In many cases I still feel relatively clear. I had to make this choice many years ago for a cat (Rumples) with whom I had shared my life for a long time. As I continue in practice and attempt to contemplate my moral responsibility, however, these decisions are not always so easy—at least for the large number of animals in the middle, in the gray zone.

The essential guiding factor we must keep always at the forefront is the interest of our companion. But this is still difficult. Just what is suffering? Is it the same for a dog as it is for a cat, or for a human? For that matter, is it the same in one individual (be he two- or four-legged) as in another of the same species? How much suffering is too much? How does the process of dying and the potential gifts it brings balance the suffering it entails? This then begs the ultimate question: what right do we have to decide this for another being? If we have that right, what parameters do we use to make the decision?

These conundrums circled my mind as I contemplated euthanasia for Rumples. On one hand, I did not want to take away his independence and his autonomy. And yet, watching him in pain tore at my heart. How was I to know which choice he might make, were he given the opportunity? Of course, I could not know. I tried homeopathic remedies to encourage him to let go, but without success. Finally I opted for euthanasia, with some misgivings but with determination to ease his suffering at last. As his body rested before me following the injection, a great sense of peace pervaded the room. I felt that in this case, I had made the best decision I could make.

In the end, it is most important to be clear that we are acting in the best interest of our companion animals. It is also important to remember that, just as in any illness, each situation is different from others and requires a new consideration. If there is doubt, wait until you understand the feeling of doubt. I remember a cat who had been suffering for some time, and his guardian had tried various treatments to help him. I was the third or fourth veterinarian whom she had consulted. It seemed that nothing was going to help, and one day she decided to end his suffering with euthanasia. When I attempted to place the needle into his vein, however, this weak cat would have no part of the procedure; he resisted strongly. The guardian and I looked at one another and simultaneously realized that it was not his time. He began to improve soon after and lived comfortably for some months before he died.

I always advise guardians that they will know when the time is correct, and they will know if euthanasia by injection is the best answer, as long as they remain clear in their contemplation of the need for their friend. Many animals die rather peacefully on their own, and sometimes homeopathy can assist this process. In most cases, I believe that allowing the natural process to unfold is best—not only the animals but also the guardians gain by participating in death. In other cases, however, assistance is truly compassionate.

And everyone is an individual. Even humans have vastly different approaches to death and dying. I had a friend, Harvey, who was in his early eighties when I first met him and his wife. Christine, his wife, died of liver cancer about five years after I met them. She had been hospitalized and had received conventional chemotherapy; she suffered a lot with her illness and death. Then, perhaps another four years later, Harvey was diagnosed with pancreatic cancer. A few months later, Harvey decided to take his life. I understood this, especially since he had seen how Christine had suffered. Other people choose to hang on as long as possible; some seem not to mind the pain, while others seem to suffer greatly. And nonhuman animals are no different; their reactions to pain and death will be just as varied as ours are. Therefore we must attempt to understand our companion's personality to know what she might choose if she had the choice.

Before choosing drug injection, though, the correct homeopathic medicine may facilitate the transition to death. It is also important to verbally give the animal permission to let go, as they often hold on to the connection with the guardian. It is equally important that you truly let go when you give permission to your companion, as they often will stay around longer than otherwise when their guardian is unable to let them go. This is critical.

The transition to death is frightening to many individuals because of the unknown. This holds true for animals as well as people. For this reason the remedy *Arsenicum album* is often helpful, as the *Arsenicum* state includes a fear of death and a fear of being alone. The animal is often restless due to the fear. This remedy is often administered in high potency to dying individuals, sometimes with great effect. It will not cause death, though. It only eases the resistance to death and makes dying easier in those animals who are in an *Arsenicum* state as they approach death. The truth is that any homeopathic medicine may provide this if it is the correct remedy for the animal's state as she approaches death and she is ready to die. I have seen *Phosphorus* work beautifully as well in a dog who was clearly a *Phosphorus* individual and was ready to die. Arsenicum matches the time of death in many cases, though, and this is why it is the most commonly recommended remedy for this transition. It may even help if you take the *Arsenicum* as well to assist in your own fear of death and in accepting the coming changes.

Another remedy that is associated with the death process is *Tarentula cubensis*. This remedy is often helpful when the animal is in great pain and is struggling. This state is much more intense than the *Arsenicum* state; it is often associated with cancer, though it can be useful in any death where there is great pain. (Don't confuse this remedy with *Tarentula hispanica*, though this remedy can also help in some cases.) Finally, *Euphorbium* (*Euphorbium officinarum,* also called *Euphorbia resinifera*) may also help with cancer-associated pains; here the pains are also intense.

In addition to homeopathic remedies, flower remedies can help. Rescue Remedy is useful in any situation of fright and stress. Walnut is useful for transition, and *Mimulus* helps overcome fear of the unknown. These may be given directly or placed on the bedding near your companion's face. They may also be rubbed on the inside of the ears.

If you decide to opt for injection euthanasia, use the above flower remedies before the injection, as they will still be helpful. Additionally, the homeopathic remedy *Passiflora incarnata* is a good calming agent. It is also found in the combination formulas Calms and Calms Forte by Hylands; these are also good for relaxing and alleviating stress. Valerian root is a good calming herb that may be given as well. Give a dropperful to several dropperfuls as needed. Ask your veterinarian about giving a tranquilizer first, either by injection or orally, to help alleviate stress in animals who are reactive. Perhaps you could even give an oral tranquilizer at home before taking her to the clinic or before the veterinarian comes to your house.

Fear

Some animals are crippled by fear. This is not the caution that one may see in some cats, who are timid by nature. It is a paralyzing fear that causes the dog or cat to vanish whenever people come to visit or may cause the animal to stay hidden in some cases. Cats may have litter box problems due to fear of entering the room or area where the box is placed. Fear may also drive dogs to bite in situations where there is really no threat but they perceive a threat.

Often this requires constitutional treatment by an experienced prescriber, as the remedy options are so vast. Some remedies are broadly applicable, however, so I decided to list a few that you may try if they seem correct. Read also the section on "Aggression" in Chapter Thirteen, "Nervous System," for the connection to rabies vaccination or ketamine in some animals.

Aconitum napellus
Aconite is one of the main fear remedies. Usually the fear is gripping and may have originated from an emotionally traumatic incident. These animals seem to be fearful of almost everything and are anxious and restless as a result. Their responses are usually rapid and violent (not aggressively violent toward others so much as violent in their strength).

Arsenicum album
This is the classic "fraidy cat" who disappears when company arrives. These cats are usually friendly and loving to their family but terrified of anyone they do not know.

Calcarea carbonica
These animals are generally fearful of new situations and people. Their fear is not so evident in what they do as in what they will not do. They often simply will not go into a certain room or down a certain street. Fear of change makes a move terrifying; they may develop physical illness follow-

ing a move. Their behavior seems to be manipulative or controlling because they simply will not budge on some requests.

Lycopodium clavatum

Animals needing *Lycopodium* are timid of new situations and of strangers. I have found this remedy often effective when other, better-known fear remedies do not work.

Passiflora incarnata

This remedy may be used for its calming effect, though it will not likely stop the fear from occurring. I usually use it in low potency—3X, 6X, 3C, or 6C. Calms and Calms Forte may be used also, but don't use these for long-term administration.

Stramonium

This remedy state is one of terror that often leads to aggression. These animals may bite when they are afraid. Perhaps they hear a noise they do not understand; their fear is aroused, and they become aggressive as a defense. They may then bite an innocent bystander due to their heightened state. Bright lights and darkness may also trigger their fear.

Fear of Noises

This is a separate group of animals, and while there are too many remedies and noises to fully consider, I decided to list just a few.

Thunder and Lightning

The most well-known remedy here is *Phosphorus,* and it will help a certain percentage of animals, though perhaps less than 10 percent. These animals are generally easily startled by any noise and may leap suddenly if you drop something. Cats leave tracks on your legs if they are lying on your lap when a loud noise occurs. *Electricitas* is a remedy made from electric current; it has been helpful for some animals who have been frightened by a close lightning strike that hit their house so that they subsequently become terrified of all lightning and thunder. *Natrum carbonicum* and *Rhododendron* may also help, if they fit the animal constitutionally. The flower essence red clover has helped some animals, as has alfalfa in herbal or flower essence form.

Gunshot, Firecrackers

Phosphorus is once again a possibility (see the above paragraph). *Borax* is good for those animals that startle greatly even if the noise is a long distance away.

Rushing Water, Running Tap Water

This is considered a part of the rabies miasm (see "Aggression and the Rabies Miasm" in Chapter Thirteen, "Nervous System") and is usually connected to rabies vaccination. These animals often have other symptoms that warrant professional homeopathic care. The remedies listed for this fear are *Hyoscyamus, Lyssin,* and *Stramonium*. See the section referenced above for further information.

Fever and Infections

Conventional veterinarians and physicians have generally considered fever to be a symptom to be removed as soon as possible. It is part of the approach that sees the symptom as the disease rather than as the body's attempt to fight the disease. Homeopathic veterinarians tend to see fever as a good sign in many cases and prefer not to directly stop the fever, but to attempt to remove the need for the fever.

A corollary is that conventional veterinarians generally see a fever as meaning an infection that must be treated with antibiotics. In their eyes, this is a method of removing the cause for the fever. Actually, a fever indicates inflammation; this does not necessarily mean an infection—though this is the usual interpretation. In many cases antibiotics are unnecessary, because either there is no infection or, if there is an infection, it is a virus infection and antibiotics are useless.

There are often accompanying symptoms with a fever, and if this is the case you should look in the appropriate sections for those symptoms, as they may be a better guide to the correct remedy. If your animal develops a fever with no other symptoms (this is common in cats), a homeopathic medicine may speed the cure without need for antibiotics and without development of other symptoms.

The normal temperature for cats and dogs is 101.5 degrees Fahrenheit (38.6 degrees Celsius). I consider anything above 102 (38.9) degrees a fever, although some practitioners feel that transient variations occur and that up to 102.5 (39.2) may be normal. This is especially true for cats, as they may spike a fever due to stress upon entering a veterinary clinic. Dogs commonly run fevers of up to 104 (40) and occasionally will reach 105 (40.5). Cats commonly go up to 104.5 (40.3) and occasionally over 106 (41.1). I don't believe high fevers are harmful and especially do not worry unless the fever reaches 105 (40.5) in dogs or 106 (41.1) in cats, and only then if the fever is prolonged. I do not recommend drugs to bring the fever down, as the fever is almost always a good reaction. I have never seen damage from a high fever.

General Care for Fevers and Infections

If your companion becomes listless and it lasts for more than a day or two, you should have him examined by your veterinarian to determine if the condition is serious.

Give immune-building herbs and vitamins such as those listed above in the section "General Care for Abscesses." Astragalus and cat's claw may also be of benefit; use these individually and dose as with the echinacea or goldenseal. *Yunnan paiyao* may be used for severe fevers with known infections (see below, under "Hemorrhage"). Give one of the following homeopathic medicines according to symptoms. If the fever does not begin to subside within twelve to twenty-four hours, change remedies or see your veterinarian. Do not just keep giving the same remedy, as you may worsen the condition. If your companion worsens at any time, stop the remedy and reassess her condition, and either change remedies or seek help.

Aconitum napellus

I have found this remedy often helpful in animals with fever and no other symptoms. The fever may have come on suddenly. It is especially useful if the animal was exposed to cold wind before the fever developed and if he is restless and anxious.

Belladonna

These fevers are also sudden, but the animal is generally hotter (symptomatically, not necessarily higher temperature) and more agitated than those needing *Aconite*. The pupils may be dilated, and the animal may be irritable, even aggressive.

Echinacea
The homeopathic remedy, like the herb, is useful for infections. These animals are usually fairly ill, with poor gum color and weakness. They may need veterinary help.

Ferrum phosphoricum
This remedy is indicated for many early infections and influenza-like conditions. The patient is often fairly listless and may be anemic. (You may see pale gums. If the gums are more white than light pink, see your veterinarian.) You may see early signs of nasal or eye discharge.

Gelsemium
This remedy is most useful for weakness as a result of a prior infection from which the animal never quite recovered. It may be useful in early fevers if the prostration and weakness are profound. These animals are generally weaker than those needing *Ferrum phos.*

Pyrogenium
This remedy is often helpful for persistent fevers that weaken the animal. These patients may have back pain along with the fever, and they are often restless as a result. The gum color may be dark or muddy instead of pink.

Sulphur
This remedy is helpful in those animals who cannot mount a good immune response. They often have marginal (low) fevers that will neither increase nor go away. These animals tend to be scruffy and dirty. Don't repeat this remedy for long if you do not get a response, as it may cause an aggravation.

Fleas

If you are sitting on the edge of your seat for this one, sit back and relax, as there are no easy answers to the flea problem. The most important measure you can take is similar to that with any illness, and that is to strengthen the overall health of the animal. In general, given the same environment, healthier animals suffer less from fleas. It all comes back to good food, lots of love, and minimal stress. Cleanliness is important also, but healthy animals generally stay clean.

Success against flea infestations depends heavily upon control of the flea life cycle off of the animal. The life cycle is similar to that of the butterfly with egg, larva, cocoon, and adult stages. The following is the life cycle for *Ctenocephalides felis,* the "cat flea." This flea accounts for 99 percent of fleas on cats and 85 to 95 percent of fleas on dogs. *Pulex irritans,* the "human flea," is next in frequency on dogs, and the "dog flea," *Ctenocephalides canis,* is last, although possibly more common in the northeast United States.

Although fleas live on the skin of our cats and dogs, they lay eggs that fall off and hatch in the environment rather than on the animal. These eggs hatch into small (one-quarter inch long) wormlike larvae after two to five days at 70 to 80 percent humidity. If the humidity is less than 30 to 40 percent, the eggs will not hatch. Larvae are clear to white with a reddish-brown streak of blood pigment in their intestines; you may see the larvae where your companion sleeps. The larvae must eat adult flea feces to develop further.

Larvae are very susceptible to heat and drying; they will die if the relative humidity drops below 50 percent. Continued temperatures above 95 degrees Fahrenheit (35 degrees Celsius) will also kill the larvae. For these and other reasons, the larvae shy away from light and tend to travel downward. Thus they develop at the base of carpet pile or grasses, under furniture, and under porches.

After one to two weeks, the larva spins a cocoon, where development continues as it transforms into a "preemerged adult." It takes one to three weeks to make this transition, but these preemerged adults do not issue from the cocoon until an external stimulus triggers them to hatch. They may sit patiently in the cocoon for up to *140 days,* waiting for a host to arrive. While in the cocoon, the flea is protected from insecticides and other external threats. Once the correct stimulus occurs, the flea can break out of the cocoon and leap onto the host in less than one second. There is virtually no exposure, even to residual insecticides.

What stimuli entice these preemerged adults to emerge? Heat is the primary agent, but vibration, moisture, physical pressure, and carbon dioxide will also incite hatching—essentially, anything that tells the flea that a warm-blooded animal is available. A vacuum cleaner with a beater bar can sometimes trick the flea into emerging, thus we can use this to our advantage.

Adult fleas must live on the animal, though they can survive for one to two weeks before finding a host. Once they feed, however, they can only survive for up to four days, and most will die after two days. The adult life span may exceed one hundred days. Eggs are laid on the animal and drop onto the floor or ground, so *the highest concentration of eggs, larvae, and cocoons will be where the animal spends the majority of its time.*

The female flea must feed constantly to lay eggs, as she may lay up to twice her body weight daily in eggs. This amounts to as many as forty-six eggs per day in the first week of life, and over two thousand eggs over a one-hundred-day life span. In order to accomplish this feat she will consume fifteen times her weight in blood every day. Although this may not sound like a lot of blood relative to the host, with large numbers of fleas on puppies and kittens the impact can be severe, even fatal.

Although freezing temperatures can kill fleas in the winter, they survive in houses and in protected spaces like piles of leaves and yard waste, and in crawl spaces under houses. Additionally, other host species such as raccoons and opossums may host these fleas. Squirrels do not host this species of flea, however.

How, then, can we control this adaptable parasite? Diligence rather than toxic chemicals is our best ally. Strong chemicals only weaken your companion's health in the long run, making her more susceptible to fleas and other diseases. We now know that these chemicals can also affect us, even if they are applied to our companion animals, so the gain is not worth the risk in my opinion. These chemicals also kill other life forms and end up in our drinking water, foods, and mother's milk. DDT is still ubiquitous, even though its usage in the United States was stopped years ago.

Flea control has two main realms. First is reducing the adult fleas on the animal, including reducing egg production. Second is to reduce the stages that live in the environment, off the animal. This includes the house and the yard.

For control of adult fleas on your companion, use nontoxic materials. Shampoos can drastically reduce adult fleas and will interfere with egg-laying even if the fleas are not all killed. You usually do not need to use a chemical flea shampoo; most shampoos kill fleas if you lather well and wait ten to fifteen minutes before rinsing. Be sure to rinse well to avoid irritating and drying the skin.

Herbal rinses can repel fleas; lavender, eucalyptus, and pennyroyal work fairly well for dogs. I would not use the latter two on cats as they can be toxic to cats. You can use a lemon rinse: steep a cut-up lemon or two in a quart of boiling water and allow it to cool. Use the liquid as a rinse, or sponge it onto the coat. Skin-so-Soft by Avon is a bath oil that repels fleas. Use one to one and one-half ounces per gallon of water and apply as a rinse or spray. It is somewhat oily, thus it is better on outside animals and on animals with coarse coats. Black walnut leaves and cedar shavings can be used in bedding to repel fleas.

Flea combs are fine-toothed combs that will mechanically remove fleas. They also disrupt feeding and egg-laying. These work well on short-haired animals. You can comb first with a wide-toothed comb to make it easier for the flea comb to get through the coat. Once you catch the fleas on the comb, drop them into soapy water (otherwise they sit on the surface and can jump out of the container) and flush this down the toilet. You can also use alcohol to collect the fleas.

Diatomaceous earth is somewhat effective on the animal as well as in the house. It mechanically damages the flea's intestines and respiratory apparatus, killing the flea. The only safety concern for you or your animals is breathing the dust, so don't make a cloud when you apply the powder.

Supplements such as brewer's yeast and garlic help 20 to 25 percent of animals repel fleas, though some animals are allergic to yeast and may develop diarrhea or skin problems.

I do not recommend the following types of agents: ultrasonic collars do not work and they are audible (ninety decibels at forty kilohertz—very loud) to cats and dogs. Hearing disturbance and behavior modification has been documented. Topical or oral products for flea control may work rather well in some cases, but it is illogical to assume they are safe. Anything that can kill one species cannot be completely safe for another species. The spot-on type products all are absorbed by the body, despite claims to the contrary. They cause liver and kidney disease, sometimes gastrointestinal distress, cancer, and other serious illnesses. Do not use them. Their convenience comes at a high price. I have heard and seen problems with many of these programs, including reactions that threatened death. I don't believe these spot treatments give our companions an advantage. D-limonene (a citrus derivative) is said to be safe, but I know of several poisonings, especially in cats, and I do not recommend this product. Flea collars work poorly and are very toxic to animals and everyone they live around. Dips and other chemicals are simply too unsafe for the planet.

If you must use topical repellents, choose herbal products. Try Bug Repel (www.bugrepel.com) or Cedarcide (www.cedarcide.com). Rose geranium essential oil is also a good repellant; you can dilute in almond oil and put a very small amount on your cat or dog. Sometimes an amethyst crystal in the drinking water helps, though I don't know the mechanism. It must change the energy field.

For household control, diligent cleanliness is the most important part of the equation. Concentrate under furniture and where your companions spend the majority of their time. Vacuum daily at first, then taper to weekly. Shampoos and steam cleaners add moisture to carpets and thus may initiate hatching of fleas. This can be good if you follow closely with thorough vacuuming.

If you need to apply a flea-killing agent, boron compounds are fairly effective and very safe. Fleabusters is a company that uses one of these compounds and guarantees effectiveness for a year. They have local franchises in many cities and will apply the product or sell it for home application. Twenty Mule Team Borax is a laundry additive that is also effective and is inexpensive, though it requires application every few months. You can buy it in most grocery stores. Sprinkle it on carpets or floors and use a broom to work it into the carpet pile or into cracks between wood or tiles. Allow it to stay overnight and then vacuum. Repeat two weeks after the first application, then every few months, as needed. Although borax is very safe (I know of no instances of poisoning), it is wise to keep animals out of the room while applying the product, and try not to stir up a cloud of dust to breathe. You could also wear a mask during application. For carpets and rugs, you can rent a "steam cleaner" (actually they use hot water) from the grocery or hardware store, and run a borax solution through this unit. Use about one cup of borax for each tankful. The heat and vibration will encourage eggs and cocoons to hatch, and then the borax is right there. You also do not need to worry about borax dust in the air. For smooth floors, mopping with a solution of about a cup of borax per gallon of water works as well, though it leaves a slightly dull appearance. You can follow in few days with a sponge mop to regain the shine if desired. Maximum effectiveness is reached about two weeks after application, so be patient if you still see fleas after a few days.

Diatomaceous earth (DE) is also somewhat effective in the house and is applied in essentially the same manner. Some people mix the borax and diatomaceous earth together for application. Ask for an MSDS (manufacturer's safety data sheet) on the DE, though, as some of these have piperonyl butoxide added (a toxic chemical that immobilizes insects). As a last resort, you can use a natural pyrethrin such as a powder of pyrethrum flowers to get a quick handle on the household infestation if it is severe. Even this is toxic, though it breaks down rather quickly. I have not seen instances where the borax or sodium perborate/polyborate did not work, though, unless they were not applied correctly.

Finally, outside control is difficult, but there are some measures that help. Keep the yard cut short and clippings raked to minimize protected areas (remember that heat and low humidity as well as freezing will kill fleas). Treat dog houses or areas where animals sleep with diatomaceous earth, and use cedar shavings or black walnut leaves. There is a nematode (worm) that parasitizes fleas and kills them; this can be applied during flea season (warm, humid weather) to reduce the flea burden in the yard. Many garden and hardware stores sell these nematodes. They are also available through the catalog "Gardens Alive" (513 354 1482, www.gardensalive.com), which specializes in nontoxic gardening.

There is little that homeopathy has to offer for flea control other than constitutional treatment to improve health and resistance to fleas. *Pulex irritans* is a remedy made from the human flea, and some feel that it can improve resistance. *Sulphur* is the remedy most often associated with flea infestation, though it is by no means the only remedy for this. I have even heard it suggested that a spray made of 30C *Sulphur* in water will repel fleas. I have not tried this, however, and I am not sure of its wisdom, as the animal and the guardian are dosed with the remedy at each application. *Ledum palustre* is the big remedy for insect bites and puncture wounds and thus is recommended by some for the reaction to the flea bite. *Caladium* is a remedy for insect bites that sting and burn excessively. It may help some animals who are especially sensitive to flea bites.

Food and Garbage Poisoning

Food poisoning is usually the result of eating foods that have spoiled, allowing bacterial growth. The bacteria contain toxins that cause nausea, vomiting, and diarrhea. In very rare cases they may cause death, but usually the vomiting and diarrhea succeed in eliminating the toxins and no further illness ensues.

Dogs are natural scavengers and will eat very repulsive items that typically cause them no harm. To their advantage, they have the ability to vomit at will, and they simply regurgitate anything that bodes ill. Occasionally they do suffer the consequences, however. Cats rarely have this problem due to their discriminating palate, as they cannot detoxify chemicals as well as dogs and thus they avoid suspicious foods entirely.

If your dog has gotten into garbage or you suspect food poisoning, take him to a veterinarian if he is severely listless or painful. Most cases readily respond to homeopathic treatment. The response is usually rapid, so you will know soon if you need help. If you are not sure that this is from spoiled food, or if there is any possibility of other poisons, have him examined as soon as possible to determine if other help is needed. This is especially true if antifreeze poisoning is a possibility. *If you suspect antifreeze poisoning, take him immediately to a clinic* (see "Acute Kidney Failure" in Chapter Eleven, "Urinary System," for more information).

In the first hour or so, the patient usually vomits several times or has watery diarrhea, sometimes with gas and abdominal pain. Do not give medicines like kaopectate or paregoric to stop the vomiting or diarrhea, as these bodily reactions are eliminating toxins. Once the initial attacks calm down, you can offer water in small amounts, or let him lick an ice cube to moisten the mouth. As he improves, you may want to give an electrolyte replacer like Pedialyte if the diarrhea or vomiting were severe. You can use a dilute sea-salt solution instead of Pedialyte. Use an unrefined sea salt, and put one-quarter teaspoonful salt in a quart of water. Rice water is also helpful; soak two tablespoons of brown rice in a quart of water for an hour to overnight. Give one of the following remedies as soon as you are aware of the food poisoning:

Arsenicum album

This is first alphabetically and first in effectiveness. This is almost always my choice for food poisoning. I have used it quite successfully on myself, friends, and patients, and the results are usually dramatic. These animals often have diarrhea and nausea or vomiting at the same time. They may be quite ill, even fearful that they are severely ill and may die. This is a keynote in people.

Carbo vegetabilis

Carbo veg is also a good choice. These patients are more severely affected and may become cold and weak. These animals usually have severe, foul gas as well. They often develop dry heaves. This is a severe state, and if you do not see rapid improvement, you may need veterinary assistance.

Crotalus horridus

The vomiting here is violent and persistent, and affected animals may vomit blood or "coffee grounds" materials. Unless you know this is food poisoning, take your companion to a veterinarian if you see this. If you are sure food poisoning is the culprit and you have this remedy, you can try it, but don't wait too long if you do not see improvement.

Nux vomica

Nux is useful for any toxic conditions, and food poisoning certainly qualifies. Consider this remedy if the animal becomes fidgety and irritable as the condition arises. Straining diarrhea is common, and the animal often continues to strain after emptying the bowel. Retching may occur as well, often without producing vomit. Rich foods may bring about this condition.

Veratrum album

This state is similar to that of *Arsenicum*, though somewhat more severe. There may be coldness and weakness along with the persistent nausea and vomiting. Usually there is not the excessive gas as with *Carbo veg*. If *Arsenicum* does not work, this is often the second choice.

Grief

Any time there is a loss, companion animals may suffer from grief in the same manner that we do. This is especially true with the death of a family member, whether human or nonhuman. It may also occur when a member of the family leaves the household. This could be from a difficult situation such as divorce, but it may also occur when a child leaves for college or to begin life on her own. The most important homeopathic remedy for immediate effects of grief is *Ignatia*. This remedy can be very helpful to individuals in grief. It will not block the experience of grief, but it can lighten the load somewhat and allow the individual (two- or four-legged) to accept and integrate the changes in his life. *Ignatia* can even help in some cases when the grief is in the past but the person has not finished letting go. There are other remedies for illness that results from unresolved grief, including *Natrum muriaticum* and *Phosphoric acid*, but this state is usually a chronic condition that warrants expert homeopathic care. Grief is often at the heart of a sudden occurrence of chronic disease. I have seen this often in animals that develop diabetes, for example.

Heart Disease

These conditions are too severe for home treatment, but I will give a few suggestions for supplements and herbs that support heart function. See a veterinarian for diagnosis and treatment of any heart illness. Homeopathy is often effective but should be used under the guidance of an experienced practitioner.

The amino acids L-taurine and L-carnitine have been associated with heart disease (cardiomyopathy) in cats and dogs, respectively. Supplement cats with L-taurine (125 mg daily) and dogs with L-carnitine (125 mg per twenty-five pounds daily) if heart illness occurs. Double the dose for the first two weeks. L-propionyl carnitine may be more effective for heart issues than other forms. These have specifically been associated with dilated cardiomyopathy, a condition wherein the walls of the heart balloon out and function poorly, and the correct amino acid may greatly improve the condition. There is no harm, however, in supplementing any animal who has heart disease with the species-specific amino acid. Taurine may also stabilize cardiac arrhythmias.

Coenzyme Q_{10} is a supplement that greatly benefits the heart muscle. I recommend supplementing all animals with heart problems with "Co Q_{10}." If you can get this in an oil base—usually in a gel capsule, like vitamin E—it is more effective than the dry form. Give about one milligram per pound of the oil form, and up to twice this amount in the dry form. Other helpful supplements include vitamin E (5–10 mg/pound daily, mixed tocopherols), lecithin (one-fourth teaspoonful per ten pounds daily), and germanium (1–2 mg/pound daily). Essential fatty acids may also be very helpful. Give flax seed oil (one-fourth teaspoonful per ten pounds daily) and evening primrose or borage oil (125 mg per ten to twenty-five pounds daily).

An herb that can stimulate improved cardiac function is hawthorn, known as the homeopathic remedy *Crataegus*. Use this under the direction of an herbalist, if possible. You may also give about three to five drops of the tincture per ten pounds, two to three times a day. If your companion is on digitalis, use only under the direction of a veterinary herbalist. Dandelion is a mild diuretic and kidney- and liver-cleansing herb. If the heart is not pumping adequately and fluid is building up in the lungs or other areas, this herb may help reduce the fluid and reduce the load on the heart. You may be able to use dandelion in lieu of Lasix (furosemide) or other chemical diuretics. Make a tea by pouring one cup of water over one teaspoonful of dried herb and allow it to steep until cool. Give one to two dropperfuls per ten pounds, two to three times a day. Alternately, give about five drops of the tincture, two to three times a day.

The homeopathic remedy *Iberis* may be helpful in hypertrophic cardiomyopathy. *Adonis vernalis* can help with dilated cardiomyopathy or other cases of weak heart muscle. *Strophanthus* (tincture or low potency like 3X or 6X) and *Apocynum* can help heart function also; *Apocynum* is especially good for fluid in the chest (chest dropsy) resulting from heart disease. It can improve circulation, possibly even with aortic thrombosis. Use in low potency.

Heartworm

Heartworm disease is a potentially fatal infestation of worms that inhabit the heart and the large blood vessels that leave the heart. Mosquitoes transmit infective larvae to susceptible dogs, so the higher the numbers of mosquitoes, the greater the likelihood of heartworm infestation. Dogs are the primary host, though cats can be infested if they do not have good immune systems; humans also rarely become infested. I will limit my discussion to dogs, though the same principles apply to cats, with the exception that the latter are uncommonly affected and treatment options are limited, as Immiticide is not safe in cats (see below).

Dogs do develop some immunity to heartworm larvae, though we do not fully understand the extent to which this happens. In a study about twenty years ago at Auburn University, researchers found that stray dogs from Mississippi had strong resistance to infestation. I suspect that most dogs develop some immunity if they are exposed, as they would be, even on monthly preventives. Thus dogs over five years old are less likely to develop problems (if they are living in an area where exposure is likely); this matched my experience when I lived and practiced in North Carolina— I mostly saw young dogs with the disease.

Once a heartworm larva–infested mosquito bites a susceptible dog, those larvae begin to mature into adult worms; this takes about six months. For the first six to eight weeks of this maturation process, the larvae are susceptible to the drugs we use for prevention. Up to six or seven weeks postbite, they are 100 percent susceptible, and at eight weeks postbite, they are still about 95 percent susceptible. The preventive drugs thus work for infestation that occurred *prior to administration.* You can see that monthly administration is unnecessary and excessive. Six to seven weeks is equally effective, and even eight weeks is close and may be sufficient if you are not in a heavily impacted area. Further, as Interceptor (not Heartgard or other preventive drugs) is dosed at five to ten times the level needed for heartworm prevention in order to attain intestinal worm prevention, you can cut the dose if your dog does not have intestinal worm problems. The simplest reduction is to cut the tablet into four pieces, and give one-quarter tablet as a dose rather than the full tablet for your dog's size. This does not work with Heartgard, as it is dosed for heartworm prevention only, and a second drug added to Heartgard Plus for roundworm and hookworm prevention. I don't recommend Revolution.

Thus, one option, especially with young dogs in the southern United States or anywhere else where mosquito counts and heartworm disease are high, would be to give the first dose of preventive four or five weeks after you see the first mosquito of the season, then continue at six- or seven-week intervals until you give a dose after the last mosquito. If you are in an area with mosquitoes all year, just continue the dosing, but increase the interval from monthly to every six or seven weeks. In the winter, if mosquito levels are low, you can go to every eight weeks. Every seven weeks is as good as every six weeks, but some people find every six weeks easier to track. This was part of the genesis for using preventives monthly, as it is easy to remember. Since these drugs are not without damaging impacts, however, minimizing their use is important. They can cause nausea and diarrhea, liver disease, and even autoimmune disease. No drug is benign.

In heartworm endemic areas, it is important to test for heartworms. You can do this yearly if you use preventives, or twice yearly if you opt for no preventives or if you push the limits of dosing to eight weeks or more. Here is how testing works: the antigen tests (the most common test) look for small heartworm particles in the blood. It usually takes about three months post–mosquito bite for these to become positive, though in uncommon cases it may take five to seven months. Thus, if your dog was bitten in June with an infested mosquito, the soonest you would pick up the infestation in your dog would be September. So if you are testing once a year, it is best to wait at least three or four months after the end of the mosquito season; this way you maximize your likelihood of finding any infestations from that year.

This has another benefit. While heartworm infestations are typically treated with an arsenic compound (Immiticide), requiring hospitalization, there may be another option. Studies at the University of Georgia found that, in infestations where the worms were less than eight months post–mosquito bite, they could clear the worms with monthly administration of Heartgard (Interceptor was not effective, and I do not know if they tested other drugs—they had not as of their initial publication). Thus, if you test twice yearly, you will pretty consistently catch an infestation early enough to be treated with monthly Heartgard alone, without having to use the arsenic drug. You will need to continue the Heartgard for at least eighteen months, maybe longer, but still this is better than the Immiticide. This is a much safer option. It is even feasible to use twice-yearly testing without preventive, then start the preventive if you get a positive test. This is especially attractive in low to moderately impacted regions, or in dogs over five or six years old in regions where heartworm is common, as they probably have some immunity. There is some risk here, but I think the risk is well balanced by the reduced drug levels, especially where heartworm prevalence is not high.

Another option for prevention, especially in low prevalence areas, is to use a remedy (nosode) made from heartworm-infested blood. While there are no studies demonstrating its effectiveness, I have had many patients on this without developing infestations. I have seen dogs on the nosode who developed heartworm disease, though they were not using the potency and frequency I recommend. It is important to use the 30C potency and give it once every week or two when mosquitoes are around (use weekly when the mosquito numbers are higher). Keep your dog inside at dawn and dusk, when mosquito numbers are higher, and use herbal repellents (see the section on "Fleas," above). If you opt for the heartworm remedy, you should test your dog at least once a year, and understand that the effectiveness is unknown, though it does provide some protection.

Finally, it is possible in some cases to treat heartworm disease with homeopathy, though you should work with an experienced homeopath, as this requires skill and experience.

Hemorrhage

Hemorrhage may occur for many reasons, and most of them indicate a need to investigate the cause. Spontaneous hemorrhage indicates a deficiency in clotting ability; this may occur for several reasons, including poisoning (rodenticides), autoimmune platelet diseases, and deficiency in clotting factors. The last category encompasses such syndromes as hemophilia and Von Willebrand's disease, which we generally consider to be genetic deficiencies. Bleeding disorders like these may also be connected to thyroid deficiency, which is mostly an autoimmune disease (the body's immune system attacks itself). See the section below on "Thyroid Disease."

Bleeding may also occur after injuries, during infections and abscesses, and after some drugs and vaccinations. In most of these situations the cause is apparent and thus treatment is generally simpler. Vaccinations often increase the bleeding tendency by impeding clotting function, though this is not a problem in most animals unless there is a concurrent injury. The bleeding susceptibility may continue for up to two weeks, so surgery and dental cleaning should not be scheduled during this period, should you choose to vaccinate (see Chapter Sixteen, "Vaccination," before you decide to vaccinate).

The following treatment suggestions are intended as a supplement to veterinary care. If your companion begins to bleed from a body orifice or under the skin, take her in to your veterinarian right away to determine the cause. Many times these can be treated with homeopathic medicine, but it is essential that you ascertain the cause of the hemorrhage. Additionally, unless the condition is simple, you should work with an experienced homeopathic practitioner.

Vitamin K and calcium are essential for proper clotting, and these may be obtained from green leafy vegetables; alfalfa is also a good source. Liver contains many ingredients that are helpful as well, since clotting factors are normally produced in the liver. If your companion has bleeding tendencies, be sure she receives adequate amounts of these foods and vitamins.

There is a Chinese herbal preparation called *Yunnan paiyao* that is often very effective at stopping acute hemorrhage, whether from trauma or other causes. This is available through Chinese herbalists and in many stores that specialize in Chinese and Asian foods. The product can be given orally as well as topically. Give one or two capsules (depending upon the severity) for dogs over twenty-five pounds. This may be repeated two to four times a day if needed. Give cats and small dogs one-quarter to one-half capsule. There is also a small red "safety pill" with each sheet of capsules that is for severe bleeding. Use this product in the short-term only. It is generally not for prolonged administration unless directed by an herbalist.

The following homeopathic remedies may be helpful as well:

Aconitum napellus

If there is bleeding with anxiety, this is the best choice. These patients are generally very restless and anxious.

Arnica montana

This remedy is especially good for hemorrhage that follows an injury. Use this first after any trauma, as it can stop bleeding as well as prevent infections and abscesses.

Crotalus horridus

This remedy is useful for bleeding due to a clotting deficiency or a severe infection. In either condition you should obtain veterinary care, but *Crotalus* may help in the interim. The blood is usually dark and thin and will not clot, or clots very minimally. The remedy has an affinity to the right side of the body.

Erigeron

This remedy is especially useful for hemorrhage from the bladder and uterus, though bloody vomitus and stool may also occur. Any movement worsens the bleeding when this remedy is needed.

Ferrum phosphoricum

For hemorrhage that accompanies a fever in weak individuals, this remedy may be helpful. See above in the section on fever and infections.

Hamamelis

Hamamelis is very similar to *Arnica* and should be used for bleeding after an injury if *Arnica* is ineffective.

Lachesis

Lachesis, like *Crotalus*, is a remedy that is made from a snake venom. It is also useful for clotting deficiencies until veterinary care is obtained. The blood is dark and thin and may be profuse. The surrounding skin may be blue-black. Symptoms may occur predominantly or initially on the left side and may move to the right side.

Millefolium
This remedy is useful for hemorrhage after injury or overexertion; the blood is bright red (with *Arnica* and *Hamamelis* it is not quite as bright). It is probably an underutilized remedy for hemorrhage. It may also be useful post-surgery.

Phosphorus
This is one of our main remedies for bleeding. If there are no other indications, this is a good remedy to start with. The blood tends to be bright red rather than dark. This remedy is also good for problems following anesthesia, so if your companion bleeds after surgery, this is the first choice.

Hyperactivity

Aberrant behavior is on the increase in nonhuman animals to a similar degree to that seen in humans. Hyperactivity, violence, and aggression all seem to occur more than ever. I have discussed this with colleagues, and many believe that domestic animals suffer from their own forms of hyperactivity and attention deficit disorder. We do not know the cause, but it seems more than coincidental that it is occurring in more than one species.

Probably many factors contribute and magnify the impact that each might have individually. Pollution, especially that of the subtle but nerve-jangling electromagnetic fields (EMF), is likely a big contributor. Cell phone radiation is now ubiquitous, as is wireless Internet radiation. These are known to cause illness, from chronic fatigue to inability to sleep to cancer. Even microchips can be problematic; I have a client who is especially sensitive to EMF pollution, and after she had a microchip put into her cat, she could not have the cat on her lap or in bed with her, as she became jangled. Fortunately, she was able to get the chip removed. Imagine what our poor cats and dogs go through with these microchips right by their heads! In the late 1980s the U.S. Environmental Protection Agency issued a statement that electromagnetic fields are carcinogenic, though industry pressure resulted in their later rescinding the report. Our bodies evolved without all these EMFs, and our bodies utilize a lot of electromagnetic energy to function. It is no surprise that external EMFs interfere with our normal bodily function, and especially with our nervous systems, which depend heavily upon biomagnetic impulses. A study with bees, for example, found that they would not return to their hives if a cell phone was placed nearby; the colony disappearance problems we now experience are likely at least somewhat connected to EMF and cell phone towers, along with new pesticides. Our bodies no doubt react similarly, though we may be less sensitive as a species. Some individuals are quite sensitive, like my client described above. Many people simply cannot be around these signals. The Santa Fe *Reporter* last year ran a story on a woman who committed suicide out of exasperation at not being able to live anywhere because of wireless Internet. Her last resort, a campground, put in wireless Internet, and she ended up living in her car but ran out of energy to live that way any longer. These frequencies do not coexist peacefully with living bodies. If you have wireless Internet, go back to wired if you are willing; otherwise turn the wireless servers off when you are not using them, especially at night, as our bodies are even more vulnerable when asleep. Your cats and dogs sleep while you are away, so remember to turn them off when you leave as well.

I believe vaccination also plays a major part in hyperactivity and aberrant behavior; this has been thoughtfully proposed by Harris Coulter in his book *Vaccination, Social Violence, and Criminality.*[1] I have heard also of connections to mercury-based dental fillings; I do not know much about this connection, although there is certainly plenty of evidence incriminating mercury fillings in many other problems. Mercury is a known neurotoxin. One certainty is that in today's world we are bombarded with many stimuli and potentially damaging agents to a degree that it is difficult to sort out the impact of each one. Though this makes proof difficult, it does not obviate the need for caution with each one. I believe that we need to carefully examine our usage of chemicals and pollutants of all sorts, as the effect is usually much worse than we first believe. The fascination with supposedly harmless X-rays in the early years of this century caused great pain and suffering as their delayed effects emerged. Many people now scoff at the proposed dangers of common pollutants today, including electromagnetic fields. Will we look back with a similar horror in the next century?

Whatever the cause, hyperactivity is real. It is often treatable with homeopathy and other holistic methods,[2] though it is too complex to offer suggestions for home treatment. I recommend stopping vaccination and providing a clean diet and environment for these animals. Eliminate all chemical preservatives and pollutants to the greatest extent you can. For more information, see Chapter Sixteen, "Vaccination," and "Aggression" in Chapter Thirteen, "Nervous System."

Liver Disorders

Although liver problems should be treated by a veterinarian, I will give a few suggestions as to supplements and possible helpful remedies. This is not intended to supplant veterinary care, however, as these conditions are truly too serious for home care without the guidance of a veterinarian. Conventional medicine has little to offer for many liver diseases; I suggest consulting a holistic veterinarian if possible.

We see more liver problems in dogs than cats, although the latter are by no means exempt from these conditions. Fatty liver is one of the more common liver diseases in cats, and it may be associated with some of the high-fat, poor-quality diets that are formulated for cats with urinary tract disorders. In dogs, chronic liver inflammation is unfortunately rather common. It is often called chronic-active hepatitis because the underlying condition is chronic but the dogs tend to suffer repeated flare-ups that resemble acute liver illness. This is a conventional recognition that acute and chronic symptoms are often different aspects of one illness.

As with many conditions, some cases of liver inflammation may be autoimmune in that the liver is attacked by the body's immune system. This may be triggered by drugs, pesticides, other pollutants, and vaccination. I suspect these causes incite most cases of liver disease in dogs, and perhaps many cats. I have seen cases where blood work before and after vaccination showed greatly increased liver inflammation a couple of months after the vaccines. One poor dog had been taken to the veterinarian for an examination because her guardian felt she was ill. The veterinarian examined the dog and took blood for analysis, and then gave her the "yearly boosters." The dog worsened over the next few weeks, and when the guardian consulted with me, the liver enzymes had skyrocketed, indicating the aggravation of the liver inflammation. The conventional assumption that vaccines are harmless (and thus it is acceptable to vaccinate a sick animal) created increased suffering for this dog and her guardian. How many other dogs and cats and their guardians suffer similarly?

Pesticides may also cause direct liver damage. Organochlorine and organophosphate compounds are commonly used for flea and tick control on and off of animals. These chemicals are highly poisonous to the liver; they include such formulas as diazinon, chlorpyriphos, lindane, chlordane, malathion, fenthion, and dichlorvos. Corticosteroids ("cortisone") may also cause liver damage—even at normal dosage recommendations.

The major blood indicators of liver disease are alanine aminotransferase (ALT; the old acronym was SGPT), alkaline phosphatase (ALP; also "alk phos" or "alk p" for short), gamma-glutamyltransferase (GGT), aspartate aminotransferase (AST; old acronym SGOT), and bilirubin. The first four are enzymes and increase as the liver cells are damaged by inflammation. ALT and AST are more specific to liver cell damage, while ALP and GGT may indicate bile duct obstruction. Bilirubin is a blood pigment that is processed into bile by the liver (conjugated) and thus may increase in either condition; it may also increase with damage to blood cells. Conjugated bilirubin, also called direct bilirubin, is usually predominant with liver-associated bilirubin increases, while unconjugated or indirect bilirubin usually predominates with red blood cell damage, such as hemolytic anemias.

Liver disease is generally diagnosed with the assistance of blood testing, though in severe cases the accumulation of bilirubin discolors the gums and even the skin. The yellowish color is called jaundice or icterus. When this occurs, liver illness is usually the culprit, though severe blood cell destruction may also cause jaundice. If jaundice occurs due to liver disease, the condition is often critical.

Any animal with liver disease should be under the care of a veterinarian. The following supplements may prove helpful, though. I use low doses of most supplements for animals with liver disease. This is because even though supplements assist the liver it must also process them, and it is important to minimize the work load on the liver to allow healing. Don't use higher amounts unless your veterinarian advises you to do so; more is not necessarily better. This is especially true for niacin, one of the B vitamins, as it may damage the liver at high doses.

Milk thistle and its active compound, silymarin, is a potent liver protective and healing compound. I have heard anecdotal evidence that it has saved the lives of people who have eaten deadly mushrooms. It is especially useful in acute attacks, though I generally recommend it for all animals with liver ailments. There are many formulas available, so the best approach to dosage is to use it according to label recommendations for humans. For cats, use about one-eighth of the recommended human dose. For dogs up to twenty-five pounds, use one-eighth to one-fourth the human dose; for dogs between twenty-five to seventy-five pounds, give one-half the human dose, and for dogs above seventy-five pounds, give a full human dose.

Nutramax Laboratories now makes a product (Marin) for cats and dogs. You can get this from your veterinarian or online.

Turmeric (the spice) is a potent liver-specific antioxidant and is useful for most animals with liver inflammation. Give a pinch twice a day to cats and one-fourth teaspoonful per twenty-five pounds twice a day to dogs. Vitamin E (5 mg/pound mixed tocopherols, once a day) and vitamin C (5 mg/pound, two to three times a day, using natural vitamin C if available) are antioxidants and also can help. Superoxide dismutase (SOD) is another very potent antioxidant that is often beneficial. It usually comes in tablets with 2,000 IU or 125 mg of elemental SOD. Give one tablet per ten to fifteen pounds daily, and if giving more than one tablet, split the daily total into two or three individual doses. Coenzyme Q_{10} is another antioxidant and immune booster; give about one milligram per pound daily. The B vitamins provide good support overall and should be administered to all animals with liver disease. Give about ten milligrams of a multi-B per twenty to twenty-five pounds daily (for cats and for dogs up to twenty-five pounds, give 10 mg). Choline is a related vitamin that may be included; give about one milligram per pound daily.

Amino acids may also support the liver by two methods. First, giving a broad-based amino acid supplement reduces the liver's work by avoiding the need for protein metabolism and elimination of the resultant by-products. A protein drink such as those used by bodybuilders often meets this need, but be sure to get one without artificial preservatives or other chemicals. Secondly, certain amino acids have specific liver healing properties. L-methionine, L-cysteine, L-glutathione, L-arginine, and L-carnitine all help detoxify the liver. If not in the general amino acid supplement, these should be given separately. Give L-cysteine as follows: cats and small dogs, 12.5 mg; medium dogs 25 mg; and large dogs 50 mg. For all others give cats and small dogs 125 mg, medium dogs 250 mg, and large dogs 500 mg. All doses are once a day. S-adenosyl methionine (SAM-e), a particular form of methionine, is useful for depression and some liver disorders. It is more of a liver tonic than a detoxing agent, though it is helpful. It is available in health food stores at dosages for humans, though occasionally you may find a lower dosage (90 mg) product. Veterinarians sell Denosyl, a form made for cats and dogs, in appropriate doses. You can also find Denosyl online, as well as Denamarin, a combination with silymarin.

Fatty liver disease most commonly occurs in obese cats who stop eating;

the body then sends fat to the liver for processing, but these cats do not process fats well. The resultant buildup obstructs the liver cells and causes an inflammation. If your obese cat stops eating, be sure to feed her something by syringe, if necessary. A good formula is a protein powder, like Goatein, plus green foods like spirulina or chlorella powder. A green drink, like Pure Synergy (from the Synergy Company) or Berry Greens (from New Chapter) can also be mixed with a protein powder. Give two to three dropperfuls, three to six times daily. For fatty liver disease, the amino acids L-arginine, L-methionine, and L-carnitine are especially helpful. Lecithin is also particularly beneficial, as it helps fat metabolism. Give one-fourth to one-half teaspoon of lecithin per ten pounds daily. Leafy green vegetables provide nutritional and detoxification support and should be fed to all animals with liver disease. *Chelidonium* is very good for fatty liver; other possible remedies include *Phosphorus*, *Antimonium crudum*, *Arsenicum album*, *Phytolacca*, and *Iodoformum*, though these should be administered under the guidance of an experienced homeopath. You can start with *Chelidonium* and the protein powder–green food formula, but if this does not help within twenty-four hours, seek help.

Combination herbal remedies often work better than individual forms; you can find these at health food stores. Use one-eighth the human dose per ten to fifteen pounds. Two products that I like are Bupleurum Liver Cleanse, by Planetary Formulas, and Thistle Cleanse, by Zand, though there are many others that can help.

The following homeopathic medicines have specific benefit to the liver and thus can be used in conjunction with other therapies. They are not a substitute for the correct constitutional remedy, although I occasionally will use these in low potency along with the constitutional remedy. Though this is not purely classical homeopathy, it is often quite beneficial, and the liver-specific remedies do not usually interfere with the action of the main remedy. As these are supportive only, the mental picture may not fit in all cases, so I recommend trying one at a time for a couple of weeks to a couple of months to see if it helps. Use them in low potency (3X, 6X, 3C, or 6C) one to three times a day.

Berberis vulgaris

While we mostly associate *Berberis* with kidney disease, it is a good liver detox and supportive herb as well. There are usually fairly severe back pains, especially in the mid-back, when *Berberis* is indicated. The kidney and liver often become affected together, since both are involved in toxin elimination, so this remedy, like dandelion *(Taraxicum)*, is a good choice when both organs are involved.

Carduus marianus

This remedy is made from milk thistle (see above), and I have used it successfully as support in animals that cannot handle the herbal form for whatever reason. There may be vomiting of green material (bile). The patient may also experience severe colic and cramping along with the liver attacks.

Chelidonium majus

This is the remedy that is most known for liver support. It may even provide help with jaundiced animals and with fatty liver disease. These patients tend to be angry (anger is the emotion related to the liver, according to traditional Chinese medicine) and domineering; they may also be rather disobedient. Hot drinks, hot foods, and hot applications or baths may soothe these animals. The mental picture may not always be present if this is not the constitutional remedy, yet the remedy may provide support. If these mental and general (better warm) signs are present, the remedy will probably be very beneficial.

Cholesterinum

As the name suggests, this remedy is made from cholesterol. It is especially helpful when there is a bile duct obstruction or with fatty liver, though it may be helpful with any liver ailment. These patients may produce copious amounts of urine before an attack of liver inflammation.

Lactuca virosa

These animals are typically restless and ill-humored. They feel a weight in their abdomen from liver inflammation. This remedy can be good for chronic hepatitis and advanced liver disease. There may be colic or loud rumbling sounds in the abdomen. Passing stools brings great fatigue. They may be worse from touch or in a warm room.

Myrica

Bayberry (the herbal name for *Myrica)* has a "marked action on the liver, with jaundice." There may be foul mucus in the mouth, throat, or stool. These animals are sore and often lame; they are weak and depressed as well. Gloominess and despondency can alternate with irritability. If you see this mental state in an animal with jaundice (icterus), *Myrica* may be your remedy. They are worse in the morning and after sleep, and better in the open air.

Phosphorus

This major remedy has a lot of affinity to the liver. Use in low potency, as above, unless you are certain it fits your animal's picture well.

Rumex crispus

Rumex is yellow dock, another good liver detox agent as an herb, or you can use a low potency like 6X. The tincture is pretty strong-tasting, so the low potency is better for compliance.

Taraxicum

Dandelion is a very good liver and kidney detoxing agent. Use a tincture of leaf and root, and give three drops per ten pounds, two to three times daily. You can also use *Taraxicum* as a low potency; this is the homeopathic form of dandelion.

New Puppy or Kitten

The first consideration regarding the important step of taking in a new companion animal is whether or not you really have the time and space to give him a good home. If you are contemplating getting a large dog, for example, do you have the room he needs to run and play? Will you have plenty of time to take him for long walks? In any animal-care situation, it is important that people are home enough to provide company. This is especially true if you live in an apartment or in a house where you cannot let the animal out to explore the yard and find entertainment. As I grow in age, practice experience, and wisdom, I find that I am more concerned about keeping animals, especially keeping them indoors—imprisoning them. I do not think cats should be kept strictly indoors, even though we just lost a cat two days ago to a coyote as I write this. There are extenuating circumstances, such as inner-city living, but in most cases cats can handle outdoor life. I basically feel the same with dogs, though they are somewhat more prone to roam than cats, being a species that roams for a living. But freedom is as essential to nonhuman animal health as it is for humans, and we may be doing a disservice by containing these animals. See Chapter Seventeen, "The Bigger Picture," for more information.

Many health problems occur because animals are simply bored, even greatly stressed, because they live indoors and alone for most of their lives. If you cannot provide a healthy mental environment, your animal will become ill. This is almost without exception. I have visited friends in apartment buildings and heard the lonesome cry of a kitten late in the evening, triggered by my walking by the door of her apartment. The guardians were not home much. It saddens me to think of the thousands of lonely animals locked in spaces by themselves. This is really unfair. These are conscious beings who need love and caring in much the same manner as we do. We really should not take in a companion if we cannot provide a good home. By contrast, the more you can interact with your companion dog or cat, the more rewarding your relationship will become. I am constantly amazed at the stories I hear from my clients. These beings are capable of many emotions and behaviors that enrich our lives immensely.

Getting a new kitten or puppy for children is often a good experience for this reason, but the children must be old enough to understand how to relate to animals. Many young children are very rough and injure animals inadvertently. Generally, children under three to five years may be too young for animals unless parental supervision is close. If you wish to teach your child responsibility in having him care for a companion animal, be realistic about his ability according to his age. Help him as much as needed; don't allow the animal to suffer because the child is not responsible. I suggest that the child be about eight to ten years old, maybe older, before you place much responsibility in his hands. Read also Chapter Seventeen, "The Bigger Picture," if you are interested in examining the pet animal culture, and Chapter Fourteen, "Reproductive System," for my concerns about breeding.

When you bring the puppy or kitten home, the change of household and the separation from his mother may engender great stress at first. The Bach flower essences Rescue Remedy and Walnut can be helpful. The former is good for any stressful situation, while the latter is helpful during times of transition. New Home–Group Living, by Pet Essences (www.petessences.com), is also helpful. If the newcomer is going to be sleeping alone, a radio or ticking clock may help alleviate feelings of loneliness. Of course, lots of love and reassurance is also very important. The first few days and weeks are critical in his adjustment to a new family, and a good start goes a long way toward a healthy relationship and a healthy life.

The two most important factors in maintaining good health are good food and avoidance of stress. The best food in my opinion is a home-prepared diet, but it must be balanced. If you simply cannot prepare foods, there are many sources of frozen, raw meat–based diets now available. Though they can be pricey, they provide a good option. Otherwise, use the best commercial food you can get, and supplement with lots of "table foods." These will give a lot of the ingredients that are missing from canned or dry foods. Any heat or processing destroys many enzymes and other nutrients, and it also destroys the life force of the food. In any case, be sure to use foods with human-grade ingredients, and organic if possible. See Chapter Eight, "Digestive System," for more information.

Avoidance of stress includes both mental stress, as discussed above, and physical stress. Physical stress comes from pollution and chemical poisoning, drugs, food additives (colorings, preservatives, etc.), and vaccination. While puppy and kitten vaccination may be helpful in animals who are exposed to diseases, most animals are not at risk for most diseases for which they are vaccinated, and the risk from vaccination is thus greater than the risk of the disease. Additionally, yearly vaccination is completely unnecessary, as it provides no additional protection. It can only cause harm. Rabies vaccination is required every one to three years according to state law, but this is a legal rather than a medical requirement. If you have the time and energy, please help change these requirements in your region. See Chapter Sixteen, "Vaccination," before you decide on immunizing your companions.

Other potential stressors include microchips and spaying and neutering. Basically, I do not recommend microchips, as I feel their potential damage outweighs their potential use, though there is an argument for their use in free-roaming animals. I would not do this to animals directly under my care, however. See the section above on "Hyperactivity," in this chapter, for a bit on microchips. Spaying and neutering may be a necessity for now, but read Chapter Fourteen, "Reproductive System," for more information on this topic. Chapter Seventeen, "The Bigger Picture," may also help place this within a moral context.

For more information on general care of animals, especially providing a good home and preparing foods at home, see Dr. Pitcairn's book on dogs and cats, Anitra Frazier's book on cats, and Helen McKinnon's book on food preparation. These are listed in the appendix.

Overheating (Heatstroke, Sunstroke)

These are uncommon but may occur if an animal is tied or otherwise restrained in the sun or in a hot space such as a car. Of course, these situations are best avoided rather than treated, and you should never leave an animal in a parked car in the sun. Even with the windows open, the car will quickly overheat. The dog's body temperature also rises rapidly under this condition, and brain damage (including death) may occur rapidly. Overheating may also occur if you take your dog for a long run in hot, humid weather, especially if he is not acclimated to such conditions.

Cats and dogs do not normally sweat as humans and horses do, so the only mechanism for rapid heat reduction is panting. Overheated animals immediately begin panting, sometimes intensely. The mucous membranes and skin become deep red as the body shifts circulation to superficial areas to increase heat loss. Nausea, dizziness, and weakness quickly ensue if the body temperature does not drop. Furthermore, continued high temperature may impair the temperature-regulating center in the brain. This may limit the ability to cool the body, greatly increasing the danger. At this time the skin may become cool and the animal is usually faint or may lose consciousness.

Overheating is an emergency situation. Veterinary care is best but time is critical, as brain damage may occur in a very few minutes. Rapid cooling is necessary to avoid damage. Rinsing or immersion in cool water is the most effective method to bring the body temperature down. Don't use ice water or even extremely cold water, as this may worsen the problem by one of two mechanisms. First, the cold water may cause the surface blood vessels to constrict, reducing the heat transfer out of the body. Secondly, extremely cold water may induce shivering, the body's method of countering cold body temperatures, and this can dramatically increase body heat, especially in conjunction with the first reaction.

One of the following homeopathic medicines may help combat the potential damage from overheating.

Aconitum napellus
Anxiety is usually strong when this remedy is needed. These animals will

be quite restless and fearful. There is congestion to the head, which may cause a headache and nausea. There may be hemorrhage from the nose. Consider this remedy first, just as the condition begins to appear.

Belladonna
The *Belladonna* state is more intense than that of *Aconite* in that these animals have greater physical changes. The ears and gums are usually intensely red, the pupils may be dilated, and the dog is generally agitated. The restlessness here is more violent compared to the anxious quality of the *Aconite* restlessness.

Gelsemium
This remedy is especially known for weakness. These patients will become weak and dizzy, possibly to the point of collapse. Their muscles often tremble from the weakness. They may alternate between flushes of heat and cold, clammy skin. This is a typical heat exhaustion sign.

Glonoinum
This is the classic sunstroke remedy. These patients develop a pounding headache with weakness and irritability from overexposure to sun. The jaws may clench together. The animal's ears and gums may alternate between paleness and redness, possibly with a bluish cast. The heart often pounds violently.

Natrum carbonicum
These patients are constitutionally averse to the sun. There is generally great debility and exhaustion from heat and exposure to the sun. This remedy may be more effective for animals who become sick due to oversensitivity to sun heat rather than those who have truly become overheated.

Selenium
This mineral is necessary for muscle function and strength. Similarly, the homeopathic remedy made from the mineral is useful for weakness and debility. Any heat increases this debility. As with *Natrum carbonicum*, this remedy is especially useful in animals who are extremely sensitive to overheating. *Selenium* is often indicated in older animals.

Veratrum viride

This remedy, like *Glonoine,* is indicated in very violent conditions. If your companion suffers from violent congestion and furious delirium as a result of sunstroke, one of these two remedies is probably needed, although *Belladonna* should also be considered. When *Veratrum viride* (not to be confused with *Veratrum album)* is needed, there are often strong muscle twitches, possibly accompanied by severe vomiting. The animal then may suddenly become weak and may even collapse.

Surgery

While surgery is an invasive and even drastic measure, it is often a necessary solution to some conditions. There are some steps you can take to improve your companion's comfort and speed her recovery.

Before any surgery (except emergencies), take time to have her in good condition. For a week or two prior to surgery, give her extra vitamins C, E, A, and B. For vitamin C, give her about 10 mg per pound twice a day, using natural C if available; for vitamin E, give 5–10 mg per pound mixed tocopherols once a day; for vitamin A, give 75–100 IU per pound daily; and give about 10–15 mg of B vitamins per ten to twenty-five pounds daily. Continue this for a week or two after surgery as well.

Other antioxidants can help also. Superoxide dismutase (SOD) is very useful. Give 2,000 IU or 125 mg elemental SOD (usually one tablet) per ten to twenty pounds daily, split into two to three doses. Coenzyme Q_{10} may also benefit the surgical patient. Give 1 mg per pound daily.

On the day of surgery, give *Arnica* 30C and Rescue Remedy (the Bach flower essence) before surgery and after surgery. These may be combined in a small dropper bottle by putting five to seven drops of Rescue Remedy and a few pellets of *Arnica* into the bottle. Fill the bottle with water and then give several drops to the patient by mouth. If your veterinarian is cooperative, ask her to give this formula immediately after surgery and every hour or two thereafter for the first day. Continue for a few days, gradually lengthening the interval between doses. This helps with pain and surgical stress. *Passiflora incarnata* 3X or 6X may also be helpful during the trip to and from the clinic as well as presurgery, as it often provides a calming effect. Calms Forte, a combination calming remedy by Hylands, is also helpful here. *Hamamelis* and *Bellis perennis* are similar to *Arnica* and may relieve postsurgical pain if the latter does not prove sufficient.

You may also use the following protocol for postsurgical treatment (use the *Arnica* and Rescue Remedy presurgically): during the initial period, usually the first day, use *Staphysagria* for incisional pain. The next period, usually the second day, use *Calendula* for deeper trauma, still in the abdominal wall. Finally, use *Bellis perennis* for the deep abdominal trauma. This will usually be the third day. These periods may vary with different animals; some may move through faster than others. Use the remedy that provides the best relief, which may be any one of the remedies listed in this paragraph and the previous one. You may also try Traumeel, a combination remedy for trauma, in the postoperative period.

If your animal has undergone a major abdominal surgery, like a major organ removal, cancer removal, or bowel resection, use *Calcarea fluorica* in low potency (6X, 6C) once or twice a day. This may reduce postoperative adhesions. If adhesions do develop, *Thiosinaminum* in low potency can help. For postneutering bleeding into the scrotum, which occasionally occurs in dogs, *Bellis perennis* is the most helpful, though *Hamamelis* and *Arnica* may also help.

If your patient awakens slowly from anesthesia, the remedy *Phosphorus* will often speed his recovery. In this situation you may alternate the *Phosphorus* with the *Arnica* preparation. If the recovery is especially difficult and his postsurgical weakness is profound, try the remedy *Acetic acid*. Of course, you will again need the cooperation of your veterinary surgeon here, as your companion will be hospitalized during the recovery period. For postsurgical bleeding, *Phosphorus* once again comes to our aid. *Millefolium* may help if *Phosphorus* is ineffective. If profound weakness occurs following bleeding during surgery, *Strontium carbonicum* may help.

Calendula ointment or gel is useful topically to ease incision pain and to speed healing. If the incision seems especially painful, try the remedy *Staphysagria* by mouth. For orthopedic surgery to repair broken bones, see also the section on "First Aid for Broken Bones" in Chapter Twelve, "Musculoskeletal System."

In some animals, the drugs and anesthesia can result in headaches and nausea in the postanesthetic period. If your animal seems like she has a hangover, try *Nux vomica*. Anesthetics can cause problems in some animals. Ketamine is especially troublesome and should never be used, in my opinion. Tiletamine (Telazol) carries the same risks. See the section on "Aggression" in Chapter Thirteen, "Nervous System," for more information on some risks with ketamine. Propofol can cause heart-muscle contractility issues and heart failure; humans (and presumably other species) occasionally die from this. I am also aware of two cases wherein propofol may have caused recurrent collapsing, possibly via the same mechanism. I prefer mild tranquilization and masking patients with inhalant anesthetics like sevofluorane to these injectable drugs.

Thyroid Disease

As with liver disease and heart problems, thyroid illness should be treated by an experienced homeopathic veterinarian. These conditions are serious, sometimes life-threatening, and warrant expert help.

The thyroid glands are located in the neck, on either side of the trachea (windpipe). They produce thyroid hormone, a substance that stimulates body metabolism. Decreased thyroid hormone, or hypothyroidism, results typically in overweight, sluggish animals who are chilly and often have a poor coat. This condition is rather common in dogs and rare in cats. It is much more common than it was when I graduated from veterinary school thirty years ago. Hyperthyroidism, an excess production of thyroid hormone, occurs in cats and is rare in dogs. When this occurs, the individual typically eats ravenously, though she loses weight as the food passes rapidly through the intestines and exits as diarrhea without providing much nourishment. These patients tend to be restless, hyperactive, and warm-natured. Hyperthyroidism was virtually nonexistent when I graduated from veterinary school. It may be a somewhat normal compensation for decreased kidney function, as the increased thyroid hormone levels improve blood flow to the kidneys.

For the hypothyroid dog, as with all conditions, it is important to provide good food such as a home-prepared diet. A few supplements may be useful. Kelp provides trace minerals including iodine, an essential part of thyroid hormone. Give one tablet per ten pounds daily. The amino acid L-tyrosine is the other major ingredient, as it forms the base for the thyroid hormones; low levels of L-tyrosine have been associated with hypothyroidism in humans. Give 125 mg per twenty-five pounds once or twice a day.

If you need to give thyroid hormones to your dog, the most commonly prescribed form is a synthetic hormone, but it contains only one of the two major forms of thyroid hormone (T_4). There are medications made from raw thyroid glands that contain all of the thyroid hormone forms, and these provide a more balanced replenishment. Armour Thyroid is the best choice here. Many practitioners feel that these work better than the synthetic drug. This is my choice in those cases that require hormone replacement. I also recommend underdosing, since full hormone replacement stops the brain (pituitary gland) hormones that tell the thyroid gland to produce thyroid hormone. Full supplementation to a normal dog may make him unable to produce thyroid hormone because of this feedback loop. Similarly, full supplementation will limit the ability of a hypothyroid dog to regain any function of his thyroid gland. By contrast, minimal dosing is usually adequate to keep him relatively symptom-free, yet still leaving room for improved function of the gland. Hypothyroidism is rarely a serious disease, although in a few dogs it is associated with bleeding disorders. In most cases, however, undersupplementation is quite safe.

In cats, hyperthyroid disease is much more dangerous and is more difficult to treat. Relatively few supplements provide benefit. Good food is essential, and digestive enzymes may improve digestion, allowing the cat to reap greater benefit from her food. Kelp or other seaweeds can help normalize thyroid function, even though the thyroid hormones are high already. The *Brassica* family of vegetables (broccoli, cabbage, cauliflower, brussels sprouts, kale, turnips) contain a compound that can slow an overactive thyroid gland. If you can get your cat to eat these, they may help. Some cats like these vegetables (I live with one cat who loves broccoli), so don't give up before you try. Some supplement manufacturers produce dehydrated broccoli (and other cruciferous vegetables) in capsule form; these can also help. Use one-half to one capsule per cat daily.

Conventional treatment offers three options. The first is a drug to destroy thyroid tissue, thus reducing hormone output. In my experience, this is poorly effective and the drugs are very liver- and kidney-toxic. I do not recommend this approach. The second route is surgical. Removal of the gland will reduce or eliminate thyroid hormone. Usually only one side is affected. Most surgeons recommend removal of both glands due to the propensity of recurrence on the unaffected side following removal of the affected side. With this approach, however, hormone replacement is necessary. Additionally, the parathyroid glands are removed also. These glands control calcium balance within the body, and this is critical. I suggest one-sided removal (if you choose surgery), as it avoids these postsurgical complications, and holistic and homeopathic treatment can minimize recurrence. I know colleagues who find this approach very satisfactory. The third treatment choice is radioactive iodine therapy. The iodine goes directly to the thyroid gland and destroys part of the gland, reducing hormone output. The reported success with this treatment is quite good by conventional standards. I have concerns about the long-term effects of the radioactivity, and this would not be my first choice. Radioactive iodine is one of the most highly radioactive elements known. In fairness, however, I have had clients who chose this for their cats and who are quite pleased with the outcome. I have had other cases where complications followed the treatment, though.

Additional note on radioactive iodine therapy: Since I wrote the first edition of this book, I have seen a number of cases wherein the radioactive iodine treatment produced only short-term improvement and produced long-term damage. One of the cats I alluded to above, from the time of the first edition, had appeared to improve nicely and partially resulted in my more positive impression, but after the book went to press she relapsed and ended up dying in short order. I know of at least two cats who suffered from burned urinary bladders as a consequence of excreting the radioactive iodine, and other cats who became severely ill following treatment, probably from immune system damage. These cats did not recover. As of this edition, I do not recommend radioactive iodine treatment. I do know that those using the procedure claim very good treatment success, but this has not been my experience. Perhaps my client base is biased against the treatment, since I don't see the ones who respond well, but perhaps also the reported successes are overstated, since they may be based upon short-term evaluations.

I would choose homeopathic or other holistic methods first if one of my cat companions were affected with hyperthyroidism. These are generally safer and sometimes can be effective. If this did not work, however, my next choice would be surgical removal of the affected side along with continued homeopathic support.

Thyroid disease is generally autoimmune in origin. That is, the body's own immune system attacks the body and causes these changes. The large number of animals with thyroid disease are part of the vastly increased volume of autoimmune diseases we see today compared to twenty years ago. Thyroid diseases have been associated with vaccination and drug use. Monthly heartworm preventives as well as "sulfa" drugs are known to occasionally trigger autoimmune thyroid disease.[3] I do not generally recommend vaccines and drugs for most animals, and they are especially risky for animals with thyroid disease. See Chapter Sixteen, "Vaccination," for more information.

Further thyroid damage results from the too-ubiquitous presence of thyroid damaging or limiting elements. Many nuclear power plants release radioactive iodine. Chlorine and fluorine are present in most municipal water supplies in the United States, even though most European countries and many countries worldwide have banned fluoridation. These elements compete with nonradioactive iodine for uptake into the thyroid gland. Radioactive iodine obviously damages the gland, and fluorine and chlorine insert themselves into thyroid hormones but produce inactive forms. This is why kelp and other seaweeds are so important for hypothyroid and hyperthyroid animals, as it provides healthy iodine in sufficient quantity. It is better as a preventive than for treatment, but still helpful in the latter situation. Incidentally, fluoridation carries great risk in addition to thyroid problems, including bone cancers. It has been a great mistake.

Vaccine Reactions

This section only covers acute reactions to vaccination. These are generally responses that occur within the first day or so. Before you choose to vaccinate, please see Chapter Sixteen, "Vaccination," for information about vaccine safety and effectiveness.

Common acute reactions to vaccines include swelling of the face, especially around the eyes; hives; breathing difficulty; fever; vomiting; diarrhea; trembling; and weakness. Behavior changes may also occur regularly. Fear and aggression are the most common behavioral reactions. Seizures and even paralysis may also occur following vaccination, though less commonly.

If your animal experiences one of these reactions, contact the veterinarian who administered the vaccine. If the reaction includes facial swelling or breathing difficulty (the latter often follows the former) you should take the animal to the clinic right away (see also "Allergic Reactions" above). With the other responses, you may usually attempt home treatment. Seizures warrant veterinary attention if they last more than a few minutes or if they repeat more than two or three times. One of the following homeopathic medicines may help if your companion has a reaction to vaccination. If you do not get a good response, see your veterinarian. Consider consulting a homeopathic veterinarian also, as these reactions may indicate a need for further treatment.

Aconitum napellus

Aconite's jurisdiction is usually the early stages of inflammation. Fever is a common indication for this remedy, especially if accompanied by anxiety or fear. These animals are usually restless. Seizures after vaccination may also respond to Aconite.

Apis mellifica

If facial swelling occurs following vaccination, this is the first remedy to consider. Diarrhea after vaccination may also respond, especially if the animal is thirstless (most animals with diarrhea are thirsty).

Antimonium tartaricum

This remedy may be needed for diarrhea after vaccination. Respiratory difficulty may also respond, although Thuja is usually the first choice for vaccine-induced breathing problems.

Arsenicum album

This remedy may also be of assistance for those animals that develop breathing difficulty, diarrhea, or vomiting following vaccination. Fear is common as well, and this is generally my first choice for fearful animals when the fear arises following a vaccination. Back pain following vaccination may respond to this remedy.

Belladonna

This remedy may successfully treat seizures that occur after a vaccination. These animals tend to be agitated and restless, with dilated pupils. They may be very aggressive as well. An animal who repetitively turns in circles following vaccination may also respond to Belladonna. Intense fevers come under the sphere of this remedy also.

Pyrogenium

This remedy may be useful for persistent fevers following vaccination, especially if the animal is experiencing pain along the back. It is also sometimes given routinely following vaccinations, but see the note below under Thuja regarding this usage.

Silicea (Silica)

This remedy may be helpful for diarrhea following vaccination, especially if the patient is weak, rather delicate, and sensitive to noises or to brushing the coat. Some cases of seizures may also respond to *Silicea*.

Thuja occidentalis

Thuja is one of our best remedies (along with *Silicea*) for adverse effects from vaccination. Asthmatic breathing, eye inflammation, diarrhea, urinary problems, and rear-leg weakness or paralysis are some of the conditions that may respond to *Thuja* if they occur following a vaccination. This is often the first remedy given, even for chronic diseases, if vaccination is suspected to be the cause. Many practitioners routinely give this remedy following vaccinations, though it probably has minimal effect when used in this manner. It is foolish to assume that we can give vaccinations and then simply remove any negative impact with homeopathy. It is much better to avoid the vaccination.

Worms (Intestinal)

Worms and animals are almost synonymous in our "cultural mind." There is much myth and fear around this topic. Cats and dogs harbor four main types of intestinal worms: roundworms, hookworms, tapeworms, and whipworms. The southeastern United States is the most worm-prevalent region in this country due to the warm, humid climate.

According to a study some years ago by the Centers for Disease Control, 90 to 95 percent of puppies have roundworms regardless of whether or not the mother has worms when she is pregnant. The roundworm and the dog (presumably also the cat, perhaps to a lesser extent) may be said to coexist. The larval stages of the worm may lie dormant in the mammary gland and then pass to the puppies in the milk. Since the maturation period is about three weeks, a three- to four-week-old puppy may have a heavy worm burden in some cases. Most puppies (according to the CDC study) clear the worms on their own by puberty. In some cases, however, the worm burden causes illness and even death. This is more common with hookworms than roundworms.

Hookworms may be transmitted to puppies in the same manner as roundworms, and since the maturation period is also three weeks, a three- to four-week-old puppy may have a worm load of both hookworms and roundworms. Hookworms are especially deadly because they attach to the intestinal wall and suck blood. Large numbers of hookworms can easily deplete the blood supply of a small puppy or kitten, causing death. Roundworms, by contrast, primarily compete with the host for nutrients in food, and though they can be serious, it usually takes longer to deplete the host compared to a hookworm infestation. The scruffy, pot-bellied puppy is a typical picture of a roundworm infestation. Adult roundworms are about two to three inches long and one-sixteenth inch wide or a little wider, and they are tapered at the ends. You may see them in stools, and occasionally in vomitus. Hookworms are tiny and almost impossible to see with the naked eye.

Many veterinarians recommend routinely deworming puppies at three to four weeks of age to prevent health problems. While I am reticent to give any medicine on a routine basis, this practice has some merit, especially in regions with high worm populations like the southeastern United States. Since it takes a mature worm to produce eggs that can be found on fecal flotation tests, puppies can develop trouble before worms are detected. In most cases this is unlikely to happen, especially if the mother and puppies are rather healthy and the mother is on a good diet. Worms, like most "invaders," are opportunists; they need a weakened host if they are to occur in great numbers. When puppies or kittens become overloaded, though, they can die rather quickly.

If your puppies or kittens are not in full health, and especially if you live in the southeastern United States, you might consider giving one dose of pyrantel pamoate (Nemex and Evict are two brand names) at three to four weeks of age. I do not recommend routine dosing after this time; rather I suggest that further treatment be based upon a fecal flotation to identify which worms, if any, are present. If you choose not to give the routine deworming, keep a close eye on the puppies or kittens as they move through the three- to eight-week age bracket, as this age is the most susceptible to worm-related depletion. Additionally, I recommend that you have a fecal analysis done on a group specimen at four to six weeks of age and deworm only if necessary.

Whipworms occur mostly in the southeastern United States. They have a three-month life cycle rather than the three-week cycle of roundworms and hookworms. Whipworms generally affect young adult dogs, and they may cause severe intestinal distress. Fecal analysis and deworming is appropriate.

Tapeworms are rather common and rarely cause problems in animals, though their appearance is rather unsightly. You generally see tapeworm segments attached to the hair around the anus, or you may see segments in fresh bowel movements. Occasionally you may see the segments on furniture or rugs where your companion has just been resting. Fresh segments are one-quarter to one-half inch long and a little less than one-eighth inch wide. They are obviously flat, and they may stretch and retract. When dry they resemble a grain of rice.

There are primarily two types of tapeworms in cats and dogs in the United States. *Dipylidium caninum* is commonly called the "flea tapeworm" because fleas ingest the eggs of this worm. When the host animal then ingests the flea, the host becomes infested with a tapeworm. Flea control is essential to prevent reinfestation. The other type of tapeworms are transmitted when carnivores catch and eat wild animals. *Taenia* and *Echinococcus* are two worm genera that may infest various prey species. The worm larvae generally inhabit the abdomen of the prey animal, and the predator ingests the larvae during consumption. Reinfestation is common if the host animal is an active hunter. Treatment is only necessary if you see tapeworm segments, and then it is not usually necessary for the animal's health as tapeworms rarely cause problems. Modern drugs for tapeworms are relatively safe and effective, though I have heard anecdotal reports of problems in rare cases.

If an adult animal has persistent or repeated worm infestations, this is a sign of chronic illness and you should consider constitutional homeopathic treatment. Any worm appearance other than tapeworms in an animal over two years of age is probably a sign of illness. While constitutional treatment can be very effective in these cases, most worm problems in puppies and kittens do not respond well to homeopathy, in my experience. To some degree, this may be that there is a place for worms in puppies and kittens, possibly to stimulate the developing immune system. For this reason, I recommend minimal worm treatment to allow nature to take her course, unless the animal is ill from the worms. As the CDC study showed, most animals handle the worms on their own. Those that become overwhelmed may need drug therapy. Those that simply cannot shake the worms need nutritional and homeopathic (or other health-strengthening methods) treatment to develop the ability to eliminate the worm burden as health improves.

Tapeworms are an exception to the need for constitutional treatment, possibly since they are of little consequence. About 50 percent of animals respond nicely to the homeopathic remedy *Granatum*. I usually give this in very low potency (3X, 6X, 3C, 6C) twice a day for five days. Sometimes the worms reappear and drug treatment is necessary if you wish to eliminate the worms. Garlic in the food may also reduce the worm burden. Gentle Dragon, an herbal intestinal cleansing product, may help in some animals with worms by cleaning the intestinal environment and making it less hospitable to worms. Though the manufacturer makes no claims for worm treatment, the product may diminish the numbers of worms with any type of intestinal worm.

I have focused upon conventional deworming medications here, as my experience with herbal deworming preparations has been mostly unsatisfactory. Additionally, many herbal preparations do contain toxic ingredients, and herbal deworming requires two to four weeks of administration. While there may easily be effective herbal preparations of which I am unaware, I tend to simply use conventional drugs here in acute phases, and homeopathy and supportive treatment to support overall health and reduce susceptibility.

Pinworms, a common problem in children, do not affect cats or dogs. Sometimes parents are told that their children's pinworm infestation came from the family cat or dog, but this is incorrect.

Part Three
IMPORTANT SUPPLEMENTAL INFORMATION

Chapter Sixteen
VACCINATION

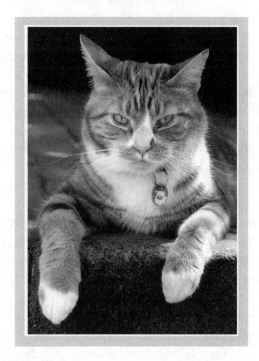

Introduction

Fortunately, since I first wrote this book and this chapter, we have made some progress on the vaccine front. Most veterinary schools and most leading veterinary organizations now offer much more conservative vaccination recommendations than a decade ago. Most experts differentiate core vaccines, such as feline panleukopenia virus, canine distemper and parvovirus, and rabies virus, from noncore vaccines like the feline leukemia virus. The latter vaccines are not typically recommended in most circumstances. This change somewhat follows my recommendations, although we do not agree totally here. Furthermore, most experts now recommend booster vaccines every three years rather than yearly. This is just how I began backing away from vaccinations twenty years ago. It is really "baby steps," and it is unnecessary to give triennial (every three years) vaccinations, but it is a big step in the right direction. As I explain in this chapter, vaccine boosters are almost totally unnecessary, but at least the profession as a whole is moving in the right direction. Still, we have a long way to go yet.

I have spoken with university veterinarians who admit that we do not need even the triennial boosters, yet they still teach this to students because they think it would be too confusing for students (and private-practice veterinarians) to learn that boosters are unnecessary. I suppose they think the students and clinicians will have a hard time bridging the gap between previous annual vaccination recommendations and the actual absence of any need for boosters. I disagree; I think my colleagues and soon-to-be colleagues are much more capable of change than this. But I am still grateful for the shift in recent years. Even seeing how the wider veterinary community is taking some of the same steps I took encourages my hope that the shift will continue in the direction I have taken.

Current recommendations, however, as taught by universities, still weigh heavily upon overvaccination. Until the universities begin teaching vaccine practices based upon current immunological knowledge, we who do not wish to use vaccinations, or wish to use them based upon current guidelines, must stand firmly. Hopefully, this chapter will help you in this area. And unfortunately, many clinicians "in the field" have yet to adopt even these basic guidelines, and they still vaccinate yearly. It takes time for new information to filter down, apparently. But you can check such Web sites as the American Veterinary Medical Association and the American Animal Hospital Association, as well as the American Association of Feline

Practitioners, if you need to give your local veterinarian evidence to at least back away from annual vaccinations. You can, of course, also show her this chapter from my book (or buy her a copy!), though obviously my views are much further away than those of the associations above.

To be clear up front, I do not recommend vaccination in almost all circumstances, just in case you have not yet read this chapter from my previous book. I only mention the above as assistance in bringing your local veterinarian along the path toward understanding how much our profession overvaccinates and the possible dangers of vaccination. This is a long distance for many veterinarians, so the information from the sites mentioned above can be a bridge between where your local veterinarian may be now and where you will be once you have integrated the information in this chapter.

Fortunately, there is widespread vaccine awareness among holistically oriented veterinarians and guardians today. In addition to moving away from excessive vaccination, emphasis has shifted toward alternative procedures to ensure animal health. Diet and decreased reliance upon drugs and pesticides are part of this shift, though not directly related to vaccination and specific disease protection. Titer testing and nosode use, however, are directly related. Many people today express interest in both as a part of protecting their companion animals or their patients. Unfortunately, there is a lot of confusion and even downright misinformation out there. In the current version of this chapter, therefore, I have added a more complete discussion of nosodes as well as an entirely new section on titers. I actually overlooked the titer issue in the first edition, so I am grateful now to be able to provide some clarity on this important issue, as titer testing can be helpful for veterinarians and guardians who would like some assurance of protection against those major diseases for which we vaccinate. Understanding just how and when titers can help—and when they do not—is critical. Nosodes as well can reassure some guardians of assistance in protecting their companions, although, as I discuss toward the chapter's end, they are not simply a replacement for vaccines but must be used according to their best effectiveness and safety.

In addition to adding the nosode and titer sections, I have also fleshed out certain parts of the original chapter, including adding new information about vaccine damage. Another shift by the conventional veterinary community has been research into vaccine damage. While I do not like animal experimentation, the fact that university researchers and others are beginning to examine the vaccine damage question is a huge step. I believe this will further result in decreasing our dependence upon vaccination in the future. I have added a few examples of these research findings to this chapter, as they support my previous conclusions nicely. I encourage anyone who has read the first version of this chapter to read the chapter again, not only for your own edification but also to assist you when you talk with others about vaccines. So let's start from the beginning.

The Vaccine Quandary

Veterinarians and animal guardians alike are seriously questioning the current guidelines for vaccination of animals. Not only holistic veterinarians, but also increasing numbers of conventional practitioners and leading veterinary immunologists believe we are overemphasizing immunization. The issue is a hot one, challenging a half-century of rapid expansion of vaccine use and the attendant income this use provides to veterinarians and vaccine manufacturers. Quite naturally, this provides an ethical dilemma as well as a mounting controversy. Personally, I do not consider the issue controversial; certainly within the veterinary homeopathic community it is not. But realizing how sensitive the vaccine issue is within the broader veterinary community, I decided the best approach for this chapter was to share my experience and what I have learned along the way about vaccination.

During veterinary school, we studied the underlying theory of vaccination: exposing animals to an organism that had been modified so that no disease would be created but immunity to that organism would develop. It made a lot of sense. It still does, at least theoretically. Vaccination would thus prevent suffering by stopping the acute expression of disease. Historically, we learned, vaccination had stopped epidemics by limiting the spread of contagious diseases. Examples in animals included reduction of rabies in most domestic animals since the 1950s, canine and feline distemper virus diseases (they are different viruses), and the feline rhinotracheitis epidemic of the late 1960s. Vaccination had led to decreased mortality, particularly in young animals who were most susceptible to disease. Domestic animals were living longer, healthier lives thanks to these vaccines and to "responsible animal owners." Our professors, in whom we had great trust, asserted that vaccination not only provided benefit to the primary host species but was a public health benefit against diseases that are transmissible to humans, such as rabies and the equine viral encephalitis viruses. Medical pioneers such as Edward Jenner (smallpox) and Louis Pasteur had gifted humans and animals with a way to reduce suffering.

We did not learn, however, that Pasteur had ultimately recanted much of his theory with the maxim, "the microbe is nothing, the terrain everything." Nor did we learn that Pasteur's success with rabies was not nearly so great as he had originally claimed.

After graduation, I witnessed firsthand the canine parvovirus epidemic of the late 1970s, and I saw the disease diminish after vaccines were introduced. (Parvovirus infection causes severe damage to the intestinal tract as well as immunosuppression. Affected animals become quite ill with vomiting and diarrhea, and many die.) How could I not champion vaccines for stopping this horrible disease that killed thousands of dogs and caused tremendous suffering for these poor animals? I saw that unvaccinated dogs would frequently get "parvo" or occasionally distemper. I observed that vaccinated animals seemed to be generally healthier than unvaccinated animals. As time passed, however, I saw more and more cases of vaccinated dogs coming down with parvo, some so soon after the vaccine that it appeared the vaccine was causing the disease, or at least making the dogs more susceptible.

I remember one client (this was in the late 1980s) who bred huskies and was having problems with parvovirus even though she was vaccinating appropriately. She had called two vaccine companies; their representatives suggested she vaccinate earlier and more often (e.g. start at four weeks instead of eight, and vaccinate every week instead of every three to four weeks). Her problems continued until, at my suggestion, she stopped using modified live vaccine and gave noninfectious (killed) vaccine at normal intervals. She had no more puppies with parvovirus after this change. When I reported to vaccine manufacturers my suspicion that the vaccine might be causing disease, I was politely informed that this was not possible.

With the introduction of the first feline leukemia virus (FeLV) vaccine during this same period of time, the veterinary community had hope that a terrible disease of cats could finally be halted (feline leukemia virus disease is similar to HIV and the AIDS syndrome in humans). Problems arose from the start, however. The vaccine, touted as safe and highly effective, did not appear to prevent the disease, and side effects were numerous and often severe. I even saw (and still see) many cases in which healthy cats, tested and found free of the virus, succumbed to the disease shortly after vaccination, as though the vaccine had initiated the disease. Again, the manufacturers assured me that this was impossible.

Studies by independent researchers, however, found the effectiveness of the vaccine to be as low as 17 percent, and typically in the 50 to 70 percent range.[1] These same researchers found the incidence of harmful side effects to be much greater than the manufacturer had reported. One study found, for example, that 32 percent of vaccinated cats died during the twenty-four months following vaccination with a feline leukemia virus vaccine. There was a 43 percent death rate of control cats in the same study; researchers vaccinated the latter group with a killed rabies vaccine as a "placebo." Both groups were then housed with feline leukemia virus infected cats to test vaccine effectiveness. While a greater percentage of control cats died, the difference was not statistically significant.[2] Interestingly, while approximately two-thirds of the control (rabies vaccinated) group who died were persistently infected with feline leukemia virus, only one-third of the FeLV-vaccinated cats that died were persistently infected. The unasked question is, why did so many noninfected cats die in both groups (one-third of rabies-vaccinated deaths and two-thirds of FeLV-vaccinated deaths)? Could it have been vaccine-induced?

Canine coronavirus appeared at about the same time as the canine parvovirus outbreak. I remember the emergence of these diseases clearly during my senior year of veterinary school, as they had just appeared, and parvo was so ominous with its fast onset and high death rate. But I remember just as clearly learning that coronavirus was relatively mild, usually causing no more trouble than a few days of diarrhea. So when a major vaccine manufacturer brought out a vaccine for coronavirus in 1984, I wondered why. The company representative reported that the virus was causing havoc "in other areas of the country." Reports of serious illness were showing up in veterinary literature. Other veterinarians in my community later reported seeing coronavirus and that it was "worse than parvo." These colleagues suggested various ways of differentiating coronavirus from parvovirus. This puzzled me. Had the disease changed so much? Was I truly not seeing the disease, or was I missing the diagnosis?

I began sending serum samples out for testing to look for the disease. I continued this for several months. While clinics around me reported case after case, I never obtained a positive report. No cases. So I researched the literature and found that the majority of the published articles about coronavirus came from the vaccine manufacturer. Then a different company announced the imminent introduction of a test for in-clinic use that would check for both parvovirus and coronavirus at one time. I was eager to get these kits so I could continue my search for the elusive virus. But when the kits became available, only parvovirus was included. I called the company and spoke with the man who developed the test. He informed me that, after months of searching, they simply could not find any coronavirus, and it was impossible to develop the test without a sample of virus. Naturally, I found that interesting.

I then called the director of the lab where I had been sending serum samples for testing. He reported that he rarely had positive tests, and these were usually in very young pups that also had parvovirus infection. I then asked him about all the positive tests my colleagues reported from examination of feces for the virus using electron microscopy (EM). He confirmed what I had heard elsewhere, that EM identification was often inaccurate, as other viruses were hard to differentiate from corona. The obvious question was, why do universities use EM instead of serology if EM is so inaccurate? His answer: the universities did not have the virus either, which they needed to develop a serological test. Coronavirus, with such a notorious reputation, seemed to be less dragon than windmill, our beloved canines not requiring the proffered protection of Don Quixote, DVM. A few years later, in fact, many of my colleagues began referring to the coronavirus vaccine as "a vaccine looking for a disease."

Incidentally, the same company that produced the coronavirus vaccine later introduced a bacterin (a bacterial vaccine) for Lyme disease, another disease that is uncommon (due to very limited geographical occurrence of the ticks that can transmit the disease). This bacterin provides poor protection and has many side effects, including symptoms that are indistinguishable from the disease itself. Unfortunately, however, veterinarians recommend the bacterin in many places where the tick carriers of the organism do not live and thus contraction of the disease is impossible.

As a result of these kinds of situations, my faith in the vaccine industry had eroded tremendously. Sadly, even my faith in the veterinary community, my colleagues, began to wane as well. I began to question the recommendations made by vaccine manufacturers, and even the American Veterinary Medical Association. The first item was the idea of yearly "boosters." It really did not make much sense. With the exception of feline leukemia virus, for which the vaccine did not appear to work anyway, I rarely saw these diseases in animals over a year of age. They were puppy and kitten diseases. Furthermore, my doctor was not sending me regular notices to come in for my boosters. Why would animals be any different?

The more I considered the issue, I saw no reason boosters would benefit animals. I changed my recommendations, which angered the colleagues in my community. Finally, through involvement in homeopathy, as well as the American Holistic Veterinary Medical Association, I found other veterinarians who also felt as I did, and in 1992 I read the following quote in *Current Veterinary Therapy XI*. This is a veterinary text akin to Conn's *Current Therapy* for human medicine. It is strictly a conventional textbook. The quote is from the section on dog and cat vaccination; the authors are Tom Phillips, DVM, of the Scripps Institute, and Ron Schultz, PhD, of the University of Wisconsin–Madison School of Veterinary Medicine:

> A practice that was started many years ago and that *lacks scientific validity or verification* is annual revaccinations. Almost without exception there is no immunologic requirement for annual revaccination. Immunity to viruses persists for years or for the life of the animal. Successful vaccination to most bacterial pathogens produces an immunologic memory that remains for years, allowing an animal to develop a protective anamnestic (secondary) response when exposed to virulent organisms. . . . Furthermore, revaccination with most viral vaccines fails to stimulate an anamnestic (secondary) response as a result of interference by existing antibody. . . . The practice of annual vaccination in our opinion should be considered of questionable efficacy unless it is used as a mechanism to provide an annual physical examination or is required by law (i.e. certain states require annual revaccination for rabies).[3] (emphasis added)

Thus, yearly "boosters" are unnecessary and provide no benefit if given (they will not increase immunity). Boosters are either a legal issue (rabies) or a manipulation issue (inducing clients to come for examinations rather than directly suggesting an examination). Or a mercenary issue.

This facet is tremendously important, and it is also decidedly clear; I believe most immunologists agree with doctors Phillips and Schultz even though the veterinary profession still operates in opposition to those facts. When I first read the quote above, I shared it with veterinarians in my community, thinking they would be interested since it came from such a respected source. The gesture, however, was met with anger and resentment. My faith in my veterinary community began to wane as I realized how attached my colleagues were to current practice and the tremendous revenue it provided. Veterinarians who declared their desire to provide the best, most up-to-date care available in fact revolted at the idea of publicizing such "heretical" information. Status quo was more important than new ideas if those ideas threatened vaccine income, even when experts deemed the old ways unscientific.

Why Do We Give Annual Vaccinations if They Are Unnecessary?

If yearly vaccination is unscientific, why did it become the accepted protocol? Some years ago, veterinary practitioners were seeing a neurologic disease they called "old-dog encephalitis." They believed this to be a form of canine distemper in older dogs to whom vaccines were administered as puppies, but not as adults. It was assumed that their immunity had lapsed, allowing development of neurologic distemper, and therefore that more repetition of vaccination would prevent the syndrome. In fact, this scenario was never proven, yet veterinarians began administering vaccines more often, eventually on a yearly basis. More likely, the so-called old-dog distemper was vaccinosis (disease as a result of vaccination). Interestingly, children who have been vaccinated for measles are more likely than unvaccinated children to show neurologic disease if infected with measles. Additionally, there have been some attempts to link measles or distemper viruses with development of multiple sclerosis in humans. Since measles and canine distemper belong to the same class of viruses (paramyxovirus), perhaps a similar mechanism is at work.

Whatever the reason for the old-dog encephalitis, it propelled vaccination into a major part of veterinary medicine. Within a decade or so, cat vaccines were also administered yearly, even though no need was ever suspected, since feline panleukopenia (distemper) vaccine is probably the most effective vaccine produced for any species. Myth simply became reality, and yearly vaccination was represented to the public as the essence of preventive health care. A further consequence was that animals' guardians were led to believe that this was all that was necessary and that they need take no other responsibility for their companion's health. This was a major step in the giving-away of power to the veterinary medical establishment, and it created a false sense of security for the guardians.

As annual vaccinations are clearly unnecessary from a medical perspective, stopping them would drastically reduce the expense of animal care as well as the trauma for the animals. I also predict that this would drastically reduce the level of chronic disease in animals (see below). This choice should be easy. Rabies vaccination is, however, mandated by state law at one- to three-year intervals. This is unfortunate, as facts are not heeded; rather, fear is the driving force. Vaccination for rabies provides lifetime immunity, probably after one but certainly after two vaccinations (in those dogs and cats that respond to vaccination; the other 5 percent will not respond even if multiple vaccines are administered).[4]

Although manufacturers license rabies vaccines for one or three years, usually they are the same vaccine but packaged with different labels. How are these claims for one- or three-year duration supported? Logic would suggest that animals are vaccinated and then challenged with live virus, and the point in time that susceptibility returns (i.e. protection wanes) would delineate the endpoint of vaccine duration of effectiveness. In actuality, animals are only kept alive for one or three years as needed, challenged, and then killed once the challenge is proven successful. Further testing is not done to determine the actual duration of immunity, as manufacturers only seek to show minimum rather than maximum duration. We need to change testing methods, and with rabies vaccination, we need to work to change state laws that currently require excessive administration.

Vaccination Does Prevent Disease, Doesn't It?

While it is clear that booster vaccination is pointless (and harmful), the question of initial vaccines is certainly more difficult and more controversial. It is generally assumed that vaccines have done much to prevent disease. As I have mentioned, however, I often saw diseases in vaccinated animals. Why was that? In part, immunization is not 100 percent effective, as some animals do not respond to vaccines. Another point that is often overlooked is the type of disease, whether acute or chronic. Only acute diseases can potentially be prevented via vaccination, as they are truly generated by an infectious organism. Acute diseases have symptoms that are constant over time, generally affect most members of a population if exposed, and will induce immunity once the individual has recovered, so that reexposure does not result in further disease. Examples in humans include childhood illnesses such as measles, mumps, and chicken pox. In cats they are limited to feline panleukopenia (distemper) and possibly the feline upper respiratory viruses (herpes, calici). Acute diseases of dogs include canine distemper, canine hepatitis, and possibly canine parvovirus. Rabies is a cross-species acute illness. We understand acute diseases as being the result of exposure to and infection by a contagious organism, although *susceptibility must precede the exposure*. As an organism seems to be responsible for the illness, it is theoretically possible to prevent the illness with a vaccine for that organism.

With chronic diseases, the primary factor is immune-system malfunction; this may be either immune-system overactivity or immunodeficiency. In overactivity diseases, the immune system attacks elements of its own body because of heightened activity and problems discriminating between host and foreign tissue. We call these autoimmune (*auto* means "self") diseases, and they include such conditions as lupus, autoimmune hemolytic anemia, pemphigus, most thyroid diseases, and the feline eosinophilia diseases ("rodent" ulcers, eosinophilic granuloma, etc.). While these autoimmune diseases are rapidly increasing in number (see below), veterinarians do not generally confuse them with acute disease and do not usually suspect them to be caused by an infectious organism. As such, vaccination is not proposed as a preventive measure.

Immunodeficiency diseases, however, we often misunderstand and place in the same category as acute diseases, as an organism may be associated with these diseases. The organism is not the cause of disease in most cases, though. It may be only a symptom, or it may worsen the disease once present, but exposure to the organism in the majority of individuals does not produce disease. Immunodeficiency is the primary cause and must be present for infection to occur, as these types of organisms are not highly contagious. Additionally, while the organisms are capable of severe damage to immune-compromised individuals, healthy individuals generally remain unaffected by the organism. *Illness must therefore precede infection.* Attempts at vaccine protection will thus fail, as the true cause is not addressed.

Some examples of immunodeficiency diseases in cats are feline leukemia virus disease, feline immunodeficiency virus disease, feline infectious peritonitis disease, and possibly the upper respiratory diseases. Immunodeficiency diseases in dogs include Lyme disease, the kennel cough complex, and possibly canine parvovirus. Examples in humans (as a comparison) include the AIDS complex and probably hepatitis B. Of course, many other chronic diseases exist, but researchers have failed to find an organism to incriminate, so these are not pertinent to this discussion.

With acute diseases, the infection itself creates the illness. These acute infections require susceptibility to the causative organism, but typically no symptoms precede the infection. As such, prevention is theoretically possible by vaccination. Whether this actually occurs is unclear. When we examine short time frames and narrow population windows, reduction in acute disease appears to result from initiation of vaccine programs. Broadening these time and number windows, however, appears to refute the credit given to vaccines. Let's look at some human diseases as examples, since the data is much more complete than for animal diseases. Please refer to the following charts for measles, whooping cough (pertussis), and poliomyelitis (polio) as they occurred in the United States and Great Britain.

The numbers of deaths from all three diseases were dropping significantly before we began vaccinating against these organisms. Yearly deaths from polio had dropped by over 50 percent before introduction of vaccination. Similarly, deaths from whooping cough diminished by 75 percent prior to vaccine use, and for measles the numbers of deaths had plummeted by 95 percent by the time a vaccine was introduced. Furthermore, the rates of reduction in numbers of deaths were not affected by vaccine use; that is,

Measles Death Rate

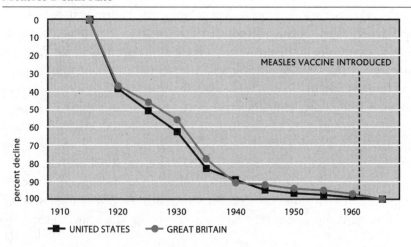

Whooping Cough Death Rate

Polio Death Rate

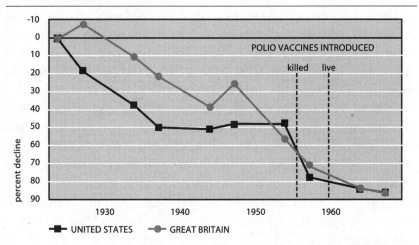

Charts reprinted with permission from *Vaccines: Are They Really Safe and Effective?* (New Atlantean Press) © 1994 Neil Z. Miller.

the diseases were diminishing just as fast before vaccination as after vaccination.

In some cases, in fact, vaccination appears to have increased the death rate. This trend occurred with polio and smallpox. With both diseases, officials reclassified the diagnostic criteria, however, so the increased numbers of cases would not show up in health records. Additionally, many European countries chose not to systematically inoculate with polio vaccines, yet polio epidemics just as surely ended in those countries as well.[5] It appears that vaccination had no positive impact upon these illnesses; rather, they diminished through natural resistance of the population. Improved hygiene also contributed to reduced infection and death rates.

Turning to veterinary medicine, let's examine a cattle disease that has a similar picture. Bovine herpesvirus I (infectious bovine rhinotracheitis) causes severe respiratory and genital infections. In the United States, vaccination has proceeded rather aggressively over the past ten to fifteen years in an attempt to reduce this disease. In Australia, however, health officials decided not to vaccinate, rather to allow natural immunity to develop within cattle populations. Interestingly, as of this date there is no difference in infection or immunity rates between the two countries—despite similar rates of infection at the outset.[6] Once again, vaccination does not appear to have made any impact, although we might have been tempted to credit vaccines if not for the comparison with conditions in Australia.

Christopher Day, a British veterinarian, compared the effectiveness of vaccination and homeopathic immunization for kennel cough among dogs housed at a boarding kennel. The kennel had been experiencing recurrent outbreaks of kennel cough prior to Day's study. Although the intent of the study was to evaluate the use of a homeopathic nosode for prevention of the disease, a curious finding was that vaccination actually increased susceptibility to the disease. This is particularly interesting in that it correlates with reports of increased susceptibility to smallpox and polio after vaccination. Incidentally, Day found the nosode to be quite effective at preventing kennel cough.[7] Nosodes are homeopathic remedies made from a product of disease such as saliva from a rabid dog *(Lyssin)* or a tuberculous lung *(Tuberculinum)*. In this case the nosode was made from phlegm of a dog with kennel cough.

In essence, vaccination is more about protecting populations rather than individuals, as Samantha McCormick so eloquently points out in the quote with which I end this section. As in the example above on bovine herpesvirus, vaccination is not necessarily an important component of herd immunity. And so Ms. McCormick's point becomes even more poignant.

> Vaccines are designed to protect populations, not just individuals, from diseases. Every individual who is vaccinated will not necessarily develop immunity. However, if enough individuals do

respond to the vaccine in a given population, the organism, whose natural host is humans, will not be able to sustain itself in that population and outbreaks will not occur or will be limited. This concept is referred to as "herd immunity." It protects both immune and non-immune members of a community. If non-immune persons fall below a certain percentage, generally around 70–90%, outbreaks of the disease will occur (Plotkin & Mortimer, 1994). This is the reason that the state claims an interest in mandating vaccines, so that the unvaccinated do not pose a threat to the vaccinated. If vaccines truly conferred individual immunity, it would be no one's business if any individual chose not to vaccinate. The risk we ask some individuals to take on, when some vaccines have dangerous adverse effects, is that a few individuals are, in effect, sacrificed, so that the rest of society may survive disease free. Unlike the virgins sacrificed to the gods in primitive societies, the victims of vaccines are not informed beforehand of their brave duty to their community. Nor are they exalted for their sacrifice.[8]

Can Vaccination Cause Problems?

Vaccination may prevent specific diseases in the short term, but the usefulness of this prevention method is uncertain. Do these diseases perhaps provide some benefit that we do not understand? Perhaps we prevent them at some sacrifice to the greater good.

From a herd or species perspective, illness represents a strengthening factor. Overpopulation generally results in a disease outbreak, which reduces the herd size and cleanses the herd (or species) by culling weaker individuals. This, of course, is Darwin's survival of the fittest in action. Diseases such as rabies and distemper have historically provided this "cleansing effect" for wolf populations when necessary (although the dynamics of wolf packs tend to limit overpopulation better than most species, and certainly far better than modern humans).

A fundamental dilemma is that vaccination, in effect, leads to weakening of the gene pool, and thus the overall health of a given population. One way this occurs is by allowing individuals to live that would otherwise succumb to disease. The benefit of the disease process was recognized, and elegantly stated, by Higinio Perez, a homeopathic physician from Mexico who practiced early in the 1900s: "It is not enough to safeguard the individual, who is a passing phenomenon. It is more important to safeguard the species."[9]

While this concept may seem harsh, particularly to the Western mind, our understanding of native or aboriginal thinking suggests that letting weak individuals die was implicitly understood to be not only acceptable but even proper. These cultures have long recognized the advantage of such a practice, and they remained in balance with their environments for incomparably longer time periods than we do today. Most modern, Western-patterned societies value the individual's right to be; therefore we make efforts to save all individuals. Our reversal of Perez's emphasis, both in human and domestic-animal realms, is conceivably a major factor in the ever-worsening health of individuals and of the species. I would even suggest it is leading to devolution of species. And, of course, the detriment to our planetary ecology is monumental.

The Chinese ideogram for crisis is formed by combining the pictograph for danger with the pictograph for opportunity. There is an old school of thought that suggests that illness is in fact a part of development, both on a physical and mental level. The crisis of illness presents an opportunity for growth. Indeed, I have a friend whose unvaccinated child made major progressions after febrile diseases. After one fever episode he began walking, and another episode was followed by initiation of talking. Vaccination may have prevented these fevers and thus the gains that followed. Perhaps this is one explanation for attention deficit disorder, hyperactivity, and other behavioral and developmental problems with children; these occur at epidemic levels today and have become more numerous over the past few decades. Is it only coincidence that this increase parallels massive childhood vaccination efforts? Apparently, vaccination is harmful not only to the species, but also to the individual.

When I first heard that vaccines may actually cause disease, I was skeptical. Of course, I knew about allergic reactions and other quick responses, but I assumed that these initial reactions were the extent of the problem. I remember a case, however, that opened my eyes. Fluffy was a sweet Persian cat who lived with an equally sweet woman.

Fluffy had recurrent bouts of cystitis (urinary bladder inflammation) that were very resistant to conventional and homeopathic treatment. Despite the fact that I liked Fluffy's guardian (and Fluffy), I hated to hear from her, as it was such a frustrating case. The bladder infections were never under control for long before they would return. One day I was reviewing the record for some clue as to what to do next when I had a stunning realization. The cystitis bouts were always about a month after the yearly boosters. I suggested to Fluffy's guardian that we no longer vaccinate Fluffy, and I never needed to treat Fluffy's cystitis again. I could only conclude that vaccines could indeed cause diseases—even a supposed infection.

Evidence for vaccine-induced damage in humans is vast. Pertussis is linked most often with problems, although all vaccines can and do cause reactions. One of the most common reactions to the pertussis vaccine is an abnormal respiratory pattern. These abnormalities tend to occur according to the typical pattern of response to stress. This pattern includes an alarm stage (the initial response), a stage of resistance (the body's attempt to negate the stress), and then a stage of exhaustion (when the bodily resources diminish).

Sudden infant death syndrome (SIDS) also occurs after DPT (diphtheria-pertussis-tetanus) vaccination, following the same pattern, with clumping of deaths during the three-week stress period following immunization. Younger infants tend to die early in the period (alarm stage), and older children later (exhaustion stage).[10] The death rate for children is eight times the average in the three days following DPT vaccination, according to some studies. Additionally, 85 percent of SIDS deaths occur during the age when children receive DPT vaccines.[11]

In 1976, Japan raised the minimum age for pertussis vaccination to two years; SIDS virtually disappeared from Japan at that time.[12] The United States was the third best in the world in infant mortality statistics in 1950. In the 1980s the country had dropped to number seventeen, and by 1994 we were at number twenty-one. Could this be related to our claims of "the most vaccinated children in history?" Japan, by contrast, was number seventeen in 1975; by 1990 they ranked number one.[13]

Vaccination: Replacing Acute Illness with Chronic Disease

Vaccinosis: a morbid condition resulting from vaccination. Does this really happen? Compton Burnett, a British physician who practiced in the late 1800s to the early 1900s, was originally a supporter of smallpox immunization. As a keen observer, however, he began to note that many chronic illnesses had begun at the time of vaccination, even though it may have occurred years earlier. Burnett also noted the ability of the remedy *Thuja* to reverse many of these vaccine-induced disease states (this especially holds true with smallpox vaccination). He coined the term *vaccinosis*. Burnett suggested that not only did vaccines create chronic disease, but that *this was how they prevented the acute disease:*

> Given a *perfectly healthy* individual who has never been vaccinated. We say to such a one, you must be vaccinated or you are liable to catch small-pox, which is often about. Let us pause to note clearly that the individual thus warned by us as being liable to catch small-pox *is perfectly healthy.* Now let us vaccinate this perfectly healthy person, and the vaccination succeeding, we say he is henceforth protected from small-pox. That is to say, this thoroughly healthy nonvaccinated person becomes more or less proof against the contagion of small-pox by vaccination, or, at any rate, it is so averred. It may be safely admitted that no one can be *more* than perfectly healthy, and any modification or altering of perfect health must result in a minus, *i.e., less* than perfect health; and *less* than perfect health must necessarily be disease or ill health of some sort and in some degree. Hence it follows that the protective power of vaccination is due to a *diseased* state of the body.[14] (Burnett's italics)

Samuel Hahnemann, in his *Organon of Medicine,* describes the interaction in the body when exposure to two or more dissimilar diseases occurs. He states that "if they are equally strong or if the first is stronger than the second, the more recent is repelled. Thus someone suffering from a grave chronic disease will not be affected by autumn dysentery or by any other mild epidemic."[15] The chronic disease prevents the acute, as with severe schizophrenics who are usually unaffected by colds and influenzas. While Hahnemann was referring to natural diseases, we can apply the same logic to vaccination and reach the same conclusion as Burnett. In this case the vaccinal, or chronic, disease occurs first and is stronger, so the acute disease is repelled. The cost, however, is a lifetime of chronic illness.

In veterinary medicine, we have noticed that whatever affinity an organism has for an organ system will surface with vaccine reactions. For example, bacteria that tend to infect the lungs will tend to create a reaction in the lungs when made into a vaccine. A good example of this in humans is the breathing difficulty induced by whooping cough vaccine. This concept was originally formulated by Richard Pitcairn, DVM, PhD. Let us look at some cat and dog diseases, including feline panleukopenia (feline distemper), canine parvovirus, rabies, and canine distemper virus, to see how this works.

With panleukopenia, major symptoms include inflammation and degeneration of the intestinal tract leading to severe vomiting and diarrhea, severe reduction of white blood cells (leukopenia) leading to immunosuppression, loss of appetite, mucopurulent nasal discharge, dehydration, and rapid weight loss. The chronic diseases we see frequently in cats correspond to many of these symptoms. Inflammatory bowel disease, an autoimmune inflammation of the intestines, is occurring at epidemic levels today. This disease was virtually nonexistent twenty years ago, yet today it is one of the most frequent diagnoses.

Another widespread cat illness is kidney failure. The panleukopenia virus has a strong affinity to kidney tissue and can persist for up to a year in cat kidneys following infection.[16] And studies done by Michael Lappin at Colorado State University found antibodies against feline kidney tissue following immunization with the cat combination ("FVRCP") vaccine.[17] Could there be a connection?

Cats are also extremely susceptible to immune malfunction and immunosuppression. The immunosuppressive state has been associated with two retroviruses (feline leukemia virus and feline immunodeficiency virus), and others are suspected. Rather than these being separate diseases, I believe they are the same, but that more than one virus can fill the niche opened by the immunosuppression (remember that with chronic diseases, the illness precedes the infection). This is probably the same in people with HIV (human immunodeficiency virus)–related viruses. Parvoviruses, which include the feline panleukopenia virus, are known to be very immunosuppressive. Additionally, I suspect the feline upper respiratory infections are a chronic state of the panleukopenia virus-induced immunosuppression and the tendency to get eye discharges.

A similar scenario now exists in dogs. While immunosuppressive states are not common in dogs, reports of their occurrence are on the rise. I believe the massive vaccination program for canine parvovirus, which began some thirty-plus years after we began vaccinating cats with feline parvovirus (panleukopenia virus), is creating this situation in dogs. If this is true, then the imminent future bodes poorly for dogs, if the problem in cats is an indication. Furthermore, we have been seeing inflammatory bowel disease in dogs over the past five to ten years. Prior to this it was virtually nonexistent. I am certain that vaccination for parvovirus and coronavirus is a major cause. I commonly see inflammatory bowel disease that arises within a month or two after vaccination for one of these viruses.

There is still another syndrome associated with parvoviruses, one that occurred first in cats and later in dogs. Cardiomyopathy is a disease of the heart muscle. The muscle may either weaken and stretch (dilated cardiomyopathy), or it may thicken greatly (hypertrophic cardiomyopathy). Either condition will limit the heart's ability to pump blood. Cardiomyopathy is usually fatal.

We have been diagnosing cardiomyopathy in cats for over twenty years, approximately the same period of time as for inflammatory bowel disease. Many (but not all) cases of the dilated form of cardiomyopathy have been associated with a deficiency of the amino acid L-taurine. The cause for hypertrophic cardiomyopathy, as well as the cause for the nontaurine-associated cases of dilated cardiomyopathy, are considered unknown. I believe that the answer may have appeared in dogs.

When canine parvovirus first erupted in the late 1970s, many young puppies died rapidly, sometimes within hours. It turned out that parvovirus was capable of attacking the heart muscle in young puppies, and this form of the infection killed the puppies rapidly.

Cardiomyopathy did not affect dogs to any degree before the parvovirus outbreak (or if it did, it was very rare), but it has appeared in the years since the outbreak. The number of cases has especially risen over the past five to ten years, coincident with the rise of inflammatory bowel disease in dogs. *The Merck Veterinary Manual* states that, "The cause [of dilated cardiomyopathy in dogs] is still unknown although viral infection and resultant autoimmune reaction against the damaged myocardium are suspect.... Since the canine parvovirus (CPV) pandemic of 1978, male Doberman pinschers appear to be highly vulnerable to both CPV and cardiomyopathy."[18] In the years since this was written in 1986, we have begun to see cardiomyopathy in many other breeds as well as Doberman pinschers.

I believe the author of this section of *The Merck Veterinary Manual* was correct, but I believe that parvovirus vaccination is even more likely to be the cause in most cases. I also believe that this explains the occurrence of cardiomyopathy in cats. Perhaps the heart muscle association of the feline parvovirus (panleukopenia virus) was not seen in natural infections, but vaccination brought it to the surface. Cardiomyopathy is an autoimmune disease, and vaccines are major causes of autoimmune disease. In my opinion, these connections are too close to be coincidence alone.

Furthermore, since writing the first edition of this book, evidence has surfaced that supports my suspicion about feline hypertrophic cardiomyopathy. Dr. Philip Fox, of the Animal Medical Center in New York City, tested about thirty-five hearts from cats with hypertrophic cardiomyopathy; the vast majority tested positive for the feline panleukopenia virus, suggesting a probable connection.[19]

For another example, let's take a look at rabies vaccination. Rabies is a neurologic disease that causes convulsions, mental confusion, paralysis of limbs, choking, rage, and aggression. Other symptoms include photophobia (fear or aversion to light); increased sexual desire; hyperesthesia (increased sensitivity to touch, sound, and other sensory stimuli); fear; desire to eat wood, cloth, and other indigestible objects; desire for solitude; or the desire to wander. Interestingly, some animals become friendlier to the point of clinginess when afflicted with rabies.

Chronic diseases of dogs and cats can readily be related to many of these symptoms. Convulsions are not uncommon; nymphomania and satyriasis are more common than ever, even in neutered animals; and eating indigestible objects is also fairly common. A syndrome we see primarily in dogs but occasionally in cats is degenerative myelopathy, a deterioration of the spinal cord that leads to painless lower-limb paralysis. This condition was first described in the late 1960s. By the late 1970s, when I graduated from veterinary school, we saw degenerative myelopathy primarily in the German shepherd dog, and it was (and still is) considered to be genetic. The age of onset was typically around ten years.

Today, the disease is common in numerous breeds, mostly large, and is occasionally seen in cats. I have seen the disease in a six-month-old golden retriever (shortly following completion of the initial vaccine series), and we commonly see it in four- to five-year-old dogs. How could this "genetic disease" cross breed lines? I would be really curious how it was genetically transmitted to cats. Maybe I missed that lecture in veterinary school! This condition may be associated with either canine distemper virus or rabies virus. The former may be more likely, but I suspect rabies may play a part in some animals, especially in cats. As rabies vaccination of cats has been emphasized only in the past decade or so, I fear this disease may become more common in cats over the next two decades.

Mentally, we see both extremes of clinginess and aggression. Aggression sometimes is noted to increase for a few days after a rabies vaccination, even with noninfectious vaccines.[20] We seem to see more and more persistently aggressive animals as well. In fact, a friend of mine, who has been practicing since 1950, flatly states that "animals were much nicer" when he graduated from veterinary school. All of the fear and aggression that we see now was rare in the 1950s.[21] I suspect that the emphasis upon vaccination for rabies, particularly for breeds such as the chow chow, pit bull, and such, serves to make these animals more likely to bite. This bite might then transmit chronic rabies to the bitten person. I also have seen many cases wherein convulsions arose following rabies vaccination, which makes sense given the virus's predilection for brain tissue and its ability to cause convulsions in active infections (see also "Aggression" in Chapter Thirteen, "Nervous System").

Finally, here is one example from canine distemper virus. This virus has an affinity to the parietal lobe of the brain, from whence the nerves of the masseter muscles and the temporalis muscles originate. These are muscles that originate on the skull, on the sides and top, and that close the mandible (lower jaw) during chewing and biting. There is a syndrome we call "chewing-gum seizures" that is a symptom of canine distemper virus infection and is caused by inflammation in the brain and nerves, with resultant muscle activity. These dogs repetitively open and close their jaws in an uncontrollable fashion, almost like chattering their teeth but not as rapidly.

Adult dogs sometimes suffer from an autoimmune disease called masseter myositis (though the temporalis muscle is equally or more affected). Its cause is considered unknown. Affected dogs initially show inflammation of these muscles, usually with difficulty chewing and opening the mouth. Eventually the muscles atrophy, leading to a skull-like appearance of the head, since the temporalis muscles provide the rounded appearance we normally see at the top of a dog's head. I have discovered that vaccination for canine distemper virus is the cause in at least some, and probably all, masseter myositis cases. Realizing that the same nerve-muscle groups were affected as with canine distemper–associated "chewing-gum seizures" led me to this conclusion, and I have successfully treated several cases now using a homeopathic medicine made from a dog distemper-combination vaccine. The same affinity exists in the vaccine virus as in the wild virus.

This concept may not make much sense from the conventional perspective that a live physical organism causes disease by infecting another organism, and thus it cannot cause disease if it is killed or modified prior to use in a vaccine. From homeopathic theory, however, we understand that a virus has a life force, which interacts with the life force of susceptible individuals. Illness then results from this interaction, which occurs on a nonphysical (energetic) level. Some form of the viral life force is present even with altered vaccine virus particles, so the life force of the vaccinated individual is still affected. Energetic illness precedes physical illness, whether it be a natural or vaccine-induced disease. The change wrought by the interaction between the vaccine life force and the vaccinated animal leads to a physical illness of some sort. This illness may only show initially as the interference with acute disease (i.e. the vaccine protection; see the quote from Burnett above), but over time the symptoms increase, and it will become more visible.

Other conditions we see frequently in veterinary medicine today are not so directly traceable to a particular vaccine. It appears that some vaccine effects are not specific to the organism in the vaccine but may be a nonspecific reaction to vaccination. When I attended veterinary school we were taught about many strange diseases—generally autoimmune diseases such as lupus, pemphigus, and the like—but were also taught that these were rare diseases we might see sporadically, if at all. We heard the adage, "When you hear hoofbeats in the backyard, don't assume it's a zebra." Today, it seems the zebras are as common as the horses, if not more common. Older practitioners affirm that these diseases were virtually nonexistent before the past few decades. Hyperthyroidism (increased production of thyroid hormones), which affects cats more than dogs, was not seen when I first graduated from veterinary school. It was not simply misdiagnosed. The symptoms are so characteristic that the syndrome would have been recognized even if the cause had been unknown. The disease did not exist. Could vaccines be responsible? Let's look at another case:

Sheba is a Siamese mix cat. She was nine years old when her guardian first consulted me. One week after vaccination, Sheba stopped eating and developed a rapid heart rate. Her conventional veterinarian suspected hyperthyroidism, although thyroid testing revealed no abnormalities. One dose of *Thuja* reversed the rapid heartbeat and the appetite problems, and her health bloomed after the remedy so that she was better than before she became ill. Clearly the vaccines had caused these problems. I believe she would have developed true hyperthyroid disease if untreated.

The status of the cat has elevated significantly since the 1960s. Prior to this most cats received little veterinary care. Since the 1970s, however, as cat status elevated, the care given to cats has climbed. This has generally meant more vaccinations. And rabies vaccination was often not recommended for cats until the mid-1980s. I believe the massive increase of vaccines in cats is responsible for hyperthyroidism as well as many other recently emerging diseases. One obvious terrible disease that is directly linked to vaccination is the emergence of fibrosarcomas at vaccine sites. This results from irritants (adjuvants) placed in noninfectious (killed) virus vaccines to increase the immune response. These cancers are extremely difficult to treat and are virtually always fatal. Other irritants (like microchips) can cause these cancers, but vaccination is by far the major culprit.

Other new and increasing diseases include hypothyroidism (decreased thyroid hormone levels) in dogs, feline immunodeficiency diseases (feline leukemia virus, feline immunodeficiency virus), feline infectious peritonitis, chronic hepatitis (primarily in dogs), renal failure, lower urinary tract diseases in cats, inflammatory bowel disease, and autoimmune blood disorders. Allergies are rampant these days, and vaccination has been linked to allergies in humans.[22] The immune systems of domestic animals have gone haywire. Sales of steroids ("cortisone") to suppress these diseases are probably at an all-time high. We have indeed traded the acute diseases for chronic, insidious, debilitating diseases.

Perhaps we have *not* eliminated the acute diseases at all, but merely changed their form into a chronic state of the acute disease. Prior to vaccination, the acute diseases were certainly life-threatening, but once puberty was reached most individuals lived a long, relatively disease-free life. Today most individuals survive or bypass the acute phase, but they (we) live relatively disease-laden lives. Vaccinations may prevent acute diseases, but if the exchange is for a lifetime of chronic disease, is that a viable option? (*Viable* is from the French *vie*, meaning "life," so the question is, will the patient live and flourish, or simply exist?)

Certainly many other stresses besides vaccines are playing a part. Studies of seals showed that consumption of pesticide-contaminated fish created an immunodeficient state that led to the 1992 outbreak of canine distemper virus, which killed vast numbers of seals in the North Atlantic.[23] Similar conditions exist in trees, such as the pine bark beetle infestation and American chestnut blight. Air pollution and acid rain weakened these trees, increasing susceptibility to disease. Perhaps the chestnut is the canary species related to air pollution. Pesticides pervade every ecological niche today, including our foods. In fact, the study with seals used fish that was being sold for human consumption.

The diet of most companion animals is equally deplorable. So many dogs and cats eat out of bags full of poor ingredients, rancid fats, and powerful preservatives; this certainly contributes to abnormal immune functioning. Many commercial pet foods contain ethoxyquin, a suspected carcinogen ruled unsafe for human consumption. I find it mystifying that a substance is labeled unsafe for humans but is acceptable for nonhuman animals. Other foods use benzene-ring compounds like BHA and BHT as preservatives. Most benzene compounds have carcinogenic properties, and they are particularly toxic to cats. Poor diet certainly plays a large part in the deterioration of our companion animals' health.

Yet vaccination is also a major contributor, as evidenced by, among other factors, the excellent response we often see to *Thuja, Silicea,* and other major vaccinosis remedies. We also see cases where the connection is clear, such as Sheba's. I see these connections almost every day in my practice. *What I discovered is that when I stopped denying vaccinosis as a possibility, the evidence was right before my eyes.* This is why I understand when other veterinarians cannot see the connection, even when it is clear. It still saddens me.

How Can Vaccination Cause Illness?

Why would vaccination be more likely than the natural disease to lead to chronic illness? The first consideration is that exposure in a natural illness, with the exception of rabies, is generally oral/nasal. This allows the body to begin local response, both nonspecific as well as specific, some hours, possibly even days in some circumstances, before the virus reaches internal organs. Specific response involves formation of antibodies at the site of exposure, while nonspecific response involves white blood cells and chemicals directed against any foreign material. Injection bypasses the local immunity and forces the body to depend 100 percent upon internal immunity.

Secondly, repetition of vaccination forces repeated responses of the immune system, leading to an excessively stimulated immune response. This is abnormal, as local antibodies (in the mouth and nose) would repel a natural reexposure without allowing penetration into the body.

Thirdly, the preparation of vaccines often breaks down the integral structure of viruses, exposing internal structures such as viral DNA or RNA (depending upon the virus) to the immune system, leading to heavy antibody production against these nucleoproteins. Since nucleoproteins are relatively similar in all life forms, the host antibodies may lose the ability to differentiate between host and virus nucleoproteins, particularly given the induced hyperactivity of antibody production. The result may be antibody-mediated destruction of host tissue, an autoimmune disease. Autoimmune diseases are occurring more frequently than ever; could this be a reason? In the past few years, doctors Scott-Moncrieff, Hogenesch, et al. at Purdue University have studied vaccination in dogs and found autoantibodies to thyroid hormones following vaccination, a possible precursor to thyroid disease, for example[24] (the authors do not state that these autoantibodies lead necessarily to disease, though this is likely). In a natural exposure, antibodies would be directed more at external structures, which are less similar to host tissues and thus less likely to induce cross-reactions. Additionally, much of the immune response would occur at the site of exposure (local antibodies).

Bacteria are much more complex organisms, thus antibody production is directed at the bacterial cell wall (the skin, in a sense) rather than against DNA or RNA, so autoimmune diseases do not so easily result from bacterins. Rather, repetition of bacterins tends to create allergic or anaphylactic reactions. The leptospira portion of the canine combination vaccine commonly produces strong allergic reactions in dogs.

Aside from the above considerations, vaccines commonly contain materials other than the organism to which immunity is desired. These materials may be added as preservatives, adjuvants (materials to stimulate immune response, usually added to noninfectious vaccines), or antibiotics. Preservatives and adjuvants include such toxins and carcinogens as aluminum (alum), mercury (thimerosal), and formaldehyde. Also, many foreign proteins are included if the organism was grown on foreign tissue such as chicken or duck embryos. Even more frightening, nonintended organisms or molecules are sometimes accidentally incorporated as contaminant "stowaways." In 1995 the *Washington Post* reported that MMR (measles-mumps-rubella) vaccine produced by Merck & Co., along with some influenza and yellow fever vaccines, contained an enzyme known as reverse transcriptase.[25] This enzyme is associated with retroviruses such as

FeLV, FIV, and HIV and has the capability to alter genetic information, leading to serious diseases such as leukemia and other cancers. Similarly, the *Seattle Times,* in a February 19, 1999, article, reported that a link is probable between polio vaccination and some types of cancer. The cause may be a virus (SV40, a monkey virus) that contaminated vaccines manufactured prior to 1963. These diseases may take years to manifest, so definitive correlation with vaccination may be impossible, masking a potentially causative relationship.

The current practice in veterinary medicine of giving annual "boosters" amplifies this cascade of events immensely. As a result, we see vaccinosis in domestic animals more clearly, and probably more commonly, than in humans. This amounts to an ongoing model that delineates the disastrous consequences of vaccination in a more obvious fashion than seen in humans. This may then provide evidence of vaccinosis that could be used to study the disease in humans, but *I am not suggesting the use of research animals for further study, as companion animals already provide enough sad evidence.*

Vaccination and Brain Damage

There is a book by Harris Coulter called *Vaccination, Social Violence, and Criminality* (see the appendix) that proposes a theory about vaccination causing psychological and behavioral changes in humans. As I found Dr. Coulter's postencephalitis syndrome to be quite compelling, I decided to see if animals provided any evidence to support the theory. I concluded that this syndrome could explain many abnormal behavior problems we see in animals, including fear, desire for solitude, aggression, rage, inability to relate to others, restlessness, and hypersexual behaviors (nymphomania, satyriasis, and masturbation—even in neutered animals).

We also see many animals with physical conditions that Dr. Coulter associated with vaccination. These conditions include paralytic states, asthma, convulsions, skin allergies, developmental problems, and poor appetite.

I would like to briefly present another case that fits quite well with Dr. Coulter's hypothesis. Dolly is a female cocker spaniel who was nine years old when I was first consulted about her condition. She had quite severe neurologic impairment, including convulsions, mental confusion, and a poor ability to relate with her guardians. She would frequently get "stuck" in corners, that is, she would get her head into a corner or into a small space such as between a chair and an end table, and she simply could not find her way out. She also had a palsy involving the facial nerves on one side, making drinking and eating difficult. This is interesting in that cranial nerve damage is another part of the postencephalitis syndrome.

A key element for me in connecting her case to vaccination was that when she was vaccinated, she became very hyperactive for a few days. On one occasion she even jumped off an eight-foot-high deck in this frenzied state. Other symptoms that pointed to vaccination were a thickened and cracked nose and foot pads, both symptoms of acute canine distemper.

Fortunately, Dolly responded dramatically to homeopathic treatment. I first tried the remedy *Helleborus*, with minimal improvement. Then, after a single high-potency dose of *Nux moschata*, Dolly's guardian remarked that "it was like she came out of a seven-year coma."

In the decade since this book was originally published, I have seen (or recognized) more and more cases of aggression, convulsions, and other brain disorders following vaccination. Additionally, in humans, there is growing evidence for vaccinations as at least one causative factor in autistic spectrum disorders, as Coulter suggested. With more awareness, more data continually accumulates.

What Steps Should You Take with This Information?

I know the above information is rather detailed and sometimes complex, but I believe in giving complete information, especially for something as controversial as vaccination. *While I include specific vaccine recommendations, this is only for those of you who feel uncertain about abandoning vaccinations altogether. I feel that vaccination is more risky than not vaccinating for most animals in most situations.* If you have read everything up to this point and still feel unsure about just what to do, here is a summary of my recommendations, starting with the most cautious position and moving forward from there.

First, remembering that booster vaccines are unnecessary, we can stop all vaccination after one year of age for virtually all diseases (see below; rabies vaccine boosters are required by law, so we need to work to change the laws so that they are in accordance with fact rather than fear). As repetition naturally increases the likelihood of problems, we can reduce side effects tremendously *with no additional risk to the patient* simply by stopping adult boosters. Of course, there will still be some risk involved with even the initial vaccinations, but no risk of contracting the acute disease once the animal is immunized by these first vaccines. See below for duration of immunity to the various diseases for which vaccines are available.

Secondly, all vaccines should be administered as single antigens. (An antigen is something that is capable of eliciting an immune response, in this case a viral or bacterial organism from which a vaccine is produced.) This means not using the polyvalent (combination) vaccines, which have become so common these days. Natural exposure to diseases is usually one at a time, and the body is probably more successful at responding to only one antigen and producing immunity without adverse effects, rather than responding to a complex of antigens. Therefore, rather than giving a group of antigens together at three- to four-week intervals, individual components should be given using an alternating schedule with a minimum of repetition (see below).

Third, only immunize for diseases that meet *all* of the following criteria:

1. The disease is serious, even life threatening.
2. The animal is or will be exposed to the disease.
3. The vaccine for the disease is known to be effective.
4. The vaccine for the disease is safe.

Let's look at some common diseases to see how this works. I'll start with feline leukemia virus (FeLV) disease. An indoor-only cat will not be exposed (criterion number two), as this virus requires direct, intimate, cat-to-cat contact for transmission. Many veterinarians recommend immunizing indoor cats against this disease, but I feel this is unethical. This disease does not fit criterion number three or four anyway, in my experience, so vaccination is unwarranted in most if not all circumstances. Most current (2009) recommendations do not include FeLV as a core (essential) vaccine. Transmission of FeLV only occurs in young cats in any case, almost without exception, so vaccination would only be warranted in young cats. Ninety-five to ninety-seven percent of cats who do become infected after exposure to FeLV recover without incident in any case. (In clusters of cats, such as in households with *a lot* of cats, this percentage may drop as low as 70 percent, but this would not pertain to most households. By "a lot," I mean more than at least twenty cats, and really thirty to fifty or more. Furthermore, FeLV infection is declining significantly, at least in the United States, but not because of vaccination, according to Richard Ford, a veterinarian at North Carolina State

University who is on vaccination recommendation committees for the American Animal Hospital Association and the American Association of Feline Practitioners.

Feline infectious peritonitis (FIP) is another disease that fits neither criteria three nor four, and rarely number two. The FIP virus vaccine has generally been found ineffective and has produced severe side effects. Among the side effects I have observed with both FIP and FeLV vaccines is induction of the clinical disease they were intended to prevent. Additionally, it is pretty clear that FIP is an immune suppression (chronic) disease, not an acute disease, so the vaccine is unlikely to help. FIP results from a feline coronavirus (FCoV) infection, but the virus's relationship to FIP illness is complicated. There are two biotypes of FCoV—an avirulent (non–disease causing) biotype one (AB1) and a virulent biotype two (VB2), the FIP virus. AB1 is contagious but rarely causes problems. Most cats only develop a transient infection, though some may become healthy lifelong shedders of AB1. In a *very* small minority of cats who contract AB1, an immunological insult or some other event (this is not fully understood) causes AB1 to mutate to VB2. (I suspect this insult is human-caused, by vaccination, medications, pesticides, or some other toxin, although researchers believe the mutations occur at random. There is a genetic susceptibility in some breeds, though, primarily Persians and Burmese, for this conversion to occur. Some lines within these breeds are worse than others.) VB2 infection results in FIP disease (the disease can have other forms that do not involve the peritoneum), which is 95 percent fatal. This conversion is rare, however. Further, *VB2 is not contagious, so cats with FIP are not contagious.* Only cats with the non–disease causing form, AB1, are contagious. Thus a cat with FIP in a household need not be euthanized or separated from other cats. There may be other cats shedding AB1, however. As with FeLV, illness occurs in only a small minority of cats.

Feline panleukopenia virus is very serious, and the vaccine is quite effective, but most cats will not be exposed to the virus, and the disease generally affects kittens only. Only those cats that are likely to be exposed would benefit from vaccination. One vaccination is sufficient (see below).

With the feline upper respiratory diseases (calicivirus and rhinotracheitis virus as well as feline chlamydia), most are not serious except in very young kittens. These kittens generally contract the disease before vaccines would typically be administered, so the vaccine is not often beneficial. Only the intranasal vaccine is effective in most cases, and it can cause illness that mimics the natural infection.

Recently a vaccine for ringworm was introduced. I have no direct experience with this vaccine, but I am certain that it will have little benefit and that it is probably unsafe. Ringworm is usually the result of immunodeficiency—a chronic disease rather than an acute illness, so the vaccine will not address the cause of disease. I strongly recommend against using this vaccine.

In dogs, canine hepatitis virus (the vaccine virus to prevent canine hepatitis is adenovirus-2) is almost nonexistent (criterion number two). Leptospirosis is extremely rare (number two) and the bacterial serotypes that cause the few observed cases are often not the same serotype as the ones used in the vaccine[26] (there is no cross-protection between different serotypes). In other words, the leptospira component in the combination vaccines rarely protects the dog against the disease (number three). Additionally, the bacterin for "lepto" is very prone to side effects (number four).

Coronavirus was never a serious threat (numbers one and two) except to dog companions' bank accounts, and the same is true for Lyme disease, except possibly in very small regions (number two). The vaccine for Lyme disease commonly causes illness, in my experience, often mimicking the disease (number four). Additional note for the second edition: Lyme disease has spread much farther than previously; at least it is being diagnosed in a much wider area. I suspect some of this is due to incorrect diagnosis, as diagnosis for Lyme disease is not entirely consistent. Further, I would still not recommend the vaccine, as it provides questionable immunity. Kennel cough disease is generally not serious (number one), and one study showed immunization to be ineffective or even counterproductive (number three).[27] Immunization for kennel cough should be limited to high-risk circumstances, if at all. As with the feline upper respiratory viruses, only the intranasal kennel cough vaccine provides much protection, though it can incite illness. Nosodes can be helpful (see below).

Recently, a horse influenza virus has developed contagion to dogs, and this virus is now spreading somewhat. It is now called the canine influenza virus. As with human influenza, the vast majority of dogs do not develop serious illness (criterion number one). Furthermore, I wonder how safe and effective the vaccine will be (criteria number three and four), since human influenza vaccination is poorly effective and often causes influenza-like illness.

Canine parvovirus and canine distemper virus present the only real threats, and most dogs will not be exposed to these diseases. Parvovirus rarely affects dogs over one year of age, and even eight- to twelve-month-old dogs generally survive the disease with minimal illness. One vaccination is usually sufficient for either virus (see below). Hepatitis virus (adenovirus type two) is a dangerous virus, although pretty rare. Consider vaccination only if your companion has a likelihood of exposure.

Rabies is another disease for which indoor cats and well-confined dogs have no exposure, so the vaccine is clinically unnecessary, although it is required by law. Even nonconfined animals have little risk of exposure, though there is some risk, and the disease is devastating. Vaccination may be of value for outdoor animals, especially in rural homes, though there is a risk of chronic illness (see "Aggression and the Rabies Miasm" in Chapter Thirteen, "Nervous System"). Once immunized, however, most animals are protected for life.

Fourth, vaccines should *never* be given to unhealthy animals. When I graduated from veterinary school, this was accepted doctrine; it was largely considered malpractice at the time. Unfortunately, however, today it is rather common to vaccinate sick animals. This has gained popularity among veterinarians for some strange reason, and it goes against the recommendations in all vaccine inserts as well as those of virtually all immunologists. It is still malpractice in my opinion—even more now than thirty years ago, as the risks are much better understood.

A bolder option is to refuse immunizations entirely, recognizing the inherent risk in administering even one vaccine into the body, and being willing to accept the risk of not immunizing. While risk does exist if animals are unvaccinated, it can be moderated significantly by feeding better quality foods (home-prepared and including fresh raw meats) and by limiting exposure until the animals are six to eight months of age. An unvaccinated animal will be significantly less likely to suffer from allergies and many health problems.

Please understand that there is a risk, albeit minimal, with not vaccinating. I have seen panleukopenia virus (FPL), for example, in adult unvaccinated cats. The cats were probably overcrowded in an apartment, thus under some stress that would have compromised their immunity, but they did become ill. But this is rare. The exposure in this case came from a sick cat who went to a veterinary clinic and was exposed there to a kitten with FPL. I also know of canine parvovirus infections in unvaccinated dogs. Again, this is quite rare. The quote by Samantha McCormick in the section above titled "Vaccination Does Prevent Disease, Doesn't It?" clarifies this somewhat. The risk is there, but I believe it is extremely small. Hopefully you understand why if you have read this chapter up to this point.

As with polio virus in humans, there is a moderate risk with exposure to vaccinated animals. Exposure of unvaccinated humans to recently vaccinated children is responsible for all of the polio infections in recent history in the United States. Similarly, exposure to recently vaccinated animals can result in illness, either in unvaccinated animals or in littermates whose vaccinations did not induce protection. This is most common with dogs, and most common with parvovirus. With puppy classes and such, dogs are much more likely to be exposed to other vaccinated dogs than are cats. Thus if you don't vaccinate your dog (or cat), it would be wise to avoid exposure to dogs for a week or two following their immunizations. This can be difficult with puppy classes, but it is possible. Nosodes can help here (see below).

I am still opposed to vaccinations in most circumstances. My position has evolved over thirty years of experience as a practicing veterinarian, from study and from personal observation. My overarching concern is that the veterinary community tremendously overuses vaccines, though there is some slow movement toward fewer vaccinations. The decision to vaccinate is an individual one, though. While I am opposed to vaccination, I do not ask that you blindly accept this judgment but that you make your own decision. I do ask that your decision be based upon facts, however, not fear.

Vaccination has become a freedom-of-choice issue. Animals, like children, have no voice. We as guardians are the voice for our companion animals, so it is up to us to make the best choice for them. *In the case of rabies, state law mandates the vaccines, and so we have no real choice other than breaking the law or asking for exemptions in certain circumstances. We can, however, strive to change the laws to a factual basis.*

Other vaccines are very heavily pushed although not legally required. Some veterinary clinics or boarding kennels require other vaccines prior to admission, sometimes even for emergencies. Guardians who question the need for vaccines are often belittled. The veterinarian will either imply that the guardian does not really care about the companion animal or that the guardian has no qualification to make such a decision. Unfortunately, however, in most cases the veterinarian himself is not making an informed decision based upon immunological science. Thus, since we as guardians are in fact morally and ethically the responsible party, we must take charge and act upon our knowledge to make a fact-based rather than a fear-based decision. This decision should not rest with someone else.

I entered veterinary medicine because of my deep care for animals, and it is their welfare I have at heart. I believe vaccination to be the source of tremendous illness and suffering in animals, and probably people. My practice involves primarily chronic disease, and I estimate that at least 75 percent (probably more) of the illnesses I treat have their roots in vaccination. Vaccination thus amounts to abuse of animals, something I cannot abide. If we do not defend our rights and those of all animals, including wild animals, we will lose our rights and perhaps even the animals.

What, then, is the best approach to protection against these diseases? First and foremost, prevention is indeed better than trying to cure disease. Rather than vaccination, however, promotion of health is the best choice for long-term well-being. This involves primarily nutrition and lifestyle choices. Good nutrition for dogs and cats is similar to that for humans in that fresh foods are best. Eating out of bags and cans is a poor substitute. As these are carnivores, fresh raw meats with small quantities of cooked grains and vegetables are the basis of a good diet. Use organic ingredients if possible. Lifestyle should include opportunities for fresh air, sunshine, and exercise—conditions that nourish mental health. With young puppies and kittens, minimize their exposure to situations where stress and the presence of unfamiliar animals create opportunities for transmission of infectious diseases.

Possibly the best use of vaccines is in an epidemic situation rather than blanket use where no risk of exposure is involved for most individuals. Interestingly, however, epidemic or other known exposures are situations when nosodes or the *genus epidemicus* (see below) appear to work well. Appropriate use of nosodes could provide adequate protection in most circumstances with a small fraction of the risk of vaccines.

Nosodes

A nosode is a homeopathic remedy made from a discharge or a similar product from an individual with the disease. It is not made simply from the causative agent; it generally contains that agent within the discharged fluid or infected tissue. It thus represents not only the infectious organism itself but also the host response. The nosode therefore carries the energy of the disease. This energetic package has the capability of, in a sense, filling the susceptibility of the patient with this modified, vibratory disease energy. In doing this, it can block receptivity to the actual disease organ and disease process.

I have seen nosodes work quite well in the exposure and stressful atmosphere of an animal shelter. Although it was not a controlled study, there was no doubt about the effectiveness. I have also seen protection in other exposure situations. Indications from these experiences as well as historical use of nosodes in epidemics suggests that nosodes work best when administered shortly before to shortly after exposure. Evidence for long-term protection seems to be lacking, but typically these diseases are a threat only in prepubertal individuals *unless* they have been vaccinated (as with measles in humans—see above). In fact, I doubt that it is possible for nosodes to induce permanent protection, as they do not work like vaccines, even though the concept is somewhat similar. One study with parvovirus in dogs, for example, showed no protection from nosodes. The study, however, was poorly designed—in a sense it was designed to fail, though that may not have been the researchers' intent. But they gave the nosodes, waited, and then exposed the puppies well after any residual nosode protection would have disappeared. Thus they found no protection.

But nosodes are not vaccines, and their protection is only transient. They require intermittent use until puberty for puppy or kitten (or children's) diseases. Alternatively, they can be administered around possible exposures, such as before and after puppy classes or during boarding. The latter works well for kennel cough prevention, for example. In my experience, overuse of nosodes may create a disease situation, however, so wise use is necessary. Do not continue them too long. In fact, it is best to not even use nosodes routinely, though some guardians are uncomfortable with no protection other than good nutrition, so they opt for regular use until puberty. As this can cause problems, *I do not recommend this approach for the vast majority of animals. Rather, dosing around probable exposure is better unless exposure risk is fairly constant.*

I recommend that you consult with a veterinary homeopath regarding nosode use for disease prevention. Nosodes are prescription medicines and should be used with appropriate guidance, so your veterinary homeopath must have direct experience with nosodes. Essentially, if you desire a vaccine-like regimen, I recommend using 30C potencies once or twice a week until the animal is six to eight months old. At this time it is usually best to stop the nosode administration. You can then go to exposure-based dosing. Some veterinarians recommend repetition of nosodes at four- to six-month intervals for the animal's lifetime, but this is unnecessary. I have seen this cause problems, especially when using high potencies (200C or 1M). Most animals have a competent immune system by the time they reach puberty, and they no longer need nosode protection.

In short, nosodes do work, and they work fairly well, in exposure situations. It is not always possible to know when an exposure has occurred, and they do not provide lasting protection, thus they require repetition. Many homeopaths (probably most) do not understand how they work, and certainly almost no conventional veterinarian or physician does. As a result, many otherwise well-meaning doctors proclaim that they do not work, or on the other hand, attempt to use them without understanding how they work. This can cause failures or problems and leads to a perception that nosodes are useless in disease prevention, which is untrue. Furthermore, nosodes will only work well in acute contagious diseases, just like vaccination (see above in the section "Vaccination Does Prevent Disease, Doesn't It?"). They will provide limited protection in chronic, immune suppression diseases like FeLV and FIP, though they do appear to provide some protection in animals who are exposed. I have even seen some apparent protection in previously exposed cats with high coronavirus titers who lived in a household with an FIP cat. This protection is far from predictable, but it can help.

A *genus epidemicus* is a traditional homeopathic remedy that matches the majority of cases in an epidemic, thus it can be used as a preventive. This has been done quite successfully in outbreaks of such diseases as cholera and yellow fever. It is equally effective for animal diseases, though you would need to consult a homeopath to see if she knows or can ascertain the best remedy for a given outbreak. This would be uncommon, as epidemics are uncommon in animals. The parvovirus epidemic of the late 1970s was the last major animal epidemic, for example.

Whether with a nosode or the *genus epidemicus,* dosing near exposure is critical. I realize I am repeating myself, but this is probably the most misunderstood aspect of prophylactic nosode use. The best method is simply administration shortly before to shortly after potential exposure. For puppy classes, give one dose of 30C before the class and a second dose upon arriving home or the next day. With boarding, dose before going to the kennel, every day in the kennel if fewer than four days total, or every two to four days for longer periods. Give a final dose after returning home. This is only for kennel cough or feline upper respiratory pathogens unless there is a likely exposure to other viruses in young animals. Even better on all counts is to keep your animals at home with a house sitter. With unknown or potentially extended exposure risk, continued repetition is feasible (e.g. in puppies or kittens up to puberty), but it is not without risk and is a secondary approach.

If You Still Decide to Vaccinate, What Vaccines Should You Use?

What should you do if vaccination still seems an appropriate choice? *If you have not read this chapter in its entirety, I suggest you do so prior to deciding to vaccinate.*

I present the following information only for those of you who cannot make the decision to avoid vaccinating a puppy or kitten. I do not recommend vaccination, but this information can limit their use for those who still wish to vaccinate. Essentially, the primary diseases for which vaccination may be warranted are canine distemper, canine parvovirus, feline panleukopenia (distemper), and rabies.

Previously, I generally supported the use of noninfectious (killed) vaccines for those who choose to vaccinate, as I feel they have less likelihood for long term damage. Dr. Ron Schultz, of the University of Wisconsin–Madison School of Veterinary Medicine, presents a strong case for the use of modified live vaccines (MLV), however, as repetition can be necessary with noninfectious vaccines. Further, the adjuvant-associated vaccine fibrosarcomas in cats warrant careful consideration of noninfectious rabies and FeLV vaccines in that species. *For this reason, you should never use adjuvanted vaccines in cats.* And maybe even in dogs, since there have been a very few rare instances of vaccine sarcomas in dogs. With modified live vaccines, one dose can have high efficacy. This primarily applies to canine distemper and canine parvovirus, as noninfectious rabies and feline pan-leukopenia vaccines are as effective as modified live versions. Rabies vaccines are all noninfectious, as far as I know, at least in the United States. I would be extremely cautious with MLV rabies vaccines in cats, as they have a tendency to revert to wild strains. Purevax, by Merial, is the only nonad-juvanted rabies vaccine at this time, and it is the one to use. Dr. Schultz's "one dose 95 percent" (one dose of vaccine at a given age will successfully immunize 95 percent of animals) suggestions are as follows:

- canine distemper (MLV): ten to twelve weeks;
- canine parvovirus (MLV): twelve to fourteen weeks;
- feline panleukopenia (MLV): ten to twelve weeks.

Thus, if you have a new puppy, one dose of modified live canine dis-temper virus vaccine at ten to twelve weeks of age, followed in two weeks by one dose of modified live canine parvovirus vaccine, stands a 95 percent chance of protecting him for life from these two diseases. Similarly, one dose (per cat) of feline panleukopenia virus vaccine will protect 95 percent of cats for life. One or two doses of rabies vaccine provide the same lifetime protection, though state law mandates regular boosters. In cats, I recom-mend panleukopenia virus vaccination only unless there is a known risk for calicivirus or rhinotracheitis virus exposure, in which case I recommend the intranasal vaccine. Intranasal vaccination mimics the natural exposure and works better than the injectable vaccine, though it may create a mild form of the disease. The intranasal rhino-calici vaccine should be given sep-arately from the panleukopenia virus vaccine. I do not recommend vacci-nation for feline leukemia virus, feline infectious peritonitis virus (feline coronavirus), chlamydia, giardia, or ringworm under any circumstances. There is now a vaccine for the feline immunodeficiency virus, but I would not recommend this either.

In dogs, I would recommend distemper virus and parvovirus vaccines only, and not combined. In rare cases you may need to dose the parvo vac-cine at an older age. A titer test can tell you if you need a booster; see below. If there is a risk of exposure to kennel cough, the intranasal bordetella-parainfluenza vaccine may be useful, though it often causes a mild case of kennel cough. I don't recommend it for most dogs, though. I do not recommend vaccination against canine coronavirus, Lyme disease, giardia, or leptospirosis under any circumstances, and I would only recommend hepatitis (adenovirus-2) vaccination if there is a definite risk of exposure (although the American Animal Hospital Association considers adenovirus-2 to be a core vaccine, the disease is quite rare, though it can be dangerous). One manufacturer has produced a vaccine for giardia, though it may no longer be on the market by the time this edition is published. It is almost universally not recommended by veterinary experts. Finally, there are vaccines against the western diamondback rattlesnake *(C. atrox)* venom and a vaccine for periodontal disease in dogs. I would recommend neither one. I have seen some harsh skin damage with the *C. atrox* vaccine, and periodontal disease is an immune deficiency. Further vaccination is likely to further depress immune function.

Finally, once again, rabies is generally mandated by law for cats and dogs, regardless of risk. This is a legal, not a medical, requirement. The medical status is not much different than with Dr. Schultz's core vaccines, as listed above. He does not give data, but approximately 80 to 85 percent of animals should be protected with one dose, and 95 percent with two doses. This protection should last for life. See the discussion on titers below. It is possible to obtain exemptions in some cases in some states, especially with animals with autoimmune or other known vaccine-compromised illness. Chronically ill animals also warrant an exemption, though not all officials will grant such an exemption. It can help to have a protective titer, however; see below. Additionally, in cats I recommend using the nonadjuvanted rabies vaccine (Merial's Purevax is currently the only one) if you must vaccinate your cat. Other nonadjuvanted single vaccines at the time of writing (to my knowledge) include Schering-Plough's Galaxy-D (canine distemper) and Merial's Recombitek (canine parvovirus). Merial currently also makes a three-way cat vaccine without adjuvant or thimerosol. Any of these products could change at any time, however, so do your research if you choose to vaccinate.

Titers (Antibody Testing)

With our awareness of potential vaccine damage, and especially as animal guardians insist upon a more conservative approach to vaccines by their veterinarians, titers have become more of an issue. As with nosodes, however, there is a lot of misinformation, or at least misapplication, regarding titer use and need. So in this section, I'll give an overview of titers: what a titer represents, what it can tell us, and when it is or is not useful. First, however, a bit about antibodies.

Just what is an antibody? An antibody is a protein, manufactured by lymphocytes, that is engineered to attach to foreign antigens and assist in their destruction and removal from the body. Remember that an antigen is anything that can induce an immune response, normally something foreign to the body. It may be an organism, like the canine distemper virus, or it may be pollens, poison ivy oils, or (in an abnormal response) food proteins. The body has basically two responses to foreign material. The first response, cell-mediated immunity, is less specific to a given antigen/foreign invader. With this immune response, once the sensory arm of the immune system recognizes a foreign antigen, the system sends cells to the area. These cells attempt to ingest and destroy the antigens by a process called phagocytosis. They also utilize other chemical and physical methods to cleanse the antigens from the body, as well as sending signals to bring in white blood cells to begin to form antibodies (also called immunoglobulins) against the antigens. This is the second, antigen-specific part of the immune system.

It usually takes about two weeks following an initial exposure for antibody production to get into high gear. Upon subsequent exposures, however, antibody levels will climb rapidly, typically within forty-eight hours. This secondary response we call an anamnestic response. The reason the anamnestic response is so rapid is that once the immune system has recognized a new antigen, it creates a population of antibody-producing cells (beta lymphocytes or ‚-lymphocytes—ß is the Greek letter beta) that are specific to this antigen. Their only job is to make antibody against, for example, canine distemper virus (CDV). For a time following activation of these cells, they continue to multiply and maintain a significant population, constantly producing that CDV specific antibody. After a few weeks or months, however, without further exposure to CDV, antibody levels will slowly drop, sometimes to very low levels. See the chart titled "Antibody Response (Titer Levels)" for more clarity.

The CDV antibody-specific ß;-lymphocytes, however, never disappear. The immune system maintains a low population of these cells, just in case. They are sometimes called memory cells because they "remember" their specific antigen, in this case CDV. If the immune system "sees" CDV again,

Antibody Response (Titer Levels)
Following Initial Antigen Exposure

After a delay, antibody levels rise within two weeks, but fall off again unless reexposure occurs.

Antibody (Titer) Level

1 week
2 weeks
3 weeks
4 weeks
weeks to months

Antigen Exposure

Time

the cells rapidly divide and multiply, producing protective antibody levels within forty-eight hours. It's a bit like firefighters. As long as there is no fire, we can forget they are around, but they are still there at the fire station, servicing trucks, taking firefighting classes, maybe even playing cards. Shortly following a fire alarm, however, they are everywhere. The anamnestic response is like this. You can test antibody titers and find very little antibody because it is not currently needed. But should reexposure occur, antibodies are everywhere, just like the firefighters. See the chart titled "Anamnestic Antibody Response" for more clarity. The line on this chart is a continuation of the previous one; the low antibody levels at the beginning follow the drop in antibody levels on the first chart.

Sometimes the circulating antibody level, as measured by a titer test, is actually below levels we consider protective. In the second chart, on the anamnestic response, this is represented by the flat line at the beginning, marked "persistent low antibody level from initial exposure." This is typically in an animal who has not been vaccinated for or exposed to CDV (using our example) in a long time, usually years. Upon reexposure, however, protective levels occur quickly. This is important, as this is often misunderstood or ignored. We'll see why in a minute as we examine titer testing.

A titer—from the word *titrate*—is an analysis of serum for circulating antibody levels against a given antigen. To assess antibody response, laboratory technicians test serum (the liquid component of blood, excluding blood

Anamnestic Antibody Response
Following Secondary Antigen Exposure

cells and clotting agents) against specific antigens to see if the serum proteins bind with the antigen. This binding we call agglutination. Here is how it works (the process is called titration): we'll continue with CDV as our example. The tech would take a given quantity of CDV and mix it with a given quantity of serum. If she found agglutination, she would then dilute the serum with equal parts of a diluent (diluting solution). If she still got agglutination, she would dilute again and retest. She would continue this stepwise dilution and testing until she reached a dilution that did not agglutinate. Then she would know she had reached the limit. The previous dilution, the last one that did agglutinate with CDV, would be the titer level. As this process has historically been done by diluting the serum to half-strength in each step, titers were (and still often are) reported in multiples of two. A serum sample that only agglutinated at the first dilution would have a titer of 1:2. A sample that agglutinated at the first and second dilutions would be 1:4, and one that agglutinated to the third dilution would be 1:8. This could go on as far as agglutination occurred. The higher the dilution at which agglutination occurs, the more antibody is present in the serum. Thus, higher titers are those that have a higher second number; the first number is always one. Titers may reach to 1:1,024 and even higher. Essentially, a titer is not a direct measurement of antibody; rather it is an inverse measurement in that it refers to the level of dilution at which the antibody is still capable of reacting to or neutralizing the antigen or virus.

In recent years, laboratories often dilute in steps of one to five, so the titer may be 1:5, 1:25, 1:125, and so on. Sometimes laboratories report the antibody level directly, in international units per milliliter (IU/ml). This is especially the case with rabies titers in most countries except the United States, as the World Health Organization utilizes antibody levels rather than titers for reporting and establishing minimum levels of protection. The numbering system is not critical, however, other than understanding what is higher or lower within a given system. Additionally, laboratories may measure the ability of antibody to neutralize live virus rather than simply the agglutination (this is the case with rabies). Again, this is not so important to know as is how your animal's test results compare with normal values and minimum protective levels.

The next step is to determine what minimum titer level is a protective level. This is complex, as it involves various factors, sometimes including animal testing. The why and how of this is not important here. The only important aspect is that laboratories or researchers determine a minimum titer that they deem protective against a given agent. It may vary, depending upon the disease organism. Essentially, however, the intent is to ascertain at what level it is clear that a vaccine (or an exposure) has induced a protective antibody response. Once this is determined, titer testing can tell if a given individual adequately responded to a vaccine. At least that is the idea, and it does work, but timing is critical.

Remember in the charts how the antibody level drops after a time if there is no reexposure? And how, upon reexposure, antibody levels rapidly climb to protective levels? This is where that comes into play. Here is why. We'll return to CDV. With at least one major laboratory, the minimum protective titer to CDV is 1:5. That is, the serum still reacts to the virus at a fivefold dilution. Now, suppose you vaccinate your puppy and then test him three weeks later. Chances are good that you would see a titer higher than 1:5, unless he is not capable of a proper immune response, which is rare. But what if you do not test him for a year? If he has not run into CDV on the street somewhere, his titer may have dropped below that 1:5 level. If we only look at that one isolated test, we might assume he is not protected, and many veterinarians would recommend a booster vaccine. Unfortunately, without testing at three to six weeks following the vaccine, we do not know if he had a response initially or not. If he did, then we know that the anamnestic response will pick up and cover him upon subsequent exposure. If he never developed a protective antibody level, then he may or may not have an adequate anamnestic response.

Now, what about the dog who was vaccinated twice, or who had a vaccine and then a street exposure somewhere? His titer will remain high much longer, months to years, so yearly titer testing is likely to find him protected, at least for a year, two years, maybe five to seven years. At some point, however, the antibody and titer level may drop. Here is the other place where veterinarians, doctors, and others err with titer testing. A common recommendation is to do yearly titers (assuming the first one shows protective levels), wait for the titer to drop below the minimum protective level, and then give a booster. But wait, you now say! What about the anamnestic response? And you are absolutely correct. He does not need the booster because the memory cells are still there, ready and waiting. The bottom line is that, if a dog ever shows a protective titer against CDV, then that dog is always protected against CDV. Are you with me? If not, refer again to the charts. A dog who at some point developed protective antibody levels against CDV will, even if those levels fall below what we call protective titer levels, regain or better those levels within forty-eight hours (often much sooner) upon reexposure. The booster vaccine is a waste of time, money, and stress.

So, are titers useful? Yes, they are. Are yearly titers useful? No, they are not. Essentially, if you have read this entire chapter, you still realize that I do not recommend vaccination for most animals for most conditions. In that case, don't worry about titers. If you vaccinate, however, you could have your veterinarian run titers three or four weeks following the vaccine. If the titer is protective, then forget it. Don't worry again about that disease. Your animal is protected. You could even test a young animal, at about six months, even if you did not vaccinate him, to see if he may have been exposed somehow and developed a protective titer. (This especially applies to outside animals, but it is also more important for them.) If so, again, relax. If not, you can decide whether you feel the risk of disease exposure is great enough to gamble with the risk (arguably more certain) of vaccine damage. Titer testing is only useful for the big diseases, like canine distemper and parvovirus, feline distemper, possibly canine hepatitis virus, and rabies. But see the next two paragraphs about rabies titers.

With rabies, I must give a cautionary note. In all likelihood, rabies titers work just the same as with other diseases. Once there is a protective titer, the animal is protected. There is an argument that this does not hold true for rabies. That argument, as best as I can determine, comes mostly from vaccine manufacturers, so I question its validity. Further, immunologists like Dr. Schultz believe that titers provide the same guidance with rabies as with other diseases. As of this writing, however, no state public health agency has gone out on a limb and officially accepted titers in lieu of their revaccination requirements. While this is not in accordance with immunological understanding, they err on the side of caution. As rabies is a threat to humans, the laws are to protect humans, even if dogs and cats (and other species) suffer from overvaccination. Everyone in the public health field is reticent to accept titers instead of boosters, in case it turns out that titers are not protective. It is a liability issue. And a shame, as there is little likelihood that titers are not accurate here, and there is so little risk for the vast majority of animals.

Should you choose to use titers in lieu of rabies boosters, you will most likely be breaking the law in your state. You will be on your own, and your local veterinarian will most likely be resistant to your choice. You can still request the titer, however. You want the RFFIT test, and you can ask your veterinarian to send the sample directly to Kansas State University (www. vet.k-state.edu/depts/dmp/service/) or Auburn University (www.vetmed. auburn.edu/index.pl/virology). These are the only laboratories in the United States (and for Canada, I believe) where rabies testing is done. The commercial labs send the samples to these university labs, and they just mark up the cost. I am totally comfortable with protective rabies titers, but the law is not on my side—yet. Work within your state to get these laws changed. Rabies vaccines do cause damage, and beyond one or two vaccines they are almost wholly unnecessary.

Summary

In summary, I hope that you understand a few things:

- While vaccination may have reduced illness in some cases with acute contagious diseases, it is not so clear what the impact has been. In diseases such as bovine herpesvirus and polio, countries where vaccination was not major saw reductions in disease to the same extent as countries that utilized vaccinations. Herd immunity (immunizing the majority of a population) is important, but this may occur as much by natural exposures as by vaccination.

- Even if vaccination is helpful, only initial vaccination is necessary. As I explained in the "Titers" section, once immunized, we are immunized for life with vaccines for acute contagious diseases. Booster vaccines are wholly unnecessary.
- Core vaccines for dogs are distemper, parvovirus, and rabies, as well as adenovirus-2 (for canine hepatitis) in rare circumstances.
- Core vaccines for cats are panleukopenia (distemper) and rabies.
- For the core vaccines, one appropriately timed vaccine provides life-time immunity in about 95 percent of animals. Rabies may require two vaccines for this.
- Vaccination for upper respiratory infections of dogs (kennel cough) and cats (rhinovirus, calicivirus) are usually unnecessary, but intranasal vaccination is best. Nosodes can work well for these as well, though.
- Diseases that are not acute contagious diseases do not benefit from vaccination. These include such diseases as feline leukemia virus, feline immunodeficiency virus, feline infectious peritonitis virus, Lyme disease, ringworm, and giardiasis.
- Vaccines can and do cause disease, sometimes severe disease. They are not the "helpful or neutral" agents that we formerly thought they were. They have great potential to do harm, and I believe the harm they do is vast. We are only beginning to understand the extent of vaccine damage. In fact, I suspect that we will abandon vaccination entirely before too long, once we as a medical society and as a general society grasp the degree of this damage.
- The more vaccinations we give, the more likely the damage, although sometimes one vaccine initiates a cascade of problems. This may result from damage passed on from parents to offspring, whether via genetic or other means.
- I do not recommend vaccination in almost all circumstances. While many may see this as extreme, I believe the risk of vaccination out-weighs the risk of disease for the vast majority of animals in the vast majority of circumstances. Arguably, those of us who do not vacci-nate our animals may depend upon the majority who do, but as explained in the first item in the summary, it is not totally clear how much vaccination plays a part. There is a risk in not vaccinating, but there is a risk in vaccinating. Each guardian must weigh these risks for herself.

- Rabies, as a public health threat, falls somewhat outside these bounds, as vaccination is mandated by law. The law, however, is based more upon fear than upon immunology, and it should be changed. Until then, any decision not to vaccinate as the law mandates should be taken seriously. It is a matter of weighing your companion animals' health against complying with the law, while not putting yourself or others at undue risk.
- Nosodes do work for immunity but must be given near exposure. They do not work like vaccines and do not provide long-lasting immunity. They can be problematic if repeated for too long.
- Titers can assess immunity, but once an individual shows a protective titer to a given illness, there is no need for further testing, as immunity is lifelong.

Chapter Seventeen
THE BIGGER PICTURE

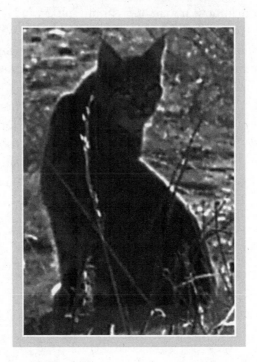

Stress and Animal Illness

Animals as Mirrors

Heroic Medicine

The Meaning of Keeping "Pets"

Animals Existing on Their Own Right

Conclusion

We are part of the earth and it is part of us. The perfumed flowers are our sisters; the deer, the horse, the great eagle, these are our brothers. The rocky crests, the juices of the meadows, the body heat of the pony, and man, all belong to the same family. . . .

I have seen a thousand rotting buffaloes on the prairie, left by the white man who shot them from a passing train. I am a savage and I do not understand how the smoking iron horse can be more important than the buffalo that we kill only to stay alive.

What is man without the beasts? If the beasts were gone, man would die from a great loneliness of spirit. For whatever happens to the beasts soon happens to man. All things are connected. This we know. The earth does not belong to man; man belongs to the earth. . . . Whatever befalls the earth befalls the sons of the earth. Man did not weave the web of life; he is merely a strand in it. Whatever he does to the web, he does to himself.

—Chief Seattle[1]

Sooner or later Nature will surely come to her own again. Nothing human is of long duration. Men and their deeds are obliterated, the race itself fades; but Nature goes calmly on with her projects. . . . When the locust swarm has passed, the flowers and grasses will return to the valley; when man has gone, the sand and heat will come back to the desert. The desolation of the kingdom will live again, and down in the Bottom of the Bowl the opalescent mirage will waver skyward on wings of light, serene in its solitude, though no human eye sees nor human tongue speaks its loveliness.

—John C Van Dyke[2]

If the earth is to remain a good place for a sane life, attention will have to be paid more to the middle ground: to the terrain of human scale and its space, the distance a man can walk or see, to the reality of flowers, houses, trees, streams—all the things in the unfashionable middle-size range, remote from molecules and planets alike. . . .

Heterogeneous, textured environments . . . as well as domesticated land and urban places, are essential for the life of the body, mind, and spirit.

—Paul Shepard[3]

This chapter is not about homeopathy, and much of it is not even really about health care, at least in a conventional sense. But it remains a critical one for me, as in it I discuss our relationship to our animal companions and some implications of that relationship. The first few sections will likely make sense, though the ideas may be new to you. I believe you will find them helpful. Some of the later sections may not be easy for some of you to read, as many concepts likely will test the bounds of your comfort and challenge your ways of relating to and thinking about companion animals. If you find these parts too difficult, save them for another time. Tear them out of your copy if you must. But read them if you can, when you can, as they are critical in the bigger picture.

From the introductory quotes, you may wonder where I am heading. I will say this much: this chapter covers a lot of territory. The older I grow and the longer my life interfaces with animals, the more I wonder if we have taken some turns that may not be working out to our best advantage. Certainly, our dominance over this planet that is our only home has gone a little too far. Within this, our relationship to animals, domestic and non-domestic alike, has also gone a little too far, at least to my way of thinking. I think we may be well served to reevaluate some of our assumptions, some of our mores regarding animals. To this end, I dedicate this chapter to wild nature generally, and to Paul Shepard specifically. Read his works about our relationship to the natural world if you want to go beyond this, especially *The Tender Carnivore & the Sacred Game* and *The Others*. Shepard's writing has helped me clarify my own discomfort with my culture's assumption of manifest destiny as it has barreled over so many other species and cultures in seeking its uncertain goals. Instinctively I knew we were not on a path that felt good, but I did not completely understand why we had gone so far off track until reading his works.

The ideas I express in this chapter, however, originate out of my own history: my own deep connection to animals in my life and my long relationship with the world out there in nature. A constant and essential healing space for me is what I call "walking in the woods," even if it might be in the desert. Out of these two aspects comes my understanding, my belief, that the world outside human control has its own value and its own song, a song that, for me, heals my soul. I suspect that song heals humanity's soul as well, though this may only reflect my bias. But a corollary is that our domestic animals—those we call pets—somehow fill this niche to at least a degree for those of us who share these needs for nonhuman energy but do not seek balms in the wilds.

One concern I have, though, is that in our dependence upon domestic animals as a source of this song, we lose connection to wildness and otherness. I am concerned that we simply cannot fulfill this need from domestication in any form. Further, I am concerned that in attempting to utilize domestic animals for this need, we are by default abandoning the wild ones out there who ultimately may be so essential to our survival, as Chief Seattle said. We are burning the very nature that we need for our nurture. We risk that "great loneliness of spirit" by destroying the Eden from whence we came.

But what about those companion animals? How has this impacted them? Certainly, as with us, they have been far more successful than their wild counterparts. Population numbers for cats and dogs no doubt far exceed those of other carnivores at any time in history. Their success is unprecedented. In this way, domestication has been a boon. Yet I worry about them, these animals who have chosen to live within our controlled environments: what have they had to lose, and do they suffer at our hands? What price have they paid for survival? And what does that say about the price we pay for our survival as we move further away from freedom and the natural world and more into security, but perhaps also into sterility?

Domestic animals, while they can and do provide a connection to the nonhuman world, also isolate themselves from the natural world in their domestication. Their choice, if you will, to be domesticated provides material gain, but possibly intangible soul-loss. They have greater security but less freedom. This especially applies to city dwellers and indoor-only animals. Do they also suffer for lack of the "wilderness song?" I suspect so. Further, in serving humans as a connection to this song, they bear the burden of our needs. This is no slight burden; in fact I now realize that this burden underlies many animals' illnesses, unfortunately. The human-animal relationship does not always nurture either party in the long run, though it is a wonderful relationship in so many ways.

As a veterinarian, of course, I live face-to-face with this relationship daily in my chosen profession. For three decades, in this capacity, I've observed illness in those animals whom we love, and for whom we expend great effort, and sometimes great expense, seeking to improve their lives—and, of course, our own. As my practice evolved into homeopathy, this observation deepened, first in consequence of my reliance upon understanding my patients' emotional states for successful homeopathic prescriptions, and secondly, since obtaining this information necessarily involves the guardian, revealing the guardian-companion relationship, often in intimate detail. From these observations came several insights, including: (1) There is often a correlation between guardian stress and animal illness. (2) Guardians and their companions often share illnesses and may receive the same homeopathic remedy, each from his own doctor, though this is by no means universal, even if it is common. (3) I see patterns in human behavior and in the human-animal interactions that appear to influence treatment outcomes in companion animals. For example, some animals just do not respond well to medical intervention of any sort, leading their caring, well-meaning guardians along a painful, often tortuous, path of seeking help. Is there some connection, some dynamic that encourages this outcome, these non-responding animal illnesses? I believe there is.

The good news is that solutions exist for these scenarios. A dose of awareness can initiate far-reaching change, both for guardians and their animals. Certainly this awareness may engender work on our parts, and sometimes deep emotional work. But such work brings balance and a lighter spirit. It is my hope that the following sections aid you in these ways.

The larger question I raise, about our choice to relate more to domestic than to wild nature, remains a dilemma. I discuss this toward the chapter's end, in potentially disquieting ways for some readers. The difficulty is that there are no easy answers to this dilemma. We find ourselves in a bit of a muddle, and it is important to examine the issue. I hope my discussion proves helpful. First, though, let's examine our direct interactions with those animals in our homes and how those interactions affect the animals, even to the point of causing illness:

Stress and Animal Illness

All relationships are complex, and the human-animal one is no different than human-human dynamics. Whereas I once assumed the human-animal interaction to be rather straightforward, I now realize how wrong my perception had been. Interfacing with our animals can have profound impacts upon them, and it often leads to disease ("dis-ease"). How this arises is not always obvious, though sometimes cause and effect are rather clear. Once I opened my eyes and my understanding, I recognize these patterns frequently. I suspect you will as well. Stress, for example, which we know causes human illness, can be just as impactful with our companions. Death, whether of a human or a nonhuman animal in the same household, often leads to grief. If a cat or dog cannot move through this grief, she'll often become ill, just as we do. The same may occur with any stressors, like divorce, children leaving home for work or college, or simply living in a household with greater than normal stress levels.

Take Ike's case, for instance. When Mary first phoned me about Ike, he had begun having seizures, and his seizures had greatly intensified in recent months. Furthermore, Ike had withdrawn somewhat from the household, spending less time in Mary's lap and more time off on his own. He also seemed overly upset, somehow, on edge and unable to relax. Mary said, "He's always watching me, as if he's trying to tell me something." I asked Mary what he might want to tell her, and she replied, "he just seems worried." I then asked Mary if there was anything going on in her house that Ike might worry about. Mary sighed deeply, and then explained that her husband, Rick, a mechanic, had injured his neck on the job a year and a half prior. His disability payments were coming to a close, his injury prevented him from returning to his work, and not only did he not know what he might do with his life, but also, without his income, Mary's income was really inadequate for their household expenses. And this all occurred at Christmastime.

Once she spoke the words, Mary clearly understood the connection with Ike's illness. He *was* worried. And it turned out that his seizures began shortly after Rick's injury, and they intensified as it came time for Rick's disability checks to stop. There was a clear connection. As with so many people, Mary knew this already on a gut level, but our discussion helped her to accept it as real, despite our cultural biases against thinking that animals have these sorts of "human" responses. Further, this understanding allowed Rick and Mary to use Ike as a "barometer" for their household stress. This alone greatly diminished Ike's stress, and his seizures lessened greatly, almost instantly. They basically disappeared from his life over the next year or two, and he has only had one or two mild seizures in the four years since Mary and I first spoke.

While many situations are not so clear, Ike's case exemplifies a rather common occurrence, whereby we deny—or simply do not recognize—how our own stresses impact everyone, human and nonhuman, who shares our life. This denial gives more power to the stress, which can lead to illness.

And simply bringing this into conscious awareness often provides great relief, even if the external stressor does not disappear, as in Ike's household. With awareness, we more easily recognize stress when it arises, and thus we more easily disperse that stress through communication and other means.

Animals as Mirrors

Sometimes our companion animals show an even more curious phenomenon, in that they appear to express aspects, often hidden or at least unexpressed, of their guardians. These situations are not so different from Ike's and Mary's, except that, whereas Mary and Rick knew that they were worried but had not completely accepted Ike's equal (or even greater) worry, in these cases guardians may not fully realize their own emotional states. Their animals may then express the guardian's unconscious emotions. Sometimes this is as simple as a dog who remains fearful, barking at slight noises, while his guardian wonders why he's on "red alert" all the time. Further inquiry sometimes reveals that his guardian holds deep fears of danger, which she may have buried in her psyche or of which she may be unaware. But she gives subtle clues, physically or psychically, to which her dog responds with heightened awareness.

Other times it's even more complex. In these situations, animals may "act out," in a sense, just as children often do when there is some undercurrent in the adult human relationship. The animal or child may then express some need or desire of one or another (adult) human in the household. Sometimes two or more animals may each exhibit different needs, different aspects.

Here's a wonderful example: Clarissa brought Arnold to me for chronic skin disease and general sluggishness. Arnold is a yellow Labrador retriever, very sweet, and although he was quite interested in our chickens and turkeys, almost as soon as he came into the old adobe house where I see patients, he lay down under the kitchen table, falling asleep right away. His skin was not bad, with only a few areas where it was red and irritated. Clarissa said he had improved greatly in the month he'd been in New Mexico and out of the humidity and heat of the Deep South, from where they had recently moved. But it was his quietness that struck me. Labs are generally pretty easygoing, but his immediately settling into slumber seemed over the top—or should I say, under the bottom.

As we talked, I found that Clarissa was in the midst of leaving a twenty-three-year relationship and marriage with a much older man. They had grown apart, somewhat due to their age difference. She had left a home in a gated community, focused around a golf course and clubhouse, and moved to New Mexico to reassess her life. Amanda, another dog, had died a couple of years previously. Unlike Arnold, Amanda was somewhat wild. She could be aggressive, occasionally bit others, and generally was a "handful." Clarissa said that Amanda constantly got in trouble in the community, whose members insisted she be muzzled when she was outdoors. Since Amanda was so disliked, Clarissa had to walk her at a nearby park, outside the gated community, where she could run free. Train tracks ran along one park edge, and Amanda loved to run alongside the trains as they sped by. One day, however, a second train came by from the opposite direction, just after Amanda had chased the first one. For some inexplicable reason, Amanda ran right out in front of the second train, probably dying instantly as she was carried away down the tracks. "We never did find her," Clarissa said. "It's like she took her own life. I don't think she could stand being muzzled any more."

I asked Clarissa if she thought Amanda might have been expressing any of Clarissa's deeper feelings. *"Yes,"* she emphatically replied. "It's like she fought against all the rules and restrictions behind those gates, and the more restrictions, the more resistant and aggressive she became. I hated that life also. I felt restricted in so many ways myself. I couldn't grow and express my deeper needs. I knew that if I did not leave that community and my husband, one of us (her husband or her) would die as well."

I remarked that perhaps Amanda *had* taken her own life, as the only way out that was open to her. Clarissa said she had wondered the same thing, but she was just not sure a dog would take such action. She could certainly believe it, though, since she felt much the same about the community as Amanda had. I could almost hear the wheels turning in Clarissa's head as she processed this information. It made sense to her, and she immediately smiled, presenting a much lighter countenance than when she had arrived.

I next asked Clarissa what aspects Arnold might represent. She knew right away: "he carries my depression, and also my inability to ask for my own needs. He isn't able to be his fullest self, and neither was I." Indeed, even Arnold's illness pattern could fit that very picture. I suspected his thyroid to be mildly underfunctioning. Further, as his most persistent skin outbreak circled his anus and involved his ears, I wondered if he had a candida overgrowth. His previous veterinarian had suspected this as well.

I was also curious about direct emotional connections to his physical symptoms, so I consulted Louise Hay's book, *You Can Heal Your Life*, in which Hay lists relationships between many symptoms or illnesses and their emotional components. My experience with her book has been that she often seems right on target. In her book, thyroid illness represents "humiliation. I never get to do what I want to do." Further, being in the throat chakra, there is also the symbolism of not speaking one's truth, not asking for what we want. And candida can represent, again according to Hay, "lots of frustration and anger. Demanding and untrusting in relationships." These could easily represent Arnold's emotional state, and also Amanda's. And, of course, Clarissa's. Could Arnold, then, still be expressing something for Clarissa? Interesting, is it not?

In a sense, Arnold expressed Clarissa's passivity, her tendency not to stand up for her needs, her own spiritual growth. She was neglecting her overt self, in a way. Amanda, on the other hand, expressed Clarissa's deep rage, not only at the external controls but also at her own inability to resist those controls, to be herself despite external resistance. Further, if Louise Hay is correct, even Arnold carried some anger, buried beneath his passive demeanor. I gave Arnold *Staphysagria*, a remedy for deep resentment at perceived (or actual) external controls, which can express either with rage or with a shut-down state like Arnold's. I also suggested that Clarissa take the remedy if it felt correct.

But I further sensed that subconsciously, subliminally, Amanda's sudden exit had triggered Clarissa's realization that she might be next if she did not take action. Her subsequent move to New Mexico and out of a relationship that no longer served her is a great beginning, and I'm sure she'll blossom here. "I feel I can breathe here, I can expand myself," she said as she left my consulting room.

A couple of months later, in late February, Clarissa phoned me. Arnold and she had been doing really well; both were emotionally much better, and Arnold's itching had almost disappeared. But then her husband sent flowers to her for Valentine's Day. This threw her off again, and Arnold also began itching a lot. We discussed how her emotional state was likely affecting Arnold, and I suggested repeating the *Staphysagria*. She e-mailed me a few days later, reporting that "I realized Arnold did not need the remedy, so I took it again, and we are both much better. Thank you."

How can this be, you may wonder? Is this just some fantasy? I don't have a definite answer, but I do feel this is real, or as real as anything else. It may be simply that, since Amanda and Arnold were exposed to the same restricting lifestyle as Clarissa, they would, as sentient beings not so different from us, develop separate but normal response patterns: passive submission or angry resistance. Clarissa seemed to be moving from passive submission to resistance; fortunately her spiritual work minimized her anger response, though I did warn her that her anger would probably surface, especially if she took the *Staphysagria*. She thought that it would be good, actually, for her to bring the anger to the surface.

But could it be more than this? Clearly there is some link, since Clarissa's redosing with the remedy improved Arnold. But I also wonder if this supports an understanding that life is a dream in which all things we see and encounter have meaning, just as in our sleeping dreams. Many cultures, especially native/aboriginal ones, as far back as human awareness, see life in this manner. Carl Jung also saw this through his work. It has only been recently in human evolution, since Western/logical thinking—since agriculture and the alphabetic languages that developed out of these farming-based societies—that we have so separated ourselves from the world around us. Modern philosophers and scientists, from Jung and Rupert Sheldrake, to quantum ("New Age") physicists and thinkers, find themselves returning to this older, experiential way of thinking. Quantum physics has shown that the experimenter's expectations influence the experiment, that we cannot so easily separate ourselves from the world around us. And if it *is* a collective dream, then why wouldn't we see meaning in our animal companions, especially since keeping animal companions has such meaning in our modern culture? Why wouldn't they provide living metaphors at times, mirroring us just as surely as our spouses and other human relationships?

You may wonder here if I mean that life is only metaphorically a dream, or if I am suggesting that it is literally a dream. Personally, I believe it is actually a dream, but seeing it as metaphor is just as helpful. To the aboriginals of Australia, however, there was no question: life is a dream, the same as our sleep dreams, or essentially the same. Only this dream is a lucid dream. They had living experiences of this over thousands of years. Some modern people also perceive life in this way, or at least aspects of this perception. We can and do guide our lives, for example, and we can affect the outcome.

We do impact our futures by what we think in our present moments. I see this in my work: if I become so busy that work becomes stressful, the overload can result in my feeling this stress when the phone rings, because I don't feel I have more to give at the time. When I feel the stress, the thought may cross my mind that I wish the phone had not rung. Sure enough, when this happens, the phone will stop ringing in the ensuing days, or ring *much* less. Then I say to myself and to the universe, wait a minute, I did not mean to *stop* ringing. And I ask for more phone calls, and soon the phone begins ringing again. Am I delusional? Maybe, but I don't think so—I've seen this over and over. So yes, life is a dream in the sense that it is malleable, that it is a fluid, responsive expression.

But life is full of metaphor as well. For example, we get messages from the universe, from the world around us. This to me further supports the dream hypothesis. A clear illustration of this happened to my wife about a dozen years ago, before we married. We were just friends at the time, and we mostly communicated by handwritten letters. I received a letter one day wherein Kathleen told of a crow who had dropped a dead rat at her feet while she was out running at a track in Seattle. The rat had a hole in its side—an exceedingly visible wound. I wrote back immediately, telling her to be careful, that crows, as very intelligent birds, did not drop their meals so readily. I told her this was a message, though I knew not the meaning. The next letter I received I could barely read. The handwriting was terrible, shaky, poorly formed. It turned out that shortly following her crow encounter but before my letter arrived, a car pulled out in front of Kathleen while she was on her bicycle. She crashed into the side of the car, breaking her right arm and a finger along with sustaining other injuries. She received my letter in the hospital and sent her reply from there, writing with her left hand. The dead rat was a warning metaphor for an impending injury, a potential death. How else to explain this except as a dream state? Clearly there is more than meets the eye here.

Returning to Clarissa's situation, her animals provide exterior messages, as does everything in her life. These messages provide opportunity for her to change. Unfortunately for Amanda, she had to leave suddenly and violently for Clarissa to notice, or at least so Clarissa would act. Arnold's message is a bit more subtle, but the consultation with me clarified the message for Clarissa, and she is making great strides now. It is the same for us all; metaphor and meaning abounds. Even a clerk at a market or a gas station can sometimes give just the right message. Have you ever experienced this? You may be mulling over some problem, go inside to pay for gas, engage in a minimal conversation as you pay, and the person says something that catches your attention. Then, as you drive away, you realize it was just what you needed to hear. I have encountered this many times. These messages come regularly; it is just that we usually do not notice. Our ancestors, however, usually did, back when they lived in nature, before separating themselves from the world around them. Even today we have many stories of those times, from not so distant cultures like those of Native Americans and Native Australians. Many Native Americans, from different nations, had dreams or visions foretelling white Europeans' arrival. These people connected to that unconscious world where such messages can be known. Robert Wolff's book, *Original Wisdom*, wonderfully describes this knowing, which he encountered firsthand with hunting and gathering people in the mountains of Indonesia. For the people of whom he writes, the dream world was their normal mode, and it was odd when they were not in contact with this aspect. Today, we still have the capacity, but we have mostly lost it, or allowed it to atrophy. We can regain this, however. The primary requirement is removing the blinders, opening our awareness to the information.

While these messages come from any aspect of the external world, naturally those animals and people with whom we spend the majority of our time will provide this feedback the most. Our domestic animals therefore engender great opportunity for growth through this mirroring; this gift, while generally unrecognized, carries vast potential for us. In suggesting that our companion animals provide meaning for our lives, though, I do not imply that this is their only reason for being. And I do not propose that they are merely aspects of our dream, our metaphor, our reality. They share this journey with us, and in that capacity can impart meaning (as long as we "listen"), but they also exist as autonomous beings in their own right. My point is just that they can give us messages, as can the clerk. We only need open ourselves to these messages. And the beauty is that if we do so, we can make changes before our animals or we have to go as far as Amanda or Arnold, or even Kathleen. We can heed the messages we receive, and if we heed them in time, we can avert tragedy.

I see another, slightly different aspect of mirroring as well, one that fascinates me but also provides frustration for guardians and veterinarians alike (when we are attached to outcome). In this scenario, companion animals seem to reflect their guardian's fears, primarily those fears about that animal's health. At least that is where the fears focus; I'm sure they go much deeper. Strangely and unfortunately, this dynamic results in the animal manifesting their guardian's fears. It's the old "you attract what you fear" cliché played out for real.

Here's an example from my practice, of lovely people with great care for the animals in their lives: Brenda was married to Robert, and they lived with one cat, Samantha. Another cat, Oscar, had died about a year or two previously. Robert worked outside the home as the wage-earner for the family. Brenda stayed home and minded the house and Samantha. Samantha was already in her teens when Brenda first called me about her. Sam was reasonably healthy, but she vomited occasionally, sometimes did not want to eat, and would occasionally cry out as if in distress, especially at night. This was not the cry of many older cats who become confused; it often came when she used the litter box or when she vomited, seemingly indicating gastrointestinal distress. Her thirst also occasionally increased, and sometimes she urinated more frequently than normal, indicating some kidney and bladder issues.

I worked with Brenda and Sam for about ten years. They had already worked with another homeopathic veterinarian before me as well as with conventional veterinarians. Samantha's record was one of the thickest I have had, with pages and pages of blood-test and urinalysis reports and Brenda's detailed monthly reports. Brenda cared deeply for Sam, as did Robert. They spent a significant part of their income on Samantha, and Brenda devoted her life to Sam's care. She kept a diary of Sam's health, with daily entries on water and food consumption, bowel and urinary output, vomiting, crying, and all other activities.

Each month we'd go over this record, covering each system and all of Sam's health issues, as well as all of Brenda's concerns about Sam. Brenda was one of the most dedicated guardians I've ever worked with, though certainly not alone in her dedicated care and her diligent record keeping.

Brenda and Robert would have done almost anything for Samantha, though they favored holistic methods and would not submit Sam to drastic conventional treatments (though I think even the constant blood tests and urinalyses are excessive and traumatic). Brenda made Sam's food with care and dedication, and she put this same devotion into all tasks involving Sam's care. Through the decade we worked together, Samantha did improve for some time, then she maintained her health reasonably well for a long time, finally dying in her early twenties. She never shook any of her complaints entirely and was never fully healthy, but she lived a long time for a cat with her ailments, for many of which, treatment options are minimal and cure is unusual. Each homeopathic remedy we tried helped Samantha, but then she'd stop responding well and we'd have to move onto another remedy. This repeated over and over. I began to wonder if I simply could not grasp her case adequately, could not see the best remedy for her. At first, I could not understand why we could not bring her back to health. After all, Brenda worked exceptionally hard for Sam; she watched Sam's every move to be sure she had all the data I needed and to be sure she knew if Sam were experiencing any difficulties.

Eventually, however, I realized that this was likely the problem rather than the solution, the root of much of Sam's troubles. I found out in time that Robert and Brenda had never really gotten over Oscar's death. They replayed his life and death often, trying to see where they had gone wrong, why he died. And they turned this anxiety onto Samantha, wanting to be sure that this time, they did not miss anything. I saw that as large as their concern was for Sam, it represented at least as large a concern for their own loss—the real loss when Oscar died, and the impending loss when Sam would die. In a sense, they focused their lives on Sam, revolving around her in some way. Perhaps, though they would not have realized this, they were even more afraid of the hole Sam would leave behind when she died than they feared how her illness impacted her. It was the hole in their own lives they may have wanted to fill in the first place by taking in Oscar and Sam.

If this description sounds cold or heartless, I assure you it is not. Certainly not on their parts: they did care deeply for their cats. And not on my part either; it's just that I recognize this pattern all too well, from seeing it repeated all too frequently, and probably from acting this out in my own life at times. *When we don't fill our own hearts and lives with joy, we often look to others for these things.* Those others may be spouses, partners, or friends, or they may be nonhuman animals. Often they are children. When they live with us, often the weight of our needs is more than they can bear. Other humans (adults, anyway) have the option of leaving the relationship. Other nonhuman animals don't so easily take this step. Cats, and less commonly dogs, do occasionally leave, but rarely (unless you consider such departures as

Amanda's). And so they remain imprisoned, sometimes literally, with no choice but to bear this burden. In Samantha's case, it was too much. The constant observation, the constant needs drained her, and she became ill. Brenda's and Robert's care did help her, and she lived to a reasonably old age, but never without illness, without dis-ease.

This pattern used to puzzle me. So often, guardians who seemed to care the most, who worked the hardest at their animals' care, also often seemed to have animals with chronic illness that simply would not improve. It seemed paradoxical until I realized that the exceptional care often arose out of an exceptional need. And it was the need that was the issue, the common thread running through these scenarios. Once I understood this, I knew that the solution was not solely in the animals' care. Rather, the solution for these cases is more in counseling guardians, as this is a family issue.

Seeing these cases as dysfunctional relationships in addition to or instead of solely as individual health problems brought me to a new understanding. And it made perfect sense. Just like in a human family, a human and nonhuman family also has identified patients who express family dynamic problems. Identified patients are the family members in whom we can identify problems, but whose problems result from dysfunctional family dynamics rather than only from within themselves. In a human-nonhuman family, these are usually the companion animals, since they have the least power in most families. This understanding has helped me in at least two ways. First, I realize that, as it involves the entire family, I won't often solve the animal's problems by focusing on his problems alone. I therefore also realize the difficulty in helping these patients, and I'm a little easier on myself and on the family in my expectations. Secondly, I know to begin discussing these aspects with guardians early on in the process. It is not always easy, but I must see if there is a willingness to open this door. And I know to refer them to a qualified counselor if things don't move along in a reasonable manner with my help alone. Often I can guide the family just fine, but sometimes they do need other help.

Nonhuman animals really are like us in so many ways. They respond to emotional stress in the same ways, within the framework of their own normal behaviors. They understand how to function in relationship to humans when these relationships remain within normal bounds. But when we demand too much, when we fight, yell, express unreasonable anger or fear, these animals will react accordingly, not so differently than we do. And if these dynamics last too long or are too intense, just as with us, nonhuman animals' coping abilities break down. If they cannot escape from the dynamic or they cannot find health-sparing ways to release built-up stress, they become ill, just as we do.

Unfortunately, life often becomes more rather than less stressful for us over time, especially as populations increase, environments and economies deteriorate, and resources diminish. This stress affects us all. Unless we somehow can change this pattern, it will only get worse, and we'll all become more and more ill. In a sense our companions can be sentries, warnings—canaries, if you will—in that the more illness we see in our animals, the more stress we know exists in our own lives. And in my thirty years of veterinary practice, I see this increase in illness not only in severity and frequency of disease but also arising in much younger animals than three decades ago. The difference is vast. By no means am I suggesting that mental and emotional stressors are solely responsible for this increase in illness. Obviously, chemical and electromagnetic pollution, poor food quality, and so many other physical impacts have also exponentially increased and incite great damage. I am simply focusing upon the less tangible concerns.

The beauty is that these less tangible problems are also more amenable to change. Certainly we can limit direct physical stressors like vaccines, pesticides, and drugs. But larger ones, like air and water pollution, as well as the exponential growth of electromagnetic pollution like cell phone, wireless Internet, radio, and television airwaves, have proven almost impossible to mitigate. Even normal power lines and wires produce these invisible stressors. It is easy to feel overwhelmed in dealing with these forces.

But our own emotional states are totally our own jurisdiction. Even if a neighbor plays his stereo loudly at three in the morning, or if our spouse has an affair, we have total control over our emotional responses. And we can make changes, even if our patterns have been damaging. We can always learn new ways. For example, we can learn to accept illness and death as part of life. This becomes more important with each passing year. Especially in light of increasing physical burdens like chemical and electromagnetic pollution, even severe illnesses like cancer increase rapidly year by year. Cancer in humans now affects almost one in every two people. Until our physical world becomes less damaging, our health and our animal companions' health will suffer. It will take decades at a minimum before this changes. We may as well accept this.

What can we do? Obviously, we can take steps in our homes and with our families to limit physical assaults on our bodies. We do this with clean, healthy food and by minimizing or eliminating chemical and physical stressors. Emotionally, learning to nurture ourselves rather than seeking this nurturance from others releases them from our needs and the subsequent stress those needs engender. Furthermore, remaining aware of illness, loss, and death can allow us to step back, in a sense, and accept these traumas as they come. In fact, they need not be traumas if we simply see them as natural outcomes. Trees drop their leaves in the autumn and regrow them in the spring. Winter arrives and grasses die, but the earth greens up again with warm weather. Without death and rebirth, we would not appreciate life. Rather than resist illness and death, we can work within these normal patterns. We can enjoy our companions while they live, help them live well while they remain, and let them go when they die. One of their greatest gifts is this one: that we learn about illness and death from their short lives. We can learn not to mourn their deaths, or to mourn and move on rather than holding on to grief. Making these changes takes practice, but we get this practice from living with animals.

A Buddhist monk had a teacup that was his favorite cup. He realized his attachment, so every time he used the cup, he envisioned the cup as broken. Using an "already broken" cup was practice for when the cup would actually break. But much more, this practice reminded him of the transience of everything. The only constant in this life is change, at least on the external level. By learning to accept change, we can begin to hold to the deeper meaning, that of simply being alive, seeing the beauty that always surrounds us. Flowers bloom so beautifully, but they don't last very long. Does this make them less beautiful? No, actually their beauty intensifies with their brevity.

Heroic Medicine

In some ways, death is easier to accept than illness. Once we know that a loved one is dying, we can let go, or at least we can begin the process. And the monk's "broken teacup" analogy can help us let go in advance, so the actual loss does not pain so sharply. But what about illness, especially illness that might result in death? A huge problem can be knowing when to let go and simply allowing death to come. Many people struggle with this, especially in Western cultures. My impression is that this has become more difficult in the past few decades.

Partly this results from advances in health technology as well as the availability of that technology. We have more options for prolonging life—or should I say, for avoiding death—at our disposal. Another part, however, relates more to our emotional fragility and possibly to loss of meaning in our lives. I suspect this relates somewhat to our estrangement from nature, as I mentioned in the introduction, and which I discuss below. But whatever the root cause, it is easy to choose to prolong life when we might better serve our companions by letting them go. We keep them here, however, for unexamined reasons, from guilt at not expending the resources to keep them alive to our inability to let go, clinging to them because *we* are not ready for the loss. Let me illustrate this with a few case examples:

Randi, a longtime client and friend, works mostly at minimum-wage jobs. When I first met her, she was waiting tables at a diner, where she adopted several of the many stray cats who lived nearby and came for food at the diner's back door. Randi has a huge heart and a small budget, so she will often sacrifice her own needs for those of her cats, family, and friends. A couple of years ago, she phoned me about Hugo, a rescue cat who had developed a facial cancer on his upper jaw. Hugo had been eating less and less for a few weeks, and his mouth smelled putrid. Randi took him to her conventional veterinary clinic a couple of weeks prior to calling me. The conventional veterinarian radiographed his face, saw a possible bone cancer on his maxilla (upper jaw), and referred Randi to a cancer specialist. The veterinary oncologist recommended surgery to remove the cancer, which would require removing most of his upper jaw on that side of his face. This would then be followed by massive radiation therapy for several weeks. The specialist hoped that, with those means, Hugo might live another six to twelve months. Hugo was about twelve to fourteen years old at the time.

As I had known Randi for about fifteen years, we had a casual and comfortable relationship. "Are you nuts?" I asked. "Hugo isn't that old, but he's surely not young either. And that's a terribly invasive surgery, incredibly painful. And then all that radiation will make him ill. All for a few extra months. Randi, it's just not worth it. And where would you get the money, anyway? I'm sure the oncologist means well, but I can't imagine Hugo would want to go through all this for a few extra months, most of which would be spent in pain or discomfort."

Randi didn't answer for a bit, but then she said yes, she agreed with me. She'd just needed my input, my reassurance in saying no. She'd gotten swept along with the momentum, from her regular veterinarian to the specialty clinic to further X-rays and procedures, to consider these drastic measures. Randi's big heart had once again almost caused her to make a decision that would have cost Hugo and her a lot of suffering, and all from a desire to prolong life despite the consequences to both.

These scenarios have become too common. As doctors, we veterinarians want to help, and we want to offer something in all cases. It can be uncomfortable to tell an anxious guardian that there is nothing we can do, or at least nothing we *should* do. For that matter, it is also uncomfortable for us to feel that we have nothing to offer. We want to remain optimistic; in part, this keeps us going. So we do what we can. And as in human medicine, technology improves constantly, as does our ability to keep bodies alive longer by doing more and more. Surgeons could have removed Hugo's upper jaw—his cheek and facial bones—and gotten him through this. Radiologists could have then bombarded his face with radiation to attempt to slow down the cancer growth. They might have given him those few extra months. It could be done. But is this enough? Is it enough that we can do something, to say it is appropriate?

I remember several instances within my conventional practice where I too encouraged treatment when it may not have been in my patient's or client's best interest. In one case, a young couple brought a dog in who was partially paralyzed from some spinal injury or condition. I felt that I might be able to help with acupuncture and medical therapy. The couple discussed their options, but they did not want the dog to suffer. I don't think they were very optimistic about the outcome. They preferred euthanasia to prolonging their companion's pain. As an optimist, I pushed a bit, and they agreed to try a few treatments. But after one or two treatments, they went elsewhere, no doubt for the euthanasia they had wanted in the first place. I felt a bit uneasy, wondering if I had served them or their dog well.

In another case, Stan, an acquaintance, brought his dog to me because Sonny had been straining to defecate. I examined Sonny and found that he had a tumor in his rectum about four inches in from his anus. We discussed Sonny's options, and I recommended a complicated procedure called a rectal pull-through, wherein I would evert the rectum through the anus and remove the last few inches of the rectum along with the tumor. I would then reattach the rectum to the anus. Stan agreed to the procedure, as it seemed Sonny's best hope of recovery.

I always enjoyed surgery, and this surgery, while challenging, went very well, and Sonny came through the surgery with no problems. I sent him home with Stan a couple of days later. I did not hear from Stan for several months, and then I saw him downtown. I asked how Sonny was doing. He replied, "He's fine now, but if I had known how hard it would be for him, I would never have done that to him." My heart sank to my stomach. I really did not know what to say. I had felt good about being able to help, and proud of the surgery. Now I did not know what to think.

Stan's reply hit me in the gut. I don't know if he was upset with me or just sorry for his own decision. I had not asked, as I just wanted to get away and so had not carried the conversation further. I was grateful for his frank response, but pained at the same time. I only wanted to help and had thought I *had* helped. Now I was not so sure. This haunted me for a long time. Was it enough that I could perform the surgery, to justify doing so? I could not say, but Stan had no doubt.

Over time, such incidents chipped and chopped away at my confidence in the rightfulness of such treatments, in what I now call heroic medicine. In my early practice years, I had little doubt; I was proud of my veterinary education and my skills. I even scoffed at the "old guys" (older veterinarians, mostly men at that time) in my community, who often recommended against newer procedures, especially expensive and dramatic/drastic ones, the heroic ones. These veterinarians instead typically recommended more conservative approaches. As one older colleague said to me during the time I worked at an emergency clinic, "My clients don't want all those blood tests and big procedures." I thought they were simply out of date, that it was because they had not kept up with the times. I though they lacked the necessary skills and knowledge. In truth, I thought they should retire, or just do vaccinations and simple surgeries, leaving medicine to those of us with the necessary skills.

Now, I find that I am becoming one of the "old guys." I see that so often our ability to perform advanced tests and procedures clouds our understanding, and we choose for our clients' and our own desires and interests rather than for our patients. I think we become inured to the pain we may inflict in the face of the power we have with modern medicine.

I see that for veterinarians, heroic medicine has often become more about our ability to provide such measures than about evaluating their appropriateness or evaluating what our animal companions need. And I see that for animal guardians, heroic medicine often represents their own needs, or at least their desires, and their own fears about their animals' suffering and death (and, by extension, their own suffering and death). We lose perspective and then make decisions that may actually increase animal suffering, or at least do not serve our patients, the ones to whom we are charged with aiding.

Further, as I discussed earlier, in relation to why we as a society keep domestic animals, heroic medicine speaks to our lacking connection to nature, to our lacking meaning in our lives. It speaks to our desperateness. And desperate times call for desperate measures, so we take those measures. We take drastic steps to prolong an animal's life so we don't have to face death so soon, so we don't have to face the loss, reflecting our inner pain, so soon.

But just because we can take these measures does not mean that we should take them. We have these animals to consider. We must always ask, what is in their best interest? And then we must act from that position. We must not make emotional decisions; here we must use reason and intuition as guides. If we put their needs first, separating our needs from our decisions, we'll make better decisions.

I'm not suggesting that all modern medicine, even all heroic medicine, is necessarily and always in error. In fact, new techniques can be very impressive and can save lives and alleviate suffering. They can be truly miraculous. They are not inherently wrong in many cases. And I don't mean to imply that those who perform such procedures do not care. I'm sure they do, just as I did when I took out Sonny's tumor (and part of his rectum). It is not a condemnation of either my colleagues or of their procedures. It's just that we so often forget to ask that critical question: is this appropriate for my patient? And in a larger sense, does it make sense to prolong life in these ways: is it really serving the animal, serving the client (aside from her desires), serving our common good, our souls, our journeys through life on this earth?

As I suggested earlier, death need not be something to fear or resist. Certainly, relieving suffering merits our efforts, but when our labor turns to life extension against the odds, it is time to reevaluate our priorities. Perhaps it is correct to continue striving for healing as long as our companions do not suffer needlessly. But consider also that letting go is a possibility. Death is not a failure. We all die eventually, but culturally we seem to have forgotten this, or at least we deem it unwelcome. Merely accepting the normality, even the beauty and goodness of death, can open the door to a different decision. And if we do not emotionally need the one whose death approaches, if we have found our own center, we can know when and how to let her go.

The Meaning of Keeping "Pets"

For me, a large part of stress, illness, even madness that so encompasses modern life arises out of our distancing ourselves from the natural world from whence we came. Maybe this only reflects my personal bias, but I don't believe we can be either fully human or fully sane without some connection to nature. I do not believe we have evolved to the point that we do not still need to feel those rhythms that the natural world generates. I suspect, then, that we populate our houses with "pets" and plants so we can still retain a bit of connection to that other, to nonhuman life forms. Nonhuman animals resonate at different frequencies than we do, therefore living with them provides some, though by no means all, of what we obtain when immersed in the natural world. It keeps us from energetic starvation, in a sense, though that is about all. I suggest that the very existence of our cultural bent toward keeping household "pets" provides an indicator of our cultural separateness from nature, of the dearth of natural-world energy in our lives. Even the term *pet* denotes this separation, as a pet is something we pet, we control, we demean. We demean them because we limit them. We want contact with the animal world, with the nonhuman world, but on our terms. We domesticate pets, we castrate them, to make them more amenable, less threatening. Perhaps pets represent not a connection to, but a fear of, nature, in one sense. Taking this a step further, I propose that the greater a culture's "pet ownership," the more insane that culture is.

Let me explain, as I know this may sound like a rash statement. One aspect of sanity in an individual is our ability to survive and thrive in the world—to provide our basic needs: food, water, and shelter (clothing I consider a type of shelter). In our modern cultures, this would entail obtaining and keeping a job, earning money to pay for these needs. In an agricultural society, this would entail having the skills and discipline to raise one's own food, make clothing and shelter, and find water. A gathering and hunting society member would have the skills and discipline to find food, (whether from animal or plant sources), find water, and make clothing and shelter. By extension, sane persons in these cultures would be able to raise a family and provide for its members, for children and grandchildren. Of course, until modern times, tribes and communities were family units, in a sense, as our hunter-gatherer and agricultural ancestors knew that it took a community to provide for everyone in the community. This was much more critical for agricultural than for hunting-gathering cultures but still true for both. By further extension, our ancestors understood that if they destroyed the land upon which they fed and clothed themselves, they would ultimately suffer and perhaps even die out. This is the basis of the Native American knowledge that we should care for the land so it still provides for the seventh generation to come. This is a metaphor for infinity; stretching our minds out to seven generations is far enough to be almost immeasurable.

Someone from a culture with this belief, that we ensure sustenance for those who will come after us in two hundred years, might think it insane, for example, to slaughter bison by the tens of thousands and leave them to rot on the prairies. They might also think it insane to so pollute land and water that to consume this water or the food from this land makes us ill, even sterile. Do you see where I am going? Only humans who have lost their deep kindred connection to nature and to the others, the nonhuman members, could carry out such deeds.

How does this relate to keeping household animals as "pets" for companionship (and entertainment) only? Until modern eras, humans rarely kept pet animals. Only the wealthy kept animals who did not earn their keep. Certainly, farmers kept stock dogs and barn cats as well as horses, mules, and so on. And many humans bonded to those animals. But the animals still had jobs, as did everyone in the farm family. Until the mid-twentieth century in the United States, the vast majority of people resided on small family farms. Resources were too dear, too hard to obtain for most families to keep nonworking animals. They mostly utilized animals as beasts of burden, for hunting, mouse killing, and so on. The animals' jobs were to protect and obtain human resources. They worked to enhance our survival; as a bonus, domesticated animals have survived while many wild animal populations have shrunk disastrously. Additionally, as our forbears lived more within nature, they interfaced with animals regularly, either domesticated or wild animals. And their lives were full; they worked long hours. They had no need for animals whose sole purpose was for relating to. And they likely knew that they would overuse their resources by feeding animals who did not contribute to those resources. Their needs were more physical, so they utilized animals to supply physical needs.

Many people today take physical sustenance for granted, as we do not struggle for the basic needs. As a consequence, we don't need animals to assist us with our subsistence. Most animals today, at least in "first world" cultures (more appropriately called "third world," since they developed third, not first), do not have the kinds of jobs they did in the past. They do have jobs, however. Their jobs today are taking care of our mental, emotional, even our spiritual needs. Some animals work hard at these new jobs, and I am not certain they are always well equipped for their roles. The mental and emotional strain on our companion animals proves at least as difficult as the physical burdens they bore in the past.

In our modern world, we have overpopulated so greatly and have become so expert at providing our physical needs that we have often lost touch with how our ancestors lived, without abundant food. Starvation always lurked around a season for them, especially when populations increased toward carrying capacity (the number of humans or animals a given ecosystem can support without degrading). Weather also ruled their lives, as one bad season could put them at great risk. Today, we can basically use and do as we choose. Obviously this primarily applies to industrialized "first world" cultures, but these cover more and more of the earth all the time.

We get our food primarily from stores, far removed from its source. So if we take a second helping of broccoli or a second cup of coffee, we don't pick the broccoli flowers or coffee beans; we don't see the numbers of beans or flowers diminish. We don't realize the limited number of servings, as the plants are not in our own gardens. And so we don't see our overconsumption. We don't notice the shrinking resources—there always seem to be plenty in the store.

We flip a switch and we have light, heat, a hot burner to cook our food, even transportation. We turn a knob and out comes water, hot or cold. However, at the rate we currently use these things, this may not last long. And the price we pay is the same one that allows us this luxury: we have no connection to the resource itself, no direct knowledge of its source and limitation, and no experience of its beauty, its energetic resonance. And we don't notice because we've mostly never known it, that we lack any connection with all those other life forms (animal and plant) from which we get our physical needs met. By the time we get the food, clothing, or whatever, it is no longer alive. We don't relate to our resources as living, resonating beings. While this allows us to survive, even thrive, at least physically, it also allows us to not notice how badly we degrade our world. We don't see the devastation required to bring us our "daily bread." It's a huge price, this lack, but it has diminished so gradually, over many generations, that rarely does one individual experience the loss. We never saw it coming, in a sense.

As a consequence of this loss, we degrade our environment: we overconsume; we pollute our water, our food, our skies. We don't much consider the second or third generation, let alone the seventh. In other words, we live in a culture that continually depletes its environment, ensuring less and less for its members over time. To me, and probably to our not-so-distant ancestors, this is an insane culture. Environmental destruction is the symptom; separation from nature is the likely cause.

Yet we also know this loss on some levels, in our souls. And that is why we live with companion animals. They connect us back to nature, even if imperfectly due to their own separation. Our hearts and souls need that connection, as we simply do not get this elsewhere, at least not nearly as much as we need. In our modern culture, with its physical surfeit, there is a tremendous dearth of other-ness, of this resonance with other life forms amidst which we evolved, and which, I believe, provides us nourishment as critical as food, water, and shelter. We won't die so quickly with insufficient "other-ness," but die we will, and catastrophically, unless we realize this. Our companion animals, then, in fact help keep us sane in the face of this dearth, this cultural insanity. I remain grateful for them daily. They provide meaning and kindredship to many who have no other humans, no family, no community. They provide joy and stress release to all who share their lives. They even absorb some of our stress, becoming ill themselves, allowing us time to understand that stress and its meaning. Without them, I think our society would implode and explode, as it would likely reach a tipping point.

But we must not forget that we probably cannot evolve quickly enough to survive only with what sustenance we derive from domesticated animals. We evolved with wildness, with a world we could not control but that we had to understand and cooperate with. Our profound loneliness and despair, manifested by such things as the Columbine shootings and the 9/11 destruction, represent not only our estrangement from other humans, from families and communities, but also our estrangement from otherness on many levels. We remain as estranged from other human cultures as we do from other nonhuman cultures. When we lived directly in the natural world, we understood that it was all one, that we were only a part of a web, as Chief Seattle said.

The following example, from Paul Shepard, I think elucidates how the disconnect impacts us. The research was with our primate cousins, and in crowded captive situations, but I suspect the root problem is as much in the separation from nature as in captivity itself.

> By the end of 1972 more than twenty species of non-human primates, mostly monkeys and apes, had been studied in their natural habitat. Ten of the same species had also been studied in zoos or other confinement. In every case the wild forms were described as generally peaceful and affectionate, sensitive to friendly, cooperative relationships, each kind with its own way of avoiding harmful physical conflict. In no species was the top-ranking individual in a group dictatorial. In all cases where the same species were studied under crowded conditions (with plenty of food and water), their social organization as well as their immunity to disease deteriorated. Maltreatment of young and violent attacks on doormats by tyrants increased as much as ten or twenty times over normal.[4]

Certainly, overcrowding greatly increased the stress in these animals. But we cannot separate out the effect of removal from their natural habitats, which no doubt also greatly affected them. Anyone who has moved from the country to the city, or even from one city to another, knows how it takes time to adjust to the change. Judy Martin, of the Navajo Nation, said that when her ancestors were forced to relocate from their homeland to an area hundreds of miles away, the people suffered an "internal injury" that has not healed yet, a century and a half after they returned to the homeland.[5] Adaptation takes time. On an individual basis, it can take months or even years to adapt to a changed habitat. For a species, even for a culture, it can take much, much longer. Here is what Shepard says:

> It is sometimes said that higher complex creatures like humans do well in a changing world. In truth, such species, with flexible, learned behavior and diverse social forms, require a stable natural environment.... It is also said that "nature is change" and

argued that such is the essence of evolution. But this observation
... distorts the fundamental aspect of evolutionary change, which
is its *tempo*. The dramatic alteration of planetary life over hundreds of thousands of years requires great stability of life cycles,
individual experience, and social organization. Without such con-
tinuity and seeming changelessness over the shorter term, life and
environment would be too chaotic for the delicate process of evolution to operate.[6] (emphasis added)

Shepard's book was published in 1973. How much faster has change
accelerated since then? How can we possibly adapt so quickly to a world
so different from the one into which we were born? It is next to impossible, or at least it is very difficult. It requires great emotional and spiritual
stability to remain calm amidst the chaos of change we experience today.

Fortunately, our companions provide a balm for this wound, this rend-
ing of our world that has left us torn asunder. With their help, we can survive until we see some way to mend that wound. But until and unless we
realize that "pets" are only a Band-Aid, only a stopgap measure, until we
see that we must look through and beyond them to the entire world, we
won't last long. We must see that everything has a value and provides for
our nourishment, even if we do not see the connection. We can no longer
afford to isolate ourselves from this larger world. There is knowledge, wisdom,
and sustenance in all human cultures and in all animal and plant species,
and we cannot afford to neglect these others any longer. Here is Paul Shepard
again:

The main thrust of modern studies of man leads by degrees toward
recognition of the universal dimensions of problems of violence,
of personal alienation, and of environmental disorder. We move
now with increasing speed toward a day when the futility of ide-
ological answers and industrial technologies will be obvious. Then
it will be necessary to make a new start by the affirmation of the
pre-men in us.[7]

Shepard was a firm believer in the hunting-gathering culture as the pin-
nacle of human development, in the sense that these societies were the most
successful in balancing themselves with their environments. With few exceptions, hunter-gatherer cultures lived for millennia within fairly stable ecosys-
tems. Depletion was not an issue, though they possibly did hunt some large

mammals to extinction. Today, of course, we have no option to return to those days. We must adapt within the environment we have created. But partly, the reason the hunter-gatherer tribes succeeded was their understanding of their place in the web, as Seattle, a hunter-gatherer chief, so wonderfully said. They also knew that they were one family; they *belonged* to the natural world. Judy Martin said of her childhood on the Navajo Reservation, "Life was safe. We did not think of 'wild animals' as wild. We were not afraid of them."[8] They were at home in the midst of nature, and they did not feel the need to protect or separate themselves from wildness, from other-ness. And so one way to return to Shepard's "pre-man" state is to return to this view, to remove ourselves from the top of the heap, so to speak. For this we need wilderness to relate to, and we need human scale, as in Shepard's quote at the beginning of the chapter. Until and unless we can restore some balance on this level, we will suffer the alienation from nature of which he speaks.

Thankfully, we have these companion animals to fill the loneliness, to assuage the despair. We can learn from them, and by respecting them, we can get by. They teach us the value of others. But we must not stop there; we must let them teach us the value of *all the others,* so we will know why we need to restore a balance with nature and not rely solely upon them. And once we stop relying solely upon companion animals for our "otherness" needs, we will have removed a huge burden from them. We will have begun the process of freeing them from captivity, releasing them to their own desires and journeys.

Animals Existing on Their Own Right

Our companions provide stability, love, joy, a touch of otherness, and in some cases, our only relationships. Theirs is a large responsibility. Do we also have responsibility in these relationships? Of course we do. Some duties may be more obvious, such as providing food and shelter for them. Others are less obvious, like providing a safe, caring, even loving environment for them. But what does this latter responsibility mean, exactly? Different people interpret this in different ways. To some, providing a safe environment means always confining them for their safety. We keep cats inside; we keep dogs inside in pens, on chains or ropes, on leashes. We keep gerbils, hamsters, rats, and birds in cages. In other words, we control their movements: we imprison them.

Now, I understand this. In a short year or two, back in the early 1980s, I lost three cats. One was shot, one killed by a car, and the third was likely stolen. Following these losses I decided that from then on, whenever the next cats showed up, I'd keep them inside—for their own good, their safety. And I did so. Slowly, over the ensuing few years, I took in three strays and an Abyssinian from a breeder who no longer wanted him. Three males and one female, and my condominium seemed more crowded with each new family member. The oldest male retreated and became somewhat edgy, especially when the youngest male reached adulthood. Still I persisted.

One time Romeo, the Abby, slipped out my open door while I brought in groceries. He disappeared into the woods behind my condo, and I could not find him, nor would he respond to my calls. I feared the worst, since he had absolutely no prior outdoor exposure, having grown up in a small cattery and then living indoors. He was about four years old at the time. But he showed up two days later, tired and hungry. I suspected he'd gotten lost or confused in the overwhelm of being outdoors, and I happily greeted him upon his return.

With time, however, I thought Romeo seemed less happy after his return than he had seemed prior to his escape. I was unsure if this was my imagination, but it seemed so. And then I wondered, or I should say it dawned upon me, that maybe he was not lost or confused that time he escaped. Maybe he had simply reveled in his freedom for as long as he could until hunger brought him home. I decided perhaps I'd been wrong in keeping these cats in after all. They seemed too stressed inside. It was not a small townhouse, yet four cats seemed too many for the space once I observed their interactions better. I was young, still away from home a lot with work and social activities, and still learning about animal behavior and their needs. (I'm still learning, of course, but I understand much more now.)

In any case, I decided enough was enough. I'd probably been keeping them in for my needs as much as theirs. Maybe *only* for my needs. Plus the more time I spent pondering human impacts upon wild animals and the environment, I began to see a connection to domestic animals. We humans tend to control everything for our own convenience, from bears to dandelions to house cats. We love bears, tigers, and lions, but we like them best in zoos or on television. Or at least in someone else's community. Let someone sight a cougar in a city neighborhood, and we want the police or wildlife officers to move it elsewhere. We love wilderness, but not too close to home.

We think we want to live close, so we carve out a section of wilderness for a new housing development. We love living there until a cougar comes up to the back fence while children play in the yard. Then we panic, and we want the animal gone. Never mind that the cougar was here first and that we moved into *her* territory. We want that cougar moved, or killed if necessary. And we have no problem with this. But I began to see an inherent problem with our assumption that we had the right to control wild animals and wild places for our needs. I became uneasy at our certainty that we "outrank" other species. I was not so certain it was that simple, that we have a moral right to go as far as we do.

From these musings, it was only a short stretch to conclude that we had no right to control even domestic animals, including "my" cats. So I let them out. I propped the front door open, propped the garage door open so they could come and go as they chose until I could install a cat door. And I will say, without a doubt, that I could see a smile on Romeo's face. He became a different cat, as did they all. I knew I was correct. I knew I had no right, no moral authority, to control these animals, that if the situation were reversed, I'd certainly choose freedom over security myself. And why would they not do the same?

I often frame this in human terms for clients who express reluctance to relinquish control with their animals: suppose someone offered you two choices for your home. The first choice would be a very nice house with all the amenities you would ever want. Great food, cooks and housekeepers, big screen HDTV with only the channels and movies you like, a great stereo with unlimited access to your favorite music, indoor swimming pool, tennis courts, yoga instructors, and so on. And maybe they even threw in a guarantee of a long life. In short, you'd have anything you would want. Except your freedom: you could never go out, except perhaps in a fenced-in yard. (Doesn't this sound like a prison, where we keep our criminals?) Or, in the second choice, you could live in a small hut, provide for yourself, and come and go as you please. You would have complete freedom, but there would be risks. You might go hungry, you might not live as long, you might even die in an accident. Which would you choose?

I've come to understand that nonhuman animals share most desires and emotions with us at a basic level. I don't mean that a cat desires to go to India to see the temples, see the Taj Mahal. Rather, I mean that a dog, a cat, a bird wants food, enjoys comforts, even enjoys relating to others but wants to be free. Herd and flock animals may differ somewhat here, but no animal wants to be confined against her will, including human animals. It simply is not in our natures. Certainly animals love cushy lives. Cats epitomize this desire; at least we picture them this way. But the cats who live in my house, while they spend plenty of time on the bed, also spend cold nights outside, even in the rain and snow. If it rains too hard, they will look out of the window, even snap at each other, as bored and edgy as any young child on a rainy Saturday. They like the comforts, but they would never trade the comforts for their freedom.

Many old homeopathic masters defined health as freedom—freedom to eat what we want, do what we want, without bodily consequences. Within reason, of course. A healthy person, for example, does not need to avoid gluten, grains, or red meat (in reasonable quantities) to stay healthy and to avoid symptoms. (I am speaking here of health issues, not moral ones, regarding meat-eating.) A healthy dog need not be restricted to lamb and emu to avoid terrible allergic skin rashes. If our health is so impaired that we must eat a restrictive diet, we lose an aspect of freedom; our poor health limits our freedom to eat certain foods. Thus, poor health equals diminished freedom.

But I think it works the other way too. I think limiting our freedom can lead to health issues. I think we are all created equally, with equal rights and freedoms. Only I do not think this applies solely to humans. In the United States' Declaration of Independence, it states that all *men* are created equal. We now understand that it should have read "all persons" or some other such non–sex discriminating word, but that document was a product of its time. I believe that nonhuman animals as well have intrinsic rights to exist, to autonomy. I'll go out on a limb here and suggest even that maybe it is time to include them, in some small ways at least, in our understanding of what it means to be a person with rights. It is time to redefine our relationship to animals from one of owner and property, or even human and pet, to some other terms that connote respect. I use *guardian* and *companion animal* in this way. Certainly these animals are currently under our care, but I think it best to no longer consider them as chattel. Terminology becomes critical, as it influences thinking. If we believe we own another being, we cannot but see that being is lesser. This thinking allowed slavery and allowed genocide and cultural annihilation, and this was with other humans. With animals, it engenders inhumane animal research, confinement feeding operations, and even "pet" confinement.

Animals do suffer from this confinement; I commonly see health consequences in animals whose lives carry few freedoms. Paul Shepard's quote about primates in captivity exemplifies this. Poultry, who are raised in horribly constrained conditions, must be debeaked so they do not kill one another. Meat animals must be on constant antibiotic therapy to avoid terrible illness due to confinement stress. Horses chew on wooden stall doors from being locked in stalls over twenty hours of the day. Can you imagine this? Think of a horse, and what comes to mind? For most people, probably a beautiful, running horse, galloping and frisking in a meadow. In nature this would be with a herd, with his family. Yet we close horses into stalls, separate from contact with others, and then we try to medically treat them so they don't chew the stalls. Pet birds we keep in cages, and they pull their feathers out. We veterinarians try to find a cause, such as lice or mites, for the feather-pulling, yet the cause is obvious.

With cats and dogs, they often overgroom or chew themselves until they develop sores. I have a client whose dogs have become hyperactive and out of control, but they are big dogs who don't even get to go for a walk daily as the guardians cannot manage this. Medical doctors prescribe Prozac and all its "cousins" to ever-increasing numbers of humans, and Ritalin to incomprehensibly large numbers of children. Yet children live such structured lives today; they are forced to be confined in child seats on car rides, even on long trips. Yes, this may save a few children from terrible deaths, but at what cost to their emotions? How many children on Ritalin simply need to run and play, just like horses, cats, and dogs? No doubt there is also an epidemic of hyperactivity and attention deficit disorder, often at least partly from vaccination and other toxins, but I suspect the overcontrolled upbringing is a large factor for some children.

James Hillman, the Jungian therapist, wrote a book (with Michael Ventura) titled *We've Had a Hundred Years of Psychotherapy and the World's Getting Worse*, wherein he wonders why we do not look at the reason we need so much psychoanalysis, therapy, and medication. He suspects the root cause rests in our culture, in job dissatisfaction because of mind-numbing repetitive work on assembly lines and such, and in the resultant lack of meaning. Further, he believes that our separation from nature also plays a part. My conventional veterinary colleagues now prescribe antianxiety drugs to more and more animals, most of whom simply spend too much time impounded indoors or even in crates. Why, I wonder, do they not question the underpinning problems? Why do they not suggest letting animals out more, going for more walks? Perhaps the most healing aspect of dog companionship can be the walk, because we humans need exercise and movement as much as our dogs. Yet we so often cannot find the time. We are way too busy. And then there is the cat, the animal supposedly so well adapted to apartment living. Perhaps, but how many of these cats really enjoy their lives? How many end up on psychoactive drug therapy?

In this area, I think we fail our faithful companions. We focus so much upon protecting them—"for their safety"—when really we do so for our own convenience, for our emotional protection. We confine them so we will not suffer the loss, the pain. We confine them so the strays don't get out of hand. And these are issues, no doubt, especially with such overcrowding of humans and their domestic (and consequently feral) animals. We do have laws restricting animals, requiring fences, leashes, and so on. But the problem, it seems, stems more from us than from them. We overpopulate, expand, and crowd further into each other and into wilderness. We are way beyond carrying capacity. And, of course, we then bump into each other, and our companion animals bump into each other.

I don't have an easy answer; I don't even think there is an easy answer—but I know that controlling others never works in the long term. As I discuss in Chapter Fourteen, on reproductive systems, I even question our right to control animals via spaying and neutering, though for now I conclude uneasily that it may be best. For now. As for confinement, I am almost totally opposed to this. Other than in heavily urban areas, I believe animals should be free. Cats should have access to cat doors, coyote risk or not. Ideally, dogs should also be free to roam. I realize that most communities restrict dog freedom, and that many even restrict cat freedom. This is wrong; it is morally inexcusable. We do not have this right.

Yes, there may be problems with allowing animals their freedom. Dogs may fight, cats may fight, cats and dogs may get hit by cars, dogs or cats may leave and not return home. It may not be as pretty as we would like, and it may not be as convenient as we like. But convenience is insufficient to justify imprisonment. A friend used to say that the height of selfishness was to ask others to change so we did not become stressed or upset—to ask others to change for our comfort. This has become the model for our relationship to animals. Can we really still condone this approach?

Until we change laws and attitudes, what can you do? If you have a yard, fence the yard in so your dog or cat can at least roam freely there. It is possible to cat-proof a fence, with floppy fence materials at the top. Walk your dogs at least twice as much as you believe they need; this will still be less than they want, but it is a start. Spend more time at home with your animals; this is especially true with indoor cats and dogs. Play with them. If you cannot do this, then reconsider bringing new animals into your home. Seek solutions that do not revolve around control, but rather revolve around adding freedom and pleasure to your animals' lives. Rethink everything you have learned about pets and about animals. See them with new eyes. Become an anthropologist, and view our culture as though you are from another planet. See if how we now envision the human-animal relationship makes sense.

Most importantly, ask yourself why you live with animals. Are you looking for sustenance that might be better sourced internally? Are you avoiding relationships with other humans because of past pains? Could you nourish your human interactions, perhaps just by opening your heart when you meet people—even the deli clerk? What about saying hello to your neighbors, to others on the street? Can you find ways to be joyful on your own, in the small things like the smell of an orange, the color of watermelon flesh? Can you even find joy in the clang of the garbage collection truck, the sounds that make up your environment—what one author called our soundscape? Can you envision relating to animals without asking them to compromise?

It all fits into that larger picture where humans really fit into the web of life on this earth. And I suspect we have made a huge blunder along the way in estimating our importance. From this came the other mistakes. Reevaluating this might unveil other options.

It comes to this: if, as I believe, humans are not in fact the center of the universe, even the apex of life on earth, but just another species trying to survive, then we have no right to control others, any more than bears have a moral right to control bobcats. This really leaves us with one option regarding domesticated animals: leave them alone. Allow them to meld back into the web, to find their own balance point in the interspecies dance, flowing this way and that as the climate waxes and wanes.

This is, of course, more a rhetorical than a realistic idea, at least now. It may not even be the morally best choice now, now that we have tipped the balance so far in favor of domestic animals at the expense of wild ones, and now that they have fewer options and skills for survival on their own. We cannot just open the doors and kick the cats and dogs outside, and we cannot simply abandon our responsibility for the imbalance we have created. Still, I think the idea that we could stop muddling so much with nature, including domestic animals and plants, is a valuable one. A hands-off approach might—probably would—prove much superior in the long run to attempted management. Whenever we "monkey around" with the nuts, bolts, wheels, and pulleys in nature, the outcome is rarely what we expect. So a managed solution to domestic animal overpopulation is unlikely to succeed. I do not have an easy answer, though I suspect that the difficult one—hands off!—might provide the best long-term outcome. But I do not know how we could make that choice.

Don't get me wrong—as I said, these animals also keep the emotional balance, the psychological balance, for now and no doubt provide a critical balm for vast numbers of humans today. They may well help us avoid enormous catastrophes. And I delight in their companionship as much as anyone. I am quite fond of the domestic animals who share my life (currently cats, turkeys, chickens, Guinea fowl, and honeybees). I am equally fond of the bobcats, the coyotes, and the hawks who have been having a heyday with the poultry in the past year. And I do not think I could stand by and watch the immense suffering that would ensue if we stopped our animal care altogether. As I said, I don't know the full answer. I just know the answer lies in a direction we currently are not pursuing, and perhaps in one we cannot even visualize just now. Still, it is a change I suspect we must make ultimately, or it will be made for us.

Conclusion

Some of you may have difficulty with this chapter, as it is as much about contemplating our relationships with animals as it is about guidelines. These are complex issues, and I realize I may seem near the fringe in the viewpoints that I express here. I have pondered these ideas for years, though, and to me we are far off course in some of the ways we relate to animals. I suspect that in choosing domesticated nature and domestic animals, we began to lose touch with a part of our selves. This has led us to depend more and more upon our domestic animals in ways that serve neither them nor us. If we do not reevaluate these relationships, to wild and domestic animals, to wild and domestic nature, we stand to lose greatly.

I recently visited several dear friends on a trip. In one household, two dogs live in the backyard, alone but for each other. They receive plenty of food but almost no attention. They strain at the fence, attempting to reach people. Theirs is a life of physical comfort but emotional starvation.

In the next household live several cats and dogs. These animals receive plenty of food and plenty of attention. Their human guardians, however, rarely clean house. Consequently the animals are flea-ridden and spend their days scratching.

I also recall visiting a friend in New York City years ago. She lives in an apartment building, as do most New Yorkers. As I walked down the hall toward her apartment, I heard a plaintive meow from a lonely-sounding kitten in a neighboring apartment. The kitten was no more than three or four months old, judging by the tenor of its meow. I arrived well into the evening; obviously the kitten's guardian was out. I imagined this young kitten all alone, all day and into the evening.

These are good, loving people whose lives do not include sufficient care for the animals whom they have chosen to bring into their homes. They mean well but do not see how the animals suffer at their hands. And this repeats millions of times in all corners of the planet. How many times do we take home a puppy or kitten only to lose interest as he grows up, as our own lives get busy or out of control? How many young couples adopt animals only to relegate those animals to the outdoors when children come into the family? What happens then?

These scenarios reminded me why I have added this chapter. They all speak to me of the disconnect, of how unaware we remain regarding companion animals' emotional and physical needs, which also represents our ignorance of the wild ones out of our control. I see it as imperative that we reconsider how and why we keep animals in our homes, and how we value (or not) wilderness and wild animals. I hope this chapter stimulates thinking and discussion, for without this, we will never verge from our present course.

There are no easy answers, and in these as well as in all decisions, we must all choose our own paths. In some areas, like heroic medicine and allowing companion animals greater autonomy, I feel strongly that I'm on the right track. We've taken these things somewhat for granted, and I believe it is imperative that we reconsider them. The same holds true in analyzing our needs versus our companions' needs when it comes to choosing for these friends who do not speak, at least not with words, and who thus find themselves with no voice in their destinies.

What you do with these thoughts is naturally up to you. I've often taken ideas to their limits, at least as far as I dare, given where society currently resides in its thinking. No longer spaying and neutering, no longer feeding, no longer controlling animals at all—perhaps in some ways ultimately the best solution, allowing a natural balance—is currently unfeasible for many reasons. But this does not mean it is unthinkable. Pondering this, even though neither you nor I are ready to take such a drastic step, still informs us. It informs me, for certain. Not that it results in definite answers, but it helps see what other choices may be becoming untenable as well.

Some will argue that the ideas expressed in this chapter suggest that I am unfeeling and uncaring, and that should you choose, for example, to forego some procedure that might save your animal friend's life, you may also be called uncaring. And nothing could be further from the truth. I care deeply for the animals who share my life, as I'm sure you do, or you would not be reading this. And choosing not to pursue treatment that, while it may be life saving, may also not be in our companion's best interest—well, this can be the most caring act of all.

And for myself, as much as I cherish "my" domestic animals, I cherish all those not in my control just as much. So if my choice to save one cat comes at the expense of a couple of bobcats, hawks, or even snakes, I think the balance has tipped, and I'm not sure that is acceptable. Even though the one cat may be "mine" in common parlance, I'm not sure it makes him more valuable than a snake or a hawk. Just imagine for a moment what it takes to feed a cat or dog for a year. How many domestic animals must die for her food? How many wild animals are displaced so we can raise those animals? Multiply this by the millions of cats and dogs we keep in the United States alone. What have we gained by this, and what have we lost as the natural world fades into oblivion? These are the sorts of conundrums I think we face as we push all of nature to the brink of extinction. How much more can she give before she collapses altogether, and us with her? She'll come back eventually; of this there's no doubt. But how this may look, we don't know. I have no idea what the world would become once it regained balance (should the collapse happen), but it would likely look much different than now. And it may not include humans. So, carefully considering our choices with companion animals may be, in the long run, in our species' best interest along with all the other species' best interests. I do not think we can afford to avoid these questions any longer.

What can you do? For starters, work toward stripping away your preconceptions and begin to see your animals more clearly. Our cultural bias colors our perceptions, and we degrade animals in our minds. Seeing them in a new light may bring the concern they deserve, may dramatically improve their lives.

Further, consider minimizing your dependence upon domestic animals for your emotional sustenance. As a culture, we spend too much time hiding in our apartments and homes, isolating ourselves behind fences and walls, including those between countries. The Dalai Lama said of our modern culture, "We can put a man on the moon, but we can't cross the street to meet our neighbors." And thus we are so lonely, so alone, so separate from others. We operate so much out of fear that we only trust those we can control: "our" cats and dogs, our horses and goldfish. This fear has devastated our world. It causes countries to make war upon other peoples; it causes us to drive by a stranded motorist or walk by a homeless person on a bitterly cold day. It drains the warmth from our hearts. We then try to renew that warmth by overdependence upon those whom we trust, whom we control.

In this I suspect we have gone past a balance point. As I watch clients and friends struggle so greatly over animal loss, as I see humans so estranged from other humans, often choosing animal relationships instead, I wonder about our choices. I have chosen animal over human relationships myself many times. I understand this. Yet it is a little too easy to make this choice, as these relationships are imbalanced. They are all in our favor. We call the shots. As much as we love our domestic animals, as much as we do for them, as much even as we sacrifice for them, we still control them. And that is a problem. We cannot derive enough nurturance from subservient beings, whether human or nonhuman. It's like eating potato chips; there simply is not enough nutrition there.

All they give is then not given freely because of this imbalance. In a sense, even their love is in their job descriptions. They really have no choice. It is their part of the bargain, for which they receive food and shelter. In choosing domestication, animals chose a subservient lifestyle in exchange for a certain security.

A few decades ago, just north of Fairbanks, Alaska, wolves went on a rampage and killed over forty dogs one winter, one by one. Residents heard nothing, but in the morning all they would find would be a collar, if anything. Biologists speculated that a hard winter had driven the wolves to kill dogs for food. Local Athabascan Indians, however, said that wolves simply hated dogs, and that was all it was about.[9] This rang true for me on one level. I wonder: do the wolves hate dogs because dogs have given up their freedoms? Many dogs that were killed had been tied up in back yards. Perhaps, even, the wolves had freed these dogs. I could see it that way.

Did these wolves understand what dogs, cats, and humans have lost? In choosing security at the expense of freedom, have we lost some part of our selves? Do we therefore have holes we cannot fill until we fill them ourselves? Are we attempting to fill them by relating to animals or other humans in unhealthy ways? Perhaps we have become desperate for love such that we seek anything that seems close. Yet, like with those potato chips, we cannot fill our need in the ways we have been choosing. We have a deep unrest that leads us to make choices that endanger our survival. Something must change.

I do not suggest it means we abandon keeping animals as companions. I merely suggest we rethink what this means, and that we bring that practice back into balance. About fifteen years ago, after another failed attempt at a human relationship, I stepped back and reevaluated my approach to relationships. I realized I had placed way too much burden on my partners. I saw that I came to a relationship from a desperate need, from a fear of being alone. I do not mean I could not be alone in the moment, as I actually enjoy solitude immensely. But I was afraid to grow old alone. I then realized that I needed to live alone and learn to nurture myself and to not expect another person or animal to fill this need. I realized that, until I could come to a relationship out of desire rather than out of need, that need would doom every relationship. I had to reach a point that I was no longer afraid of living the rest of my life alone. Since attaining this goal, I now have a successful relationship. Without the desperateness, I make better choices.

This is what I mean regarding animals and putting those relationships back into balance. Separating our needs from those relationships will almost automatically bring them into a healthier pattern. Without a desperate need, we can bring real love, not a false love that only seeks to gain something. The Buddhists say we should not love one person (or animal) more than any other because then we become trapped by that love; we need that person too much. It is a subtle concept in that of course we love our own families a bit more than others. At bottom, what they mean is that we must never let that love become a means to gaining something we should give ourselves. They also mean that we should never let that love become a need that we will sacrifice ourselves to fill. Love, in its pure sense, has no demands upon others. This is the sort of relationship to animals and to the world that can bring us back from the precipice.

And if we can, as a worldwide human culture, include wild animals and wild nature in our hearts and prayers, perhaps we may yet find a way to yield more space to that world. We may yet see that, just by being out there, just by its very existence, that world beyond human control serves as a balm, acts as a counterbalance to humanity. We might see that we feel better, that we are healthier and happier with more true wilderness—by this I mean areas totally devoid of humans—just out there living and breathing.

Finally, once we see that we gain from others by their very existence and not merely by what material gain they provide us, maybe we could even abandon our need to control or compete with others. We might begin to work together for our joint survival and our joint thriving. Perhaps we could even see that we also gain from other human cultures, by *their* very existence. If we find peace within ourselves, if we can even love ourselves, the rest is easy.

> *A way stands open into heaven,*
> *but none can enter the way*
> *except those who have heaven within them.*
>   —**Emanuel Swedenborg**

Part Four
HOMEOPATHIC REMEDIES

Chapter Eighteen
MATERIA MEDICA

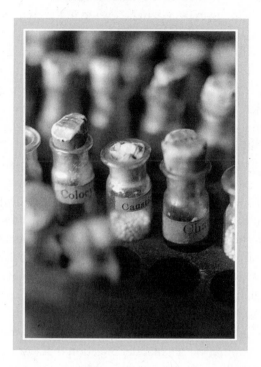

Description of Homeopathic Medicines

THIS SECTION CONTAINS A DESCRIPTION OF EACH of the medicines I have listed in the book. Since the detailed information about a remedy's effect upon a given organ or system is covered in the chapter pertaining to that organ or system, I will not generally repeat this information here.

As you know by now (if you have read the first five chapters on homeopathic principles), each homeopathic remedy is known to cause and cure a complex of physical and psychological symptoms. This pattern of symptoms, also called a remedy's picture, includes not only the remedy's local affinity and effects (from provings), but also an impact upon the entire body. This bodily impact includes mental and behavioral changes (psychological symptoms, also called the "mentals"), physical changes that affect more than one part of the body (generalities), and sensitivity to factors that may improve or worsen the animal's condition (modalities).

It is in the mentals, generals, and modalities that we often find the clues that assist us in choosing the remedy that best fits our patient's illness. These symptoms tend to be more unique to the sick individual, whereas local physical symptoms are often common to many individuals. For example, in a dog with diarrhea, the diarrheic bowel movements are often unremarkable, but the diarrhea may occur each time the dog hears thunder; the latter is unusual and is more likely to lead us to the best homeopathic remedy. Similarly, your cat may have a bladder infection that causes her to urinate several times a day. This is common to cats with bladder infections. Perhaps, however, she has also become extremely timid and hides constantly, especially from strangers, and this behavior started about when the bladder problem began. This is not common, and this is a clue that is probably essential to choosing the best homeopathic medicine.

In my description of the remedies for this section, the modalities, generalities, and mental (behavioral) symptoms constitute the majority of the information. I also refer to each section in the book where there is a description of a remedy's local indications. In some cases, I give more information about local patterns if these are not covered elsewhere.

Use the information in the *materia medica* to confirm your choice of remedy once you have read the information in the chapter that addresses your companion's main symptoms. You should have just a few remedies to consider after you have read the information about the specific illness, and hopefully the information in the *materia medica* will help you choose one remedy from the list of possibilities.

Remember that mental and behavioral symptoms are extremely important, but if these did not change at about the time of onset of the primary complaint, they may not be valuable and could be misleading. This is a tricky area. Essentially, if your companion's behavior is not too abnormal and has not changed as she became ill, place less emphasis upon the behavior. On the other hand, if the behavior is odd or strong, and if it changed or intensified along with the current problem, then it is probably an important component of the illness. The third possibility provides a confusing factor, but still needs to be considered. Sometimes the remedy that fits your companion's overall behavior—the way she has always acted—is a constitutional remedy for acute illnesses and will work most of the time when she is ill. In this case, her acute symptoms will generally (but not always) match those of the constitutional remedy. If you think she is a *Pulsatilla*, for example (i.e. her behavior and general state match those of *Pulsatilla*), and you do not see a remedy that clearly fits her acute symptoms, try a dose of *Pulsatilla*.

Finally, if you still cannot decide upon a remedy, consult with a more experienced friend, or read other books on *materia medica*. You will find suggestions for other books in the index. There are many entire books devoted exclusively to remedy description (even some ten-volume or twelve-volume sets of books), thus there is much more information than I can possibly cover, though the information here should suffice the majority of the time.

Descriptions of Homeopathic Medicines

Note: In the "Clinical Use" part at the end of each remedy, I list each section in the treatment chapters where the remedy is listed. The section is indicated with quotation marks, and the chapter is in italics. For example, under *Acetic acid*, "Bites of Dogs and Cats" and "Surgery" are sections within the chapter *Therapeutic Indications by Condition*.

Note regarding plant remedies: Many plant remedies are available as their herbal form as well as their homeopathic form. For example, the homeopathic remedy *Hydrastis* is known as goldenseal when in herbal form. You can often use the herbal tincture as a homeopathic remedy if you do not have the homeopathic form. This may especially hold true in acute circumstances. Either give one to three drops directly in the mouth, after succussing (shaking) the bottle, or dilute as with a liquid homeopathic remedy. In this latter case, use the herbal tincture as if it were a liquid remedy, and dilute into water for dosing. See the instructions in the section "Dosage: How to Handle and Administer Remedies" in Chapter Five, "Using Homeopathy at Home."

Acetic acid (Acetic acid)

The indications for most of the remedies made from acids include some form of weakness, and *Acetic acid* is no exception. Animals needing this remedy are usually profoundly weak. They often slip into this state following an injury or following anesthesia. There may be hemorrhage from various body orifices. These animals may be extremely thirsty if they have the strength to drink.

Clinical Use: See "Bites of Cats and Dogs" and "Surgery" in *Therapeutic Indications by Condition*.

Aconitum napellus (Aconite) (Monkshood)

The primary state we associate with *Aconite* is fear. These animals tend to be very fearful, even terror-stricken, in almost all situations. It is especially useful for traumatic conditions like accidents, earthquakes, and fires. Animals needing *Aconite* may pace frantically, and they often look very anxious. This fear may have come from a traumatic incident, or it may have come about seemingly on its own.

Suddenness is another element that is common to *Aconite* conditions. This remedy is useful for early stages of acute illness such as fever and colds, and these usually appear suddenly. They often follow a traumatic incident, though they may also appear following exposure to a cold dry wind. These animals are usually chilly.

Physical symptoms that indicate this remedy tend to be sudden and intense. There may be intense pain and redness, for example, or a high fever. Often the symptoms are sparse, but the few that do appear are pronounced.

The fear and the intensity of physical symptoms create a condition whereby the patient is commonly very sensitive to external stimuli such as noise, light, and touch.

Clinical Use: See "Cough" in *Respiratory System, Nose, and Sinuses*; "Conjunctivitis" in *Eyes*; "Cystitis" in *Urinary System*; "Convulsions" in *Nervous System*; and "Fear," "Fever," and "Vaccine Reactions" in *Therapeutic Indications by Condition*.

Aletris farinosa (Stargrass)

The primary general symptom that indicates *Aletris* is weakness, often profound. These animals may appear confused, and they may seem especially heavy and sluggish. The heaviness is most pronounced in the rear legs, and the right leg will often be weaker than the left leg. The patient may also be constipated and may pass a lot of gas, and she may feel better after passing gas. This remedy has an affinity to the uterus.

Clinical Use: See "Discharge from the Vulva" in *Reproductive System*.

Allium cepa (Red onion)

If you have ever peeled and cut an onion, you have a general idea of the main indications for the remedy. These animals tend to become worse in warm rooms and toward evening, and they feel better in cool open air. Their symptoms may arise in cold, damp weather. The symptoms tend to be worse on the left side, or they may move from left to right. I primarily use this remedy for colds in the early stages.

Ravenous hunger with belching and colicky diarrhea with flatulence may accompany the upper respiratory symptoms. These animals may be very anxious and melancholic, especially in the morning.

Clinical use: See "Sneezing and Nasal Discharge" in *Respiratory System, Nose, and Sinuses* and "Conjunctivitis" in *Eyes*.

Aloe (Socotrine aloes)

This remedy is made from a member of the lily family. (It is not made from *Aloe vera*—the "burn plant.") The most common indications for the remedy are liver and intestinal disorders. These animals tend to have severe diarrhea, which is very irritating.

Many animals that need *Aloe* are irritable, and they dislike others, preferring solitude over company, though they may become more cheerful in the evening. They especially dislike contradiction, so any attempt at discipline may incite an aggressive response. *Aloe* patients often have a history of a sedentary lifestyle.

The physical symptoms tend to be worse in hot damp weather and in the early morning. These animals usually improve in cool air. Their symptoms often bring about exhaustion, though they may alternate between exhaustion and activity.

Clinical use: See "Diarrhea" in *Digestive System*.

Alumina (Aluminum oxide)

The most pronounced symptoms of this remedy are dryness and weakness. The coat often appears dry and flaky, the animal may produce small volumes of tears and saliva, and the stools are generally dry. The weakness appears in the form of constipation without much urging to stool; these animals also commonly have weakness and heaviness in their rear legs. They may stagger about as a result. These patients tend to be thin and undernourished. They often crave indigestible items such as dirt, ashes, and chalk, and they often prefer dry food despite their internal dryness.

The mind is weak as well, so these animals often appear dull-witted and confused. They may take a long time in executing their daily tasks. They generally feel better in open air and worse in warm rooms, and their symptoms tend to cycle up and down, sometimes on alternate days.

Clinical use: See "Constipation" in *Digestive System*, "Degenerative Myelopathy" in *Nervous System*, and "Discharge from the Vulva" in *Reproductive System*.

Antimonium tartaricum (Tartar emetic; Tartrate of antimony and potash)

The main sphere of this remedy's action is upon the mucous membranes, especially those in the lungs. These animals produce a lot of mucus, which rattles in the lungs. They may also produce mucus in the mouth, and their stools often have mucus in them. Diarrhea and vomiting may accompany the respiratory symptoms, and there is often back pain as well.

These animals are generally quite despondent and apathetic, and they usually wish to be left alone. They tend to be worse in warm weather and warm rooms.

Clinical use: See "Cough" in *Respiratory System, Nose, and Sinuses* and "Vaccine Reactions" in *Therapeutic Indications by Condition*.

Apis mellifica (Honeybee venom)

Think of a response to a bee sting and you have a general idea of the indications for this remedy. The symptoms that are expressed tend toward redness and swelling, whether they occur on the skin, in the mammae, in the throat, or on the genitalia. There is also a tendency to shininess where the swollen areas are visible. Even if the pathological change is not directly visible, swelling is usually the mechanism. This occurs in the lungs and kidneys, for example.

The *Apis* individual may be fidgety and restless, and often does not want to be left alone. Some animals will be depressed or apathetic. Most animals that need this remedy are relatively thirstless, even when they are feverish. They are very intolerant of hot rooms and heat in general, and much prefer cool air. They may be very sensitive to touch, even to light brushing.

Clinical use: See "Itching," "Hotspots," Burns and Scalds," and "Insect Bites and Stings" in *Skin and Ears*, "Conjunctivitis" and "Corneal Ulcers" in *Eyes*, "Cystitis" and "Decreasing Kidney Function" in *Urinary System*, "Paraphimosis and Phimosis" and "Mastitis" in *Reproductive System*, and "Allergic Reactions" and "Vaccine Reactions" in *Therapeutic Indications by Condition*.

Apocynum cannabinum (Indian hemp)

Apocynum is good at reducing dropsy (fluid accumulation), especially in the chest, but also in the abdomen and even in the extremities as swelling. It is said to be similar to *Apis,* but chilly. Even the kidneys may be affected, as with *Apis*. These animals are often restless but debilitated. Urine output is decreased. They are confused and low-spirited. The restlessness tends to be worse at night. Because of chest dropsy, breathing is difficult and labored, and they must sit up, as lying down creates extreme breathing difficulty. The abdomen may be distended and painful. Watery diarrhea often accompanies other symptoms.

These animals desire and are better from warmth and worse from cold. They may feel better after a bowel movement. They may feel worse after sleep. They are often quite thirsty, and while they usually retain the water, they often feel worse after drinking.

Clinical Use: See "Lung Problems" in *Respiratory System, Nose, and Sinuses;* "Decreasing Kidney Function" in *Urinary System;* and "Heart Disease" in *Therapeutic Indications by Condition.*

Argentum nitricum (Silver nitrate)

This is the same chemical that has historically been placed into the eyes of newborn children to prevent eye infections, especially those due to syphilis. The homeopathic remedy also has a great affinity to eyes. Many of the other symptoms of this remedy are similar to syphilis as well: there may be erosions or ulcers on the genitalia, ulcers and inflammation in the mouth and throat, and severe nervous system impairment (incoordination and paralysis) similar to that seen in chronic syphilis.

These animals may be very fearful and may even be afraid to venture far from home. Situations that trigger their anxiety will worsen their symptoms. For example, these animals often develop diarrhea after a fright.

They prefer cool air and cannot tolerate much heat. Many animals that need this remedy crave sweets, though sugar often worsens their symptoms. They may have a predominance of symptoms on the left side.

Clinical use: See "Bloat" in *Digestive System,* "Conjunctivitis" and "Corneal Ulcers" in *Eyes,* and "Degenerative Myelopathy" in *Nervous System.*

Arnica montana (Leopard's bane)

Arnica is perhaps the best-known homeopathic medicine. Many people use this remedy for muscle aches, sprains, strains, and other injuries. It is useful in almost any injury, especially for blunt traumas that result in bruising, though it is also a good choice in puncture wounds to prevent the development of an abscess.

Animals that need *Arnica* are usually in great pain following an injury, and as a result they are extremely fearful of touch. This state is common shortly after trauma, but it may also exist long after the trauma, when the pain should have disappeared. This situation is a good indication for *Arnica.* Mental trauma and the resultant fear of the approach of others will also respond to this remedy.

Arnica patients tend to be restless, as they move from place to place in search of a more comfortable spot to lie. Their pain simply will not allow them to rest. Most conditions arise as a result of some sort of trauma; this includes overexertion as well as physical and emotional trauma.

See also *Bellis perennis.*

Clinical use: See "Insect Bites and Stings" in *Skin and Ears;* "Homeopathic Remedies for Dental Care and Extractions" in *Mouth, Gums, and Teeth;* "Nosebleed" in *Respiratory System, Nose, and Sinuses;* "Injuries to the Eyes" in *Eyes;* Arthritic Conditions," "First Aid for Broken Bones," and "Sprains and Strains" in *Musculoskeletal System;* "Injuries to the Brain and Spinal Cord" in *Nervous System;* "Paraphimosis and Phimosis," "Orchitis," "Injuries to the Testicles," "Labor," "Postpartum Pain," "Postpartum Infections," "Weak Kittens or Puppies," "Mastitis," and "Injuries to the Breast" in *Reproductive System;* and "Abscesses," "Bites of Cats and Dogs," "Cuts and Lacerations," "Hemorrhage," and "Surgery" in *Therapeutic Indications by Condition.*

Arsenicum album (Arsenic trioxide; the white oxide of arsenic)
Arsenicum is one of our best remedies, and it is especially useful for many acute conditions that you might face. The general symptoms of this remedy are rather specific and constant. They include chilliness, restlessness, weakness, and aggravation after midnight. These animals are almost always very thirsty as well, though they may be thirstless if they have severe chronic disease. Cold is usually intolerable, whereas heat generally improves most symptoms. Many symptoms appear on the right side when this remedy is needed, and discharges are usually acrid and burning.

Toxic conditions often respond to this remedy, whether the toxin is from a drug or vaccine, food poisoning, or a buildup of toxins in kidney or liver disease. Probably due to the toxicity, these animals often seem interested in food or water but do not actually eat or drink. They either walk away (usually with food) or they hang their head over the bowl (more common with water).

These patients are usually anxious and fearful (this drives the restlessness), and they seek order as a counter to their anxiety. They may clean themselves obsessively; this especially applies to cats. Solitude is unbearable (because of the anxiety), and many symptoms worsen when the *Arsenicum* patient is alone. Many animals needing *Arsenicum* are afraid of strangers, however. They may disappear as soon as company arrives, and they only reappear when it is certain that the strangers have left.

Clinical use: See "Itching" and "Burns and Scalds" in *Skin and Ears;* "Gingivitis and Mouth Inflammation" in *Mouth, Gums, and Teeth;* "Vomiting" and "Diarrhea" in *Digestive System;* "Sneezing and Nasal Discharge" and "Cough" in *Respiratory System, Nose, and Sinuses;* "Conjunctivitis" and "Corneal Ulcers" in *Eyes;* "Cystitis" and "Decreasing Kidney Function" in *Urinary System;* "Vestibular Syndrome" in *Nervous System;* and "Allergic Reactions," "Bites of Snakes," "Drug Reactions," "Euthanasia," "Fear," "Food and Garbage Poisoning," and "Vaccine Reactions" in *Therapeutic Indications by Condition.*

Arum triphyllum (Jack in the pulpit; Indian turnip)
This plant contains an irritating chemical; the homeopathic medicine is useful for conditions of mucous membrane inflammation. I have found good success in some cats with mouth inflammation. This is the only situation for which I have employed the remedy, but any inflammatory con-

dition may respond, whether it is the mouth, the nose, the genitalia, or the anus.

These animals may be cross and irritable, and they may lick or scratch at themselves until they bleed, more out of emotional distress than due to itching. They are usually chilly. Diarrhea may accompany other symptoms, and all discharges are irritating to the skin.

Clinical use: See "Gingivitis and Mouth Inflammation" in *Mouth, Gums, and Teeth.*

Asafoetida (Devil's dung)
This remedy has an impact upon calcium metabolism, as some of the main indications involve milk production and bone diseases. These animals may be irritable, "hysterically restless," and sensitive. They may have explosive belching and regurgitation as well as colicky, flatulent diarrhea that is forcibly ejected. Their symptoms are usually worse at night and at rest, and better with motion in open air.

Clinical use: See "Hypertrophic Osteodystrophy" and "Rickets" in *Musculoskeletal System* and "Inadequate Milk Flow" in *Reproductive System.*

Asarum europaeum (European snake root)
These patients are excessively sensitive to noise, and generally sensitive and nervous. They are especially sensitive to scratching on linen, paper, and similar fabrics with a fingernail. Penetrating sounds also disagree violently, like the ring of a spoon on a stainless steel bowl.

Clinical use: See "Injuries to the Eyes" in *Eyes.*

Astacus fluviatilis (Crawfish)
This remedy has great affinity to skin and mucous membranes. Itching, stinging pains (urticaria) are common with skin disease. The animal may be slightly delirious with the itching. The affected areas may be bright red and/or crusty, especially on the head. The cervical (neck) lymph nodes may be enlarged in conjunction with the skin eruptions. The mouth is often terribly inflamed as well, with ulcers. This often induces the lymph node swelling. The liver is often affected as well, and stools may be clay colored.

Cold air is intolerable and worsens these patients.

Clinical use: See "Itching" in *Skin and Ears* and "Gingivitis and Mouth Inflammation" in *Mouth, Gums, and Teeth.*

Aurum (Gold)

This remedy is a deep-acting polychrest. The only indication I give for acute (home) use is for cryptorchidism (retained testicle). Since this is usually treated in young animals, you may not see the many other *Aurum* signs. The typical state in an adult is one of depression, despondency, and intolerance of contradiction. The animal may moan during sleep. There may be evidence of poor bone formation or bone disease, and there may be a heart condition. They may experience pain in bright light and they may have inflammation of the eyes; they may walk with a heavy-footed step as well (*Aurum* is gold, a heavy metal).

   Clinical use: See "Retained Testicle" in *Reproductive System*.

Baptisia (Wild indigo)

When *Baptisia* is indicated, the animal is generally very ill with fevers and inflammations. Deterioration is often rapid. The patient usually has very sore muscles along with the inflammation, and discharges from any orifice are putrid. It is a good remedy for putrid, bloody, exhausting diarrhea. The gums are often brown or muddy-looking. This reflects poor circulation and septic conditions. The animal may appear intoxicated due to the intensity of the condition. These patients probably need veterinary care, but give the remedy as well to speed their recovery.

   Clinical use: See "Diarrhea" in *Digestive System* and "Orchitis" in *Reproductive System*.

Baryta carbonica (Barium carbonate)

Individuals needing this remedy are usually dull, sluggish, and timid. They border on mental retardation. If strangers come to the house, these animals will usually disappear. This remedy is very powerful, and generally used as a constitutional remedy. The only indications for acute use are for puppies and kittens that are not developing properly.

   Clinical use: See "Weak Kittens and Puppies" and "Runts, Dwarfishness" in *Reproductive System*.

BCG

(See *Vaccin atténué bilié*)

Belladonna (Deadly nightshade)

This remedy is very useful for many acute conditions. When *Belladonna* is needed, the condition is usually hot, intense, and comes on very rapidly. These animals will be restless, and they may be delirious and even aggressive. The intensity of the behavior is often due to the intense, throbbing pains that these poor animals have. They usually have dilated pupils, at least when the fever or inflammation is intense. The gums will be bright red and hot.

Belladonna individuals have a propensity to right-sided symptoms. Their symptoms often worsen after three in the afternoon and again after midnight. They cannot tolerate the heat of the sun, nor do they like cold drafts. They are often very thirsty.

Clinical use: See "Hotspots" and "Aural Hematomas" in *Skin and Ears*; "Cough" in *Respiratory System, Nose, and Sinuses*; "Conjunctivitis" in *Eyes*; "Arthritic Conditions" in *Musculoskeletal System*; "Convulsions" and "Aggression" in *Nervous System*; "Orchitis," "Eclampsia," and "Mastitis" in *Reproductive System*; and "Bites of Snakes," "Fever," "Overheating," and "Vaccine Reactions" in *Therapeutic Indications by Condition*.

Bellis perennis (Daisy)

This remedy is botanically related to *Arnica*, and its use is very similar. We primarily use *Bellis* for posttraumatic conditions. It is especially useful for bruising and pain in internal organs. When an animal has been hit by a car, for example, consider giving *Arnica* first and later giving *Bellis*. This remedy is also very useful after surgery and after childbirth. These animals, like those needing *Arnica*, do not wish to be touched because of the pain. Motion may relieve the pains when *Bellis* is indicated.

Bellis is, in a sense, the *Arnica* for deeper, interior trauma. Whereas *Arnica* works better on trauma to the exterior, like muscle bruising, sprains, and strains, *Bellis* finds an affinity to the interior surfaces of the body, like the peritoneal (abdominal) cavity, breast tissue, and scrotal/testicular tissues. Similarly, *Bellis* is a good remedy for whiplash (formerly called "railway spine"), a more internal bone injury than the *Arnica* sprained ankle, for example. There is overlap, however, so do not exclude either remedy solely upon this distinction.

Clinical use: See "Homeopathic Remedies for Dental Care and Extractions" in *Mouth, Gums, and Teeth*; "Sprains and Strains" in *Musculoskeletal System*;

"Paraphimosis and Phimosis," "Injuries to the Testicles," "Postpartum Pain," "Mastitis," and "Injury to the Breast" in *Reproductive System;* and "Surgery" in *Therapeutic Indications by Condition.*

Berberis vulgaris (Barberry)

Berberis has specific affinity to the kidney and liver, and it can help detox these organs. These animals are listless, apathetic, and indifferent. They tend to have pains in the back associated with the kidney and liver congestion. Standing and exercise worsen the pains. Symptoms tend to change or alternate, such as thirst alternating with thirstlessness, or hunger alternating with appetite loss. There may be constant urging to stool and painless, clay-colored diarrhea. The rectum and anus, however, may also burn, so you may see the patient lick the anus, especially following stools. The same holds true with the urethra, so they may lick following urination as well.

I usually use Berberis as a tincture, giving one to ten drops, three times daily, though a 3X to a 6C may also help. Oregon grape root *(Berberis aquifolium)* is in the same plant family and may work if you cannot find Barberry.

Clinical use: See "Cystitis" and "Decreasing Kidney Function" in *Urinary System* and "Liver Disorders" in *Therapeutic Indications by Condition.*

Bioplasma

This is a combination of the twelve tissue salts (cell salts), and can be used as a general tonic for any animal in a weakened or debilitated condition. Give one to four tablets, two or three times daily.

Clinical use: See "Decreasing Kidney Function" in *Urinary System.*

Bismuth (Bismuth subnitricum)

The indications for *Bismuth* are primarily for digestive system complaints. In these symptoms it is similar to *Arsenicum* and *Phosphorus* (these three elements are chemically very similar), though the vomiting of *Bismuth* is more intense. The stomach is usually painful, so the animal may cry out, especially right before he vomits. Behaviorally, these animals tend to be very clingy, as they hate to be alone. This is also similar to *Arsenicum* and *Phosphorus* but more intense. Eating and solitude may worsen the symptoms when this remedy is needed.

Clinical use: See "Vomiting" in *Digestive System.*

Borax (Sodium biborate)

This remedy has an affinity to all mucous membranes, causing inflammation and ulceration. These symptoms may occur in the eyes, in the mouth, on the genitals, or in the urethra. These areas of erosion tend to be quite painful. Behaviorally, the most striking element is a fear of downward motion. Thus, these animals may panic when you place them on the floor after holding them, or they may resist going down stairs. Sudden noises are also frightening, and these individuals may be very fearful of a gunshot, even at great distance. Sometimes soft noises are more frightening to these animals than loud ones. *Boron metallicum* may be useful if *Borax* seems indicated but does not work. *Boron,* however, is much less common and harder to find.

Clinical use: See "Gingivitis and Mouth Inflammation" in *Mouth, Gums, and Teeth;* "Entropion" in *Eyes;* "Bad Milk" in *Reproductive System;* and "Fear of Noise" in *Therapeutic Indications by Condition.*

Bryonia alba (Wild hop)

Bryonia is best known for musculoskeletal conditions that are greatly aggravated by motion. Even slight movement is often intolerable. This aggravation from motion carries over to other *Bryonia* symptoms as well. For example, these animals may suffer from constipation, a reflection of the pain of motion and exertion. These animals may be incredibly thirsty. Heat and hot weather are intolerable, and cool open air makes the *Bryonia* patient feel better. If they have painful limbs, a peculiar symptom is that pressure on the painful leg will alleviate the pain. Thus they may lie on the affected side.

Clinical use: See "Constipation" in *Digestive System;* "Cough" in *Respiratory System, Nose, and Sinuses;* "Incontinence" in *Urinary System;* "Arthritic Conditions" in *Musculoskeletal System;* and "Mastitis" in *Reproductive System.*

Caladium seguinum (American arum; Dieffenbachia seguine)

This remedy is very minor. It is useful for insect bites that burn and sting. It also has a reputation (along with *Plantago*) for inducing nausea when someone smokes tobacco, thus it has been suggested as a deterrent to smoking.

Clinical use: See "Fly Strike" in *Skin and Ears* and "Fleas" in *Therapeutic Indications by Condition.*

Calcarea carbonica (Calcium carbonate)

This remedy is made from an oyster shell, and it is one of the polychrest remedies. We generally refer to it as *Calcarea* or *Calc carb*. Individuals needing this remedy are generally overweight, big-boned, and pale, and they move sluggishly and sometimes awkwardly. It is especially useful for very young animals and for animals in middle to old age.

Poor nutrition is often a factor in these patients. They may have had poor-quality foods, or they may be unable to extract the nutrients from food because of their illness. They may especially suffer with problems of calcium metabolism, thus they may have difficulty healing wounds and fractures. Despite the supposed benefit of milk as a calcium supplement, these animals are generally averse to milk, and if they do drink milk, it usually causes problems for them. *Calcarea* individuals often have a sour smell, possibly due to their defective metabolism. These animals may crave dirt and other similar substances in an attempt to aid their nutrition.

Exertion is difficult for these animals. They prefer to lie quietly and observe life. This may also be a fear reaction, as these individuals commonly experience fear. The fears are not necessarily specific, but they are somewhat fearful of anything new or of changes in their routine. A change of residence can devastate a *Calcarea* individual. Even going on walks can be a struggle, so these animals may prefer to stay close to home. In cold weather they often prefer to stay indoors, as much because they are chilly as because of their fears. Though they can sometimes be difficult because of their fear, they are generally friendly, loyal animals.

Many symptoms of *Calcarea* patients center around problems with healing. They also develop poorly, so there are many instances of malformation of bones and body structures. There are several other *Calcarea* family remedies, three of which are in this book. All of these remedies have the element of poor nutrition, poor development, and poor healing.

Clinical use: See "Ranula" and "Abscessed or Decaying Teeth" in *Mouth, Gums, and Teeth*; "Constipation" in *Digestive System*; "Entropion" in *Eyes*, "Arthritic Conditions" and "Rickets" in *Musculoskeletal System*; "Retained Testicle," "Discharge from the Vulva," "Eclampsia," "Weak Kittens or Puppies," "Inadequate Milk Flow," and "Bad Milk" in *Reproductive System*; and "Fear" in *Therapeutic Indications by Condition*.

Calcarea fluorica (Calcium fluoride)

Calc fluor is even more extreme than *Calc carb* in the sphere of poor nutrition and poor bone structure. These animals are often asymmetric in their body form. Their bones and teeth are generally very weak and brittle, and they decay rapidly. These are very unhealthy animals—thin and malnourished, with poor coats, very pale skin, and bad teeth. This remedy state is not nearly so common as that of *Calc carb* and *Calc phos.*

Clinical use: See "Abscessed or Decaying Teeth" in *Mouth, Gums, and Teeth* and "Rickets" in *Musculoskeletal System.*

Calcarea phosphorica (Calcium phosphate)

This remedy is similar to *Calc carb,* but *Calc phos* individuals tend to be thin and undernourished rather than obese and undernourished. These are scrawny animals, though not quite as poor as those needing *Calc fluor.* Their body form is symmetrical, but they are thin and weak.

Animals needing this remedy have poor digestion and often have stomach pains after every meal. They are very chilly, especially their extremities, which may even be cool to the touch. They may crave smoked or salty foods. *Calc phos* has a stimulant effect upon bone healing and calcium deposition, so it is useful for fractures and bone growth problems.

Clinical use: See "Arthritic Conditions," "First Aid for Broken Bones," and "Rickets" in *Musculoskeletal System* and "Retained Testicle," "Pregnancy Maintenance," "Eclampsia," "Weak Kittens or Puppies," and "Inadequate Milk Flow" in *Reproductive System.*

Calcarea sulphurica (Calcium sulfate; Plaster of Paris; Gypsum)

Most animals that need this remedy have thick yellow discharges of mucus and/or pus from some body outlet. These individuals especially have the *Calcarea* family's poor healing ability, so they have infections that they just cannot shake. This remedy is especially useful for colds, nasal discharge, and eye inflammation. Recurrent abscesses may also respond to *Calc sulph.* These animals may be irritable or anxious in the evening.

Clinical use: See "Sneezing and Nasal Discharge" in *Respiratory System, Nose, and Sinuses;* "Conjunctivitis" and "Injuries to the Eyes" in *Eyes;* and "Abscesses" in *Therapeutic Indications by Condition.*

Calendula officinalis (Marigold)

Calendula is somewhat well known as a topical herb for cuts, abrasions, infections, and inflammatory conditions. It is available as a tincture, as a nonalcohol-based liquid, as a gel, as an ointment, and as a cream. All forms can be effective. The tincture should be diluted in water before use. *Calendula* is very good as an antiseptic, and it promotes healing of wounds. In some cases of deep wounds, it causes the skin to close too quickly, causing a pocket that cannot drain. This may become an abscess, or it may simply need to rupture in order to drain and heal. For deeper wounds, I recommend using *Hypericum* (St. John's wort) instead of *Calendula*. For either one, use ten to thirty drops of the tincture and one-fourth teaspoon of salt to one cup of water. This solution may be applied topically or used to rinse any wounds.

Although it is most commonly employed topically, the potentized form is very beneficial as a homeopathic remedy as well. Many conditions respond nicely to homeopathic *Calendula*. It is excellent at relieving pain of wounds and lacerations, and stimulates healing at least as well when used orally as when applied topically. It is a specific for healing torn muscles.

Clinical use: See "Homeopathic Remedies for Dental Care and Extractions" in *Mouth, Gums, and Teeth;* "Injuries to the Eyes" in *Eyes;* "Torn Muscles" in *Musculoskeletal System;* and "Abscesses," "Cuts and Lacerations," and "Surgery" in *Therapeutic Indications by Condition.*

Cantharis (Spanish fly)

This insect contains a chemical that irritates skin and mucous membranes. Even the urinary bladder and the urethra are affected, causing inflammation that resembles cystitis and inducing frequent attempts to urinate. The irritation in the region of the genitals may incite sexual behavior, and the Spanish fly has some aphrodisiac properties.

Homeopathically, this remedy can treat these conditions. Many of this remedy's indications center around the skin and mucous membrane irritation. The burning and inflammation is intense and often arises suddenly. It may be accompanied with blisters in the mouth or in the vagina. Burns, mouth irritation, frequent urging to urinate, and hypersexual behavior all fall within the realm of *Cantharis's* action.

Behaviorally, these animals are sometimes very irritable as well. The irritative impact upon body tissues apparently extends to the brain, causing emotional distress. In the provings, many people reported that there was a burning sensation in the brain. As a consequence, the animal needing *Cantharis* is generally violently restless. The resulting mania often has a sexual component.

Clinical use: See "Insect Bites and Stings" and "Burns and Scalds" in *Skin and Ears* and "Cystitis" in *Urinary System*.

Carbo vegetabilis (Vegetable charcoal)

This remedy is made from ashes (charcoal, or carbon) from burnt vegetable matter. You might think of this as a state after the fire has burned out all of the energy. These animals are usually sluggish and cold, sometimes over-weight, and exhausted. The head may be warm, and they may desire air or even to sit in a draft (as though wanting to fan the flames to find the last bit of fire). Collapse is common, and they may have blue gums because of poor circulation and their internal coldness. The mouth and tongue may feel cold to the touch. Flatulence is common because their digestion is poor; they don't even have the energy to digest foods. *Carbo veg* may be useful anytime an animal is weak, cold, and blue, whether from illness or trauma.

Clinical use: See "Bloat" in *Digestive System* and "Weak Kittens or Puppies" in *Reproductive System*.

Carbolic acid (Carbolic acid; Phenol)

Carbolic acid (the chemical) is an anesthetic as well as an antiseptic. The remedy is useful for severe infections that result from wounds. It is similar in some ways to *Carbo veg* in that it is useful for animals that are cold and extremely weak. Remember that weakness is common to all remedies made from acids. The breath is putrid, and there may be intense inflammation of the mouth. The indications for acute use are posttrauma.

Clinical use: See "Insect Bites and Stings" in *Skin and Ears* and "Cuts and Lacerations" in *Therapeutic Indications by Condition*.

Carduus marianus (Milk thistle; St. Mary's thistle)

This herb is a powerful liver stimulant and cleanser. I have used the home-opathic remedy in low potency occasionally as a liver tonic when the animal could not handle the herbal form. Homeopathic indications include despon-dency, vomiting bile, and constipation with hard knotty stools.

Clinical use: See "Liver Disorders" in *Therapeutic Indications by Condition*.

Caulophyllum (Blue cohosh; Squaw root)
Any midwife knows this herb for its actions in tonifying the uterus. Blue cohosh can induce or speed labor when it is not progressing normally, as can the homeopathic remedy. There may be exhaustion and nervousness when *Caulophyllum* is needed. I use the remedy almost exclusively for uterine complaints—usually pregnancy and postpartum conditions.

Clinical use: See "Discharge from the Vulva," "Pregnancy," "Labor," and "Postpartum Conditions" in *Reproductive System*.

Causticum (Hahnemann's tinctura acris sine kali; Potassium hydrate; obtained by distilling slaked lime with potassium sulfate)
This remedy is indicated for weak, broken-down animals; it is often indicated in older animals. Weakness, chilliness, and paralysis often call for this remedy. It is a very deep remedy and should be used mainly under the supervision of an experienced homeopath, except for the two indications I have listed in the book. Don't give this remedy before or after *Phosphorus*, as there could be a bad reaction in rare cases.

Clinical use: See "Burns and Scalds" in *Skin and Ears* and "Incontinence" in *Urinary System*.

Cedron (Simaba cedron)
This remedy has a reputation for antidoting snake bites and insect stings when the tincture of the bean is applied topically. The affected animal may have pains in the temples and behind the eyes. It may be more useful in tropical climates.

Clinical use: See "Bites of Snakes" in *Therapeutic Indications by Condition*.

Chamomilla (Chamomile)
This remedy is sometimes administered in low potency as a calming agent; the tea is also useful for this. The animal that needs the homeopathic remedy is usually young, often during teething (three to six months old for cats and dogs). The behavior that indicates *Chamomilla* is irritability and restlessness in an animal that seems to want consolation but then resists petting. Only carrying the animal will calm her, and she must be carried constantly; the whining and restlessness reappear as soon as she is put down.

Clinical use: See "Diarrhea" in *Digestive System* and "Bad Milk" in *Reproductive System*.

Chelidonium majus (Greater celandine)

Chelidonium is a remedy that is very organ-specific. It has a great affinity to the liver and bile duct. It is occasionally very helpful in liver inflammations, though it should not be chosen over the constitutional remedy if the latter is known. *Chelidonium* may help an animal through a crisis, however. The homeopathic indications include lethargy and despondency with a heaviness to both the mental state and the physical movement. The animal may also be quarrelsome. He generally prefers hot food and drinks. The stools may be clay-colored if there is a bile duct obstruction. He may be so severe that he is jaundiced; you may see that his gums, eyes, or even his skin are yellow. The skin discoloration is often easiest to see in the ears. These animals need veterinary care, but *Chelidonium* may be helpful in addition.

Clinical use: See "Liver Disorders" in *Therapeutic Indications by Condition.*

Chimaphila umbellata (Pipsissewa; Ground holly; Wintergreen)

This remedy has an affinity to the urogenital systems. These animals must strain to urinate, especially before the urine begins to flow. A *Chimaphila* condition often arises from cold damp weather or from sitting on cold stones. Animals needing this remedy are likely to be thin and poorly nourished or worn out. The main indication is for prostate problems.

Clinical use: See "Prostate Affections" in *Reproductive System.*

China officinalis (Cinchona officinalis) (Peruvian bark)

We commonly call this remedy *China.* It is pronounced "keena" because it comes from the bark of a Peruvian tree, and *kina* means bark; the Peruvian Indians called this *kina-kina* or bark of barks because of its medicinal qualities. This is the substance from which we isolated quinine, the well-known malaria drug. *China* is the substance that Hahnemann first proved and found that its symptoms simulated those of intermittent fever (malaria). Thus we owe a great deal to this remedy for so clearly indicating its action to Hahnemann and starting him on his path to discovery.

One of the main general symptoms of this remedy is debility over time from disease, and especially from loss of fluids. This fluid loss may occur through diarrhea, vomiting, suppuration, hemorrhage, or excessive urination. As with malaria, the *China* state has a tendency to periodicity, or alternating up-and-down periods. Thus these animals will have good days alternating with bad days, but as the condition continues the strength diminishes.

Many symptoms are worse at night, from cold air and drafts, and from exertion. Warmth and lying quietly can improve the condition. An odd modality is that light touch aggravates, while hard pressure ameliorates most symptoms.

These animals are often very ill and may become morose and apathetic. The despondency may alternate with cheerfulness as the physical symptoms cycle up and down. Many organ systems are affected: liver, kidneys, intestines, lungs, and so on.

Clinical use: See "Diarrhea" in *Digestive System*, "Decreasing Kidney Function" in *Urinary System*, and "Drug Reactions" in *Therapeutic Indications by Condition*.

Chininum arsenicosum, Chininum muriaticum, Chininum phosphoricum, Chininum sulphuricum (Quinine arsenite, Quinine muriate, Quinine phosphate, Quinine sulfate)

I have grouped these remedies together because I have found them to be very similar in their indications and usage. I often use these remedies in cats with chronic kidney failure, as the *China* element has the characteristic of weakness from loss of fluid. When an animal in kidney failure (with excessive urination) becomes weak, one of these remedies is often helpful. They are all compounds of quinine. Read the description of *China* above and the descriptions of *Arsenicum album, Natrum muriaticum, Phosphorus,* and *Sulphur*. The combinations will give an approximate picture of these three *Chininum* remedies (e.g. *China* plus *Arsenicum* = *Chin ars*).

Clinical use: See "Decreasing Kidney Function" in *Urinary System*.

Cholesterinum (Cholesterol)

This remedy mostly shows an affinity to liver disorders, especially when there is a fatty degeneration. The liver is congested, there may be jaundice (icterus), and there may be opacities in the eye. Liver or gallbladder colic will often respond to this remedy. There may be profuse urination before the attack. Touch, jarring, sudden motion, and bending worsen the pain when *Cholesterinum* is indicated.

Clinical use: See "Liver Disorders" in *Therapeutic Indications by Condition*.

Cicuta virosa (Cowbane; Water hemlock)

The *Cicuta* state is one that often involves brain damage or severe brain malfunction. These animals have a tendency toward violent spasms, convulsions, jerking, and twitching. The head and spine may be bent backward. The pupils may be crossed, or more commonly they are divergent (the opposite of crossed). I list the remedy primarily for the unfortunate situation when your companion may have had a head injury. You should seek veterinary treatment, but this remedy may help greatly if the symptoms fit. If you can observe behavioral symptoms (i.e. if the injury is not so severe), the animal may want to completely avoid company, preferring to be alone.

Clinical use: See "Injury to the Brain and Spinal Cord" in *Nervous System* and "Eclampsia" in *Reproductive System*.

Cina (Wormseed)

In some ways this remedy state is similar to that of *Chamomilla*. The patient is usually young, irritable, and dissatisfied. But whereas carrying calms the animal that needs *Chamomilla*, the *Cina* animal is not calmed, though she may ask to be carried anyway.

These animals are often fat and scruffy (like a wormy puppy), and their complaints often accompany a worm infestation. This remedy is more for the effects of worms than for elimination of worms. The puppy (or less commonly, kitten) may twitch and jerk, and may even bite. These puppies are generally from one to six months old, when they are most affected by worms, and roundworms are most common in *Cina* pups.

Clinical use: See "Cough" in *Respiratory System, Nose, and Sinuses.*

Cinnabaris (Red sulfide of mercury)

This remedy is a mercury and sulfur compound. It has elements of *Mercurius* and *Sulphur* in its disease picture. There is the redness and thirst of *Sulphur* and the great inflammation of *Mercurius*, especially in the genitalia. These animals may have eye inflammation as part of their symptom picture. The symptoms are generally better in open air and worse with touch and in the evening. The patient is sometimes irritable, and he may be sad after eating; he also may start from sleep. The main indication for acute use is for penis and preputial inflammation.

Clinical use: See "Discharge from the Sheath" and "Paraphimosis and Phimosis" in *Reproductive System.*

Clemetis erecta (Upright virgin's bower)

These animals are generally very sleepy and confused. Their symptoms often worsen at night, especially in a warm bed. Glandular swelling is common, and the glands are usually hard and painful to touch. The breasts may be affected similarly, though the testicles are perhaps the organ with which *Clematis* has the most affinity.

Clinical use: See "Orchitis" in *Reproductive System.*

Cocculus (Indian cockle)

One of the most prominent *Cocculus* symptoms is motion sickness, especially from riding in a car, so we often use this remedy for animals that develop nausea in cars (though it is not the only remedy that can help). The other sphere of action is weakness and paralysis, sometimes affecting only one side of the body. The limbs may tremble. These animals are often very sad, confused, dull, and generally inward; it may be difficult to communicate with them. Cold is uncomfortable for these animals—they prefer to rest quietly in a warm room.

Clinical use: See "Regurgitation and Vomiting" in *Digestive System* and "Degenerative Myelopathy" in *Nervous System.*

Coccus cacti (Cochineal—an insect that feeds on cactus plants)

Like *Cantharis,* many of *Coccus cacti*'s symptoms involve mucous membranes. With this remedy there is a great production of mucus, often thick. The state may come on after a cold exposure. Lying down, especially at night, often worsens the symptoms, so these animals may be restless. The indication for acute use is for a mucus plug that obstructs the urethra, usually in male cats.

Clinical use: See "Urethral Obstruction and Catheterization" in *Urinary System.*

Colchicum (Meadow saffron)

This remedy has an affinity to joints and to the gastrointestinal system. The pains are intense when *Colchicum* is needed. Motion aggravates the symptoms, and the joint pain is so intense that touch may cause the animal to cry out in great pain. These patients may deteriorate rapidly, possibly in part due to the difficulty in dealing with the intense pains. They become weak and may collapse, though they will show signs of restlessness as well.

Their pain is such that it is hard to become comfortable. The pain often makes them very irritable also. A keynote symptom for *Colchicum* is nausea, and especially when the nausea occurs at the sight or upon the smell of food. Sometimes even thinking of food induces nausea, as when an animal is called for supper and she immediately begins to drool or lick her lips (in preparation for vomiting rather than as a Pavlovian response). These individuals are chilly and sensitive.

Clinical use: See "Bloat" in *Digestive System* and "Arthritic Conditions" in *Musculoskeletal System*.

Colocynthis (Bitter apple)

This remedy is similar to *Colchicum* in its affinity to the digestive tract and to the joints. When *Colocynthis* is needed, however, the pains are not quite as intense. The intestinal pain, however, is strong enough to cause the patient to bend forward, as this sometimes relieves the pain. You may see your companion lying on her abdomen with her head very low. She may even lie across a pillow or a similar object as pressure will relieve the pains. The cramping abdominal pains often appear suddenly; they may be brought on by anger (or any other intense emotion). The animal is often irritable during the pain as well. Cold usually worsens *Colocynthis* symptoms, and warmth relieves the discomfort.

Clinical use: See "Diarrhea" in *Digestive System*, "Arthritic Conditions" in *Musculoskeletal System*, and "Paraphimosis and Phimosis" in *Reproductive System*.

Conium maculatum (Poison hemlock)

Poison hemlock is the substance that Socrates drank in order to carry out his death sentence. Poison hemlock induces a paralysis that starts in the legs and gradually ascends, ultimately paralyzing the heart and lungs, causing death. There is a sensation of heaviness along with the paralysis. One of the more common symptoms of *Conium* is a numbness or paralysis that originates in the rear legs of animals. There is no pain; the animal just stumbles or walks as though the legs are heavy.

Conium also has an affinity to glands. Stony hard inflammations of the lymph nodes, breasts, prostate gland, and testicles may respond to this remedy. Animals needing *Conium* often move and act slowly, and they are weak, dull, and confused. Light is often intolerable, thus they may stay in dark places. Older animals are more likely to need this remedy than younger ones. They gradually but continually deteriorate. This remedy is more commonly indicated in chronic diseases, thus you may not use it often. There are some acute indications, however, as I have listed. If you believe your companion has chronic symptoms that call for *Conium*, I suggest that you work with an experienced homeopathic prescriber.

Clinical use: See "Injuries to the Eyes" in *Eyes,* "Degenerative Myelopathy," "Coonhound Paralysis," and "Injuries to the Brain and Spinal Cord" in *Nervous System,* and "Paraphimosis and Phimosis," "Orchitis," "Injuries to the Testicles," "Prostate Affections," "Mastitis," and "Injury to the Breast" in *Reproductive System.*

Copaiva (Balsam copaiba)

This is another plant remedy that is effective for mucous membrane irritation and the resultant mucus discharges. The discharge is usually quite foul, and it may appear from any orifice. Animals who need this remedy are often very sensitive to noise and startle readily at almost any sound. *Copaiva* is similar to *Sepia,* though not as well known.

Clinical use: See "Discharge from the Vulva" in *Reproductive System.*

Crotalus horridus (Timber rattlesnake venom)

Crotalus is made from the venom of the timber rattlesnake. Many snake venoms induce hemorrhage, and this is one of the main acute indications for this homeopathic medicine. The blood is dark, and it oozes slowly and continuously when *Crotalus* is indicated. Many septic and gangrenous wounds may respond to this remedy also. Mentally, these animals may be sad and despondent or they may be somewhat delirious. In either case there may be a desire to escape. Symptoms may occur on the right side of the body.

Clinical use: See "Aural Hematomas" in *Skin and Ears* and "Food and Garbage Poisoning" and "Hemorrhage" in *Therapeutic Indications by Condition.*

Croton tiglium (Croton oil seeds)

Croton oil is a skin and mucous membrane irritant. It produces a rash that is similar to a poison ivy rash; the homeopathic medicine is sometimes effective as a treatment for the latter. Poison ivy and poison oak rarely (if ever) affect cats or dogs—though they will certainly bring the oil to their guardians, where it does have an impact. But cats and dogs may develop a rash that looks like poison ivy, and this may respond to *Croton*. Another area of *Croton*'s affinity is the intestines, and diarrhea will sometimes respond to this remedy; the diarrhea is usually yellow. The least amount of food or drink may worsen the *Croton* state. The mucous membranes may be red and inflamed when this remedy is indicated.

Clinical use: See "Diarrhea" in *Digestive System.*

Drosera (Round-leaved sundew)

This remedy is primarily used for coughing. It has been successfully employed for whooping cough. These animals may be irritable, and they are anxious at night and when alone. In this they are similar to *Arsenicum* animals, but the *Drosera* cough is often more severe. The symptoms worsen at night and when the animal lies down.

Clinical use: See "Cough" in *Respiratory System, Nose, and Sinuses.*

Dulcamara (Bittersweet; Woody nightshade)

The big keynote for this remedy is aggravation from dampness, especially cold damp weather or climates. A *Dulcamara* illness often follows when an animal is chilled after being warm, such as too-rapid cooling following exertion. Coughs, diarrhea, and skin conditions may all ensue.

Clinical use: See "Cough" in *Respiratory System, Nose, and Sinuses.*

Echinacea (Purple cone-flower)

Many people know about this as an herbal remedy for fevers and infections. The herb stimulates the immune system so the body can better resist infection. The homeopathic medicine is even more powerful in this, but it must be used according to homeopathic indications. It is especially useful for serious infections where the body is weak and has been worn down by the infection. There is often a lot of damage to the tissue at the site of the infection. The animal will be so tired that he appears confused, though he may be irritable if forced to do something against his will.

Clinical use: See "Discharges from the Vulva" and "Postpartum Infections" in *Reproductive System* and "Bites of Snakes" in *Therapeutic Indications by Condition.*

Equisetum (Scouring rush; Horsetail)

Horsetail's primary affinity is to the urinary bladder. The patient who needs *Equisetum* typically has continual urging. With each successive urination the volume is less, but the urging grows stronger. The urging is stronger immediately following urination. The pain is worst at the end of urination, so the animal may quickly move to lick her genitalia immediately following urination. There may also be involuntary urination at night, in alternation with the inflammatory urging. The urine may have mucus, and the patient is sometimes better in the afternoon and while lying down. Horsetail contains a lot of silica, so this remedy has similarity to *Silicea,* and may be helpful if *Silicea* is indicated but seems not to work well.

   Clinical use: See "Cystitis" and "Urinary Incontinence" in *Urinary System.*

Erigeron (Horseweed; Canada fleabane)

This little remedy is mainly employed for hemorrhage from any bodily orifice. The blood is bright red, and the bleeding is worse with motion and better if the animal lies quietly.

   Clinical use: See "Hemorrhage" in *Therapeutic Indications by Condition.*

Eucalyptus (Blue gum tree; Fever tree)

The oil from these trees irritates mucous membranes, causing much mucus production. The homeopathic medicine may be useful for conditions when the body produces a lot of mucus. The stomach, the lungs, and the kidneys are especially affected. The patient generally wants to move around and exercise.

   Clinical use: See "Bloat" in *Digestive System* and "Decreasing Kidney Function" in *Urinary System.*

Eupatorium perfoliatum (Boneset, Thoroughwort)

Boneset has great affinity to the bones, and can be helpful with pains associated with broken bones, as well as bone pains from other causes like influenza in humans. The pains are violent and aching, and the patient constantly shifts in an attempt to get comfortable, which is difficult as the movement does not help even though the pains compel movement. Moaning and crying are not uncommon. They are frequently much worse between seven and nine in the morning. This remedy has much affinity to damp climates with associated liver and general organ sluggishness, and malarial symptoms, but as I am mentioning the remedy mainly for its bone pains, I am not including those symptoms in this summary. You can find these in any good *materia medica.*

Clinical use: See "Panosteitis" and "Broken Bones" in *Musculoskeletal System.*

Eupatorium purpureum (Gravel root; Joe-Pye weed; Queen of the meadow)

Like *Eup per,* above, *Eup pur* is good for dampness-induced conditions with restlessness. This remedy, however, has a kidney and bladder focus along with the liver impact. These patients tend to be dull, depressed, and sleepy, and may sigh. Bladder symptoms include straining and pain, and the pain extends to the back if the kidneys are also affected. There is often protein in the urine. Thirst is decreased, sometimes absent. Homesickness is marked in humans, so if a urinary disorder follows a move, this remedy may be useful. There may be swelling associated with kidney disease, and the remedy can be useful for early kidney shutdown. Stools tend to be loose and may contain bile (greenish to yellow-green). The prostate may be affected in males, along with the urinary system.

Animals needing Eup pur often worsen every other day, alternating good and bad days.

Clinical use: See "Cystitis" in *Urinary System,* "Arthritis" in *Musculoskeletal System,* and "Prostate Affections" in *Reproductive System.*

Euphorbium (Euphorbium officinarum, Euphorbia resinifera)

When *Euphorbium* is indicated, the patient is in a heightened state, such as a manic state. There is often cerebral (brain) congestion, with the result that the patient is anxious, panting, and extremely restless. He may cry out. You may even see convulsions and intermittent loss of consciousness. Nighttime is worse, and he may startle easily or from his restless sleep. The pains in the *Euphorbium* state are severe and burning, "as if a live coal were on or in the part." This remedy can be especially useful in some cancers, especially as death approaches. Like *Tarentula cubensis,* this remedy can help animals die when there is intense pain and anxiety.

The pains tend to be worse at rest, worse with initial motion, and better with continued motion, like *Rhus tox.*

Clinical use: See "Euthanasia" in *Therapeutic Indications by Condition.*

Euphrasia (Eyebright)

Both the herbal and the homeopathic form of this plant are primarily used for inflammation and injury to the eyes. These animals may start from sleep as if awakened by a noise. Their symptoms are generally worse from sunlight, wind, warmth, and being indoors; they may improve outside in the open air.

Clinical use: See "Conjunctivitis" and "Injuries to the Eyes" in *Eyes.*

Ferrum metallicum (Iron)

This remedy is usually indicated for young, weakly animals; exertion is very overtaxing for these patients. They are often restless, especially at night. Contradiction and discipline is difficult for these animals, and they may become quite irritable under these circumstances. Hemorrhage may accompany other symptoms. They are somewhat like animals needing *Arsenicum album,* but more irritable, and those needing *Ferrum* often prefer to be alone. Also, *Arsenicum* animals are generally thirsty, while drinking may worsen the condition of a *Ferrum* patient. The latter also do not like eggs, and if they eat eggs their symptoms often worsen.

Clinical use: See "Vomiting" in *Digestive System.*

Ferrum muriaticum (Iron chloride)

These animals may have anemia, either from reduced production of red blood cells or from hemorrhage. The spleen is often enlarged, so the remedy may come into play with autoimmune hemolytic anemias. They often cough blood or have bloody discharge from the nose. Their appetites are diminished to absent, but with great thirst; some may be thirstless. They often vomit or regurgitate shortly after eating, even while eating. Stools are dark and soft, often with blood. There may also be blood in the urine. Cramping muscles accompany many conditions when *Ferr mur* is needed.

Nighttime and morning tends to find these animals worse, and they improve with the daytime. Weakness is common, but with anxiety.

Clinical use: See "Decreasing Kidney Function" in *Urinary System.*

Ferrum phosphoricum (Iron phosphate)

Ferrum phos is especially well known for its influence upon fevers and infections, especially in their early stages. Lung and upper respiratory infections are especially in the sphere of *Ferrum phos,* and hemorrhage often accompanies the infections. Animals needing this remedy tend to be thin, weakly, and anemic. They may have the irritability of *Ferrum* alternating with the gregariousness of *Phosphorus*. Night and early morning (four to six in the morning) are times when the symptoms may be at their worst for these patients.

Clinical use: See "Nosebleed" and "Cough" in *Respiratory System, Nose, and Sinuses* and "Fever and Infections" in *Therapeutic Indications by Condition*.

Ferrum picricum (Iron picrate)

These patients are even weaker than those needing *Ferrum metallicum,* and exertion causes failure of organs when *Ferrum picricum* is indicated. One of the main indications for this remedy is senile prostatic hypertrophy (noncancerous enlargement).

Clinical use: See "Prostate Affections" in *Reproductive System*.

Fluoric acid (Hydrofluoric acid)

The element fluorine accumulates in bones, and excess fluorine in bone tissue weakens the bones. There is evidence that fluoridation of water supplies often causes damage to bones and teeth in the long run. The homeopathic medicine *Fluoric acid,* like *Calcarea fluorica,* retains this affinity to teeth and bones. These remedies have similar indications and effects, though the *Fluoric acid* state is more one of decay and degeneration in older animals as compared to the developmental origin of the *Calc fluor* state. When *Fluoric acid* is needed, the damage is generally more severe, and there is often ulceration in various body tissues. These animals are intolerant of heat and rest and are better with motion and cold. They are especially improved with cold baths, a rather unusual modality, and they may be indifferent to guardians and family members.

Clinical use: See "Abscessed and Decaying Teeth" and "Ranula" in *Mouth, Gums, and Teeth*.

Formica rufa (Red ant)

This remedy's main use is for acute treatment of itching, burning skin. It may also help some cases of arthritis, and it can reduce polyp formation, though these are chronic indications and should be treated by an experienced homeopath.

Clinical use: See "Itching" in *Skin and Ears*.

Galphimia glauca (Thryallis, a plant found in Mexico and Central America)

This remedy is fairly limited, at least in our understanding, to individuals with allergic tendencies. They may have hay fever or bronchial asthma symptoms and/or skin reactions like itchiness and eruptions, even with herpes-like lesions. There may be swelling also. These animals would usually be hypersensitive to weather changes.

Clinical use: See "Itching" in *Skin and Ears.*

Gelsemium (Yellow jasmine)

Weakness, dullness, and lassitude mark the *Gelsemium* state. This remedy is often needed after an acute illness when the animal simply cannot shake the disease and remains tired and lethargic. Paralysis also comes under the sphere of *Gelsemium's* influence. The limbs and the body may tremble with the weakness. These animals generally wish to be left alone. New tasks or new situations are difficult for these animals, and the anxiety around these situations can induce the weak state that calls for *Gelsemium.* In fact, any strong emotion or any shocking event may induce the *Gelsemium* state.

Clinical use: See "Degenerative Myelopathy" in *Nervous System,* "Labor" in *Reproductive System,* and "Fever and Infections" and "Overheating" in *Therapeutic Indications by Condition.*

Glonoinum (Nitroglycerine)

Overheating, especially from overexposure to the sun, is one of the primary causes of the *Glonoinum* state. These animals are profoundly weak, and they often have a severe headache. Raising the head and sitting in open air can improve the symptoms.

Clinical use: See "Overheating" in *Therapeutic Indications by Condition.*

Granatum (Pomegranate)

I only use this remedy for tapeworm infestations, though it has homeopathic indications of salivation, stomach pain, constant hunger, and itching feet. All symptoms are better after eating dinner.

Clinical use: See "Worms" in *Therapeutic Indications by Condition.*

Graphites (Black lead; Plumbago)

This remedy is made from graphite, which is primarily carbon. As carbon is the basis of all organic materials, any carbon-containing remedy is very important, especially for deep physical damage or malfunction. This remedy is often best given under the supervision of an experienced homeopathic prescriber, though there are some acute indications. These animals are usually stout or obese, and they are sluggish in movement and in their ability to heal. They have a tendency to experience skin eruptions at the bends of joints, and many skin eruptions discharge a honey-colored liquid when *Graphites* is needed. These animals are usually chilly, though they can be worse from heat or hot rooms and better in open air, like animals needing *Pulsatilla*.

Clinical use: See "Hotspots" in *Skin and Ears*, "Constipation" in *Digestive System*, and "Discharge from the Vulva" in *Reproductive System*.

Guaiacum (Gum guaiacum)

Guaiacum's affinity is to ligaments, tendons, and joints. It is sort of a chronic *Rhus tox* in that it is often helpful for chronic arthritides. Limbs may be contracted and stiff, with shortened muscles. The animal may try to stretch his limbs frequently. The body often smells dirty. There may also be foul secretions, like perspiration and saliva. *Guaiacum* can also encourage these discharges, so it can help with some abscesses. The neck and upper back, including the shoulders, are often stiff. These animals tend to sit down a lot and may sit quickly after walking somewhere.

The modalities are opposite those of *Rhus tox*, in that heat and motion worsens these animals. Touch also worsens the pains. Cold damp weather also worsens the pain, as does the nighttime, generally from six in the evening to four in the morning. Cold applications, however, improve local pains; this is unusual for arthritic pains.

Clinical use: See "Arthritis" in *Musculoskeletal System* and "Abscesses" in *Therapeutic Indications by Condition*.

Gunpowder (Gunpowder!)

Gunpowder is a great remedy for many septic conditions, like abscesses, tooth infections, and even bone infections following wounds, including gunshot wounds and bite wounds. I find this remedy to be remarkable for these sorts of conditons. Cat bites (in humans) often respond remarkably well. When this remedy is indicated, the wounds are often deep and painful, with reddened skin. Consider it for any abscess or bite wound. It may also help with acne and boils.

Clinical use: See "Acne" in *Skin and Ears;* "Abscessed or Decaying Teeth" in *Mouth, Gums, and Teeth;* and "Abscesses" and "Bites of Cats and Dogs" in *Therapeutic Indications by Condition.*

Hamamelis (Witch hazel)

Hamamelis is therapeutically similar to *Arnica* and *Bellis perennis* in its indications for bruising injuries and hemorrhage. Many of the physical effects that call for *Hamamelis* involve passive congestion of veins and poor circulation to the affected part, usually as a consequence of trauma. The patient is usually worse from touch and movement and better while lying quietly. The pains may be strong, and this remedy has a reputation for relief of post-surgical pain. If *Arnica* or *Bellis* do not help, consider *Hamamelis.*

Clinical use: See "Nosebleed" in *Respiratory System, Nose, and Sinuses;* "Injuries to the Eyes" in *Eyes;* "Sprains and Strains" in *Musculoskeletal System;* "Orchitis" in *Reproductive System;* and "Hemorrhage" and "Surgery" in *Therapeutic Indications by Condition.*

Hecla lava (Fine ash from Mount Hecla, an Icelandic volcano)

Hecla has an affinity to bone, especially the jawbone, and it is mostly employed for bony tumors and inflammation. The glands in the region of the bone swelling are often enlarged as well. All swellings are generally painful to touch.

Clinical use: See "Abscessed and Decaying Teeth" in *Mouth, Gums, and Teeth.*

Helodrilis (Earthworm)

This remedy has rather recently been proven by Lou Klein and is not common, so it will not be in most other books on *materia medica.* It has an affinity to the spine and to spinal injuries.

Clinical use: See "Injuries to the Brain and Spinal Cord" in *Nervous System.*

Hepar sulphuris calcareum (Chemically prepared by burning oyster shells with sulfur)

Hepar sulph is a major remedy for abscesses and painful inflammatory conditions. Many animals that need the remedy are also irritable and aggressive, perhaps because the inflammation involves the brain as well—though the pain often seems very intense to these animals, so this in itself might induce irritability. When *Hepar sulph* is needed, the patient reacts to touch with violence, giving the impression that the inflammation or wound is much more painful than you might expect from its appearance. Thus if you attempt to examine or clean a *Hepar sulph* wound or infection, your companion may snap or scratch at you. Most inflammatory conditions suppurate (discharge pus) when this remedy is needed. *Hepar sulph* patients are extremely chilly and sensitive to drafts and to the slightest cold. This state is more common in winter, when the weather is cold and dry; warmth and dampness often improve the symptoms in these patients.

Clinical use: See "Hotspots" in *Skin and Ears*; "Abscessed and Decaying Teeth" and "Homeopathic Remedies for Dental Care and Extractions" in *Mouth, Gums, and Teeth*; "Sneezing and Nasal Discharge" and "Cough" in *Respiratory System, Nose, and Sinuses*; "Hypopyon" and "Corneal Ulcers" in *Eyes*; "Aggression" in *Nervous System*; "Discharge from the Sheath" and "Mastitis" in *Reproductive System*; and "Abscesses" in *Therapeutic Indications by Condition*.

Histaminum muriaticum (Histamine)

Histaminum is derived from histamine, one of the chemicals released during allergic reactions. Histamine induces capillary permeability, which can lead to the four cardinal signs of inflammation—*rubor, calor, dolor,* and *tumor*—redness, heat, pain, and swelling. As a remedy, histamine can counteract the allergic reaction in some patients. It is mostly an acute treatment, but can be helpful for bee stings and the like. It may prevent the breathing difficulty that can follow allergic reactions, including those to vaccines. When needed, the patients tend to be restless, pacing, and irritable, even quarrelsome.

Clinical use: See "Insect Bites and Stings" in *Skin and Ears* and "Allergic Reactions" in *Therapeutic Indications by Condition*.

Hydrastis (Goldenseal)

Goldenseal is an herb with great antiseptic properties. The homeopathic remedy is especially useful for infections where there are thick, yellowish, ropy secretions. The infected areas tend to be severe, often with a lot of damage to the local tissues; there may even be ulceration and draining tracts. Cold air often aggravates these animals. *Hydrastis* has an affinity to older animals, and it is often beneficial in ulcerated, cancerous wounds.

Clinical use: See "Sneezing and Nasal Discharge" in *Respiratory System, Nose, and Sinuses* and "Discharge from the Vulva" in *Reproductive System*.

Hyoscyamus (Henbane)

Aggression with sexual overtones marks the *Hyoscyamus* condition. The patient may alternate between aggression and masturbation or mounting behavior; she may also alternate between aggression and buoyant, cheerful behavior. These animals are generally very suspicious and may attack strangers or other animals. Jealousy is common in *Hyoscyamus* animals; it may be expressed as a sexual possessiveness. They generally do not like to be alone. There is a lot of fear that underlies the aggression, as there is in *Stramonium* animals. Spasms and twitches often accompany other symptoms. This remedy is often needed for animals that have deep, chronic illness and should be treated by an experienced homeopathic prescriber, but the remedy may help in some acute situations. The *Hyoscyamus* state is often induced by rabies vaccination.

Clinical use: See "Aggression" in *Nervous System*, "Eclampsia" in *Reproductive System*, and "Fear of Rushing Water" in *Therapeutic Indications by Condition*.

Hypericum perforatum (St. John's wort)

This remedy has been called "The *Arnica* of the nerves" because of its great affinity to nerve injuries. Any wounds that involve areas with a lot of nerve endings will often benefit with a dose of *Hypericum*, as this will relieve the pain. The fingers and toes, teeth and gums, tongue, and tail are examples of areas with high nerve density. Of course, the brain and spinal cord are nerve tissue, and *Hypericum* is often helpful when these are injured. This remedy may relieve the pain of extremely painful lacerations (see also *Calendula* and *Staphysagria*). When *Hypericum* is needed, jarring, touch, and motion worsen the wound pain. This remedy is said to be useful in tetanus.

The herb (*Hypericum* tincture or St. John's wort) is very useful as a top-ical wound cleanser and antiseptic agent; it can be used in lacerations, infected ears, abscesses, and so on. When using topically, make a tea with fresh or dried herb, or put ten to thirty drops of the tincture, along with one-fourth teaspoonful of salt, into a cup of water.

Clinical use: See "Intervertebral Disc Disease" in *Musculoskeletal System*, "Injuries to the Brain and Spinal Cord" in *Nervous System*, "Postpartum pain" in *Reproductive System*, and "Bites of Cats and Dogs" and "Cuts and Lacerations" in *Therapeutic Indications by Condition*.

Ignatia (St. Ignatius bean)

Most times an animal experiences grief, *Ignatia* can be helpful. Grieving animals may not eat, may sleep excessively, and may become depressed—just the same as a human. Sighing is common and is a pointer to *Ignatia*. Animals needing this remedy may alternate between happiness and sadness, which is rather normal for grieving individuals. If they cannot shake their grief, however, this remedy will often help. There are other uses for *Ignatia*, but grief is often at the heart of the case, though the grief may be in the past.

Clinical use: See "Grief" in *Therapeutic Indications by Condition*.

Inula Helen (Elecampane; Scabwort)

Elecampane has a strong affinity to mucous membranes, especially those of the respiratory tract. It is great for acute lung conditions where there is mucus; it can help disperse the mucus and resolve the congestion. It is not for congestion related to heart and circulation issues; rather it is for con-gestion following acute viral infections like the feline upper respiratory viruses. Generally the cough is rather loose.

These animals worsen at night and lying down. They may also be itchy and chilly.

Clinical use: See "Cough" in *Respiratory System, Nose, and Sinuses*.

Ipecac (Cephaelis ipecacuanha)

Many parents keep syrup of ipecac in their medicine chest for the times when children ingest potentially dangerous substances. Syrup of ipecac will induce vomiting, so the child can eliminate the other material from his stomach. Homeopathic *Ipecac* is useful as a treatment for some cases of vomiting. The animal that needs this remedy often coughs along with the vomiting, or she may cough a number of times in a row, ending with vomiting. The coughing attack brings about the need to vomit. Nausea is often persistent. Hemorrhage may also occur when *Ipecac* is needed; blood may appear in vomitus, in urine, or as a discharge from the vulva (usually of uterine origin). Warmth and overeating may bring about an *Ipecac* state.

Clinical use: See "Vomiting" in *Digestive System;* "Cough" in *Respiratory System, Nose, and Sinuses;* and "Postpartum hemorrhage" in *Reproductive System.*

Iris versicolor (Blue flag)

This plant remedy is especially good for pancreatitis and liver inflammations. Vomiting is almost always a part of this remedy's indications. Nausea can be profound. The vomitus and the diarrhea are burning and irritating, thus the mouth or anus may be reddened. Vomitus tends to contain bile. Patients tend to be irritable and snappy. The stomach and abdomen are usually quite painful, sometimes with sharp, colicky pains. The appetite is decreased, or the animal may be hungry but unable to eat due to the nausea. These are fairly sick animals.

Nighttime is worse, especially between two and three in the morning. They are usually restless at night also. They may tend to have recurrences in spring and fall as well as during especially hot weather.

Clinical use: See "Vomiting" in *Digestive System.*

Kali bichromicum (Potassium bichromate)

The sphere of influence of *Kali bichromicum* is in the mucous membranes. Like *Hydrastis,* this remedy is often indicated when there are yellow, thick, ropy discharges from body orifices. The discharge forms crusts when either remedy is needed, but the crusts may adhere more tightly when *Kali bichromicum* is the indicated remedy. Pulling the crusts off will usually leave a raw sore, as the inflamed outer layer of the skin comes off with the crust. Animals needing this remedy may be worse in the morning. Cold is usually intolerable and may also worsen the symptoms. Behaviorally, these animals tend to be irritable and indifferent toward others; this is also similar to *Hydrastis* animals. A difference from *Hydrastis* is that the irritability is lessened after eating when *Kali bichromicum* is needed, whereas eating worsens the irritability in *Hydrastis* patients.

Clinical use: See "Sneezing and Nasal Discharge" in *Respiratory System, Nose, and Sinuses* and "Discharge from the Vulva" in *Reproductive System.*

Kali chloricum (Potassium chlorate)

This remedy has a great affinity to the mouth; it is indicated for severe inflammatory states. The breath is usually putrid. The tongue or other body parts may be cold to the touch. These animals are often very weak and quite ill when this remedy is needed. They may refuse to eat. Their behavior may alternate between cheerfulness and depression. This state is often one that is severe enough to warrant professional help from a veterinarian and a homeopath (optimally the same person), but you may try this remedy along with veterinary help if you do not have access to a skilled homeopathic prescriber. *Kali muriaticum* is a related remedy that may also help; it is easier to obtain, as it is one of the tissue salts. Tissue salts are often available (in 6X potency) in health food stores.

Clinical use: See "Gingivitis and Mouth Inflammation" in *Mouth, Gums, and Teeth.*

Kali phosphoricum (Potassium phosphate)

In the *Kali phos* state, the nerves are weak, as is the entire patient. This can be true of many phosphorus-containing remedies. The patient may also be irritable and oversensitive. Physical and mental exertion worsen these animals. Creeping paralysis, wasting diseases, and softening of the spinal cord fall under this remedy's jurisdiction. Homesickness may be an inciting cause, so if your patient develops nerve difficulty or other weakness following a move, consider *Kali phos*. They are often hungry, even shortly after eating, though in some cases the hunger disappears upon being offered food.

Pale, sensitive, irritable animals are a stereotype for the *Kali phos* picture, and worry, excitement, and exertion can bring about this condition—even slight worries, as they are so sensitive.

Clinical use: See "Degenerative Myelopathy" in *Nervous System.*

Kali sulphuricum (Potassium sulfate)

Kali sulph is often indicated for thick, yellow discharges, but these are less ropy and less irritating than those that call for *Kali bichromicum*. Another distinction from the latter remedy (and from *Hydrastis*) is that *Kali sulph* patients are worse in warmth and prefer cool open air. *Kali sulph* is similar to *Pulsatilla* in many ways (*Pulsatilla* also has bland, yellow discharges and a desire for open air). These animals are anxious and irritable, however, in contrast to those that need *Pulsatilla*. They may have an itchy, very flaky skin rash along with other symptoms.

Clinical use: See "Sneezing and Nasal Discharge" in *Respiratory System, Nose, and Sinuses.*

Kreosotum (Creosote)

Creosote is a very irritating plant oil. The homeopathic remedy is often indicated for mucous membrane irritation and the resultant discharges. Like the oil, the discharges are acrid and burning when this remedy is indicated. There is usually a foul odor to inflammations and discharges. The gums are especially affected, and the animal may lose teeth at a young age to gum inflammation and tooth decay. The *Kreosotum* state often arises as the animal begins teething. These animals are usually sickly and weak. Oddly, they are often worse from rest, so they move around a lot; this restlessness is especially bad at night.

Clinical use: See "Gingivitis and Mouth Inflammation" in *Mouth, Gums, and Teeth;* "Incontinence" in *Urinary System;* and "Discharge from the Vulva" in *Reproductive System.*

Lac caninum (Dog's milk)

While this remedy has many indications, I primarily list it for its impact upon the mammae. Animals that need this remedy may be insecure and desirous of approval and attention. Symptoms tend to alternate sides, and there is also an affinity to the throat. The remedy is very useful for sore throats in humans, especially if the pain alternates sides. Touch and jarring greatly increase the pain when there is a *Lac caninum* inflammation.

Clinical use: See "Inadequate Milk" and "Mastitis" in *Reproductive System.*

Lachesis (Bushmaster snake venom; Surucucu)

This is one of our polychrest remedies. Animals that need *Lachesis* often act somewhat like a snake: they are timid and suspicious until they get to know someone new, and they are generally happy to be left alone; they may strike out if pushed too far. The tendency to strike can occasionally become a habit with these animals. Jealousy is a common keynote for this remedy as well.

The physical symptoms tend to occur on the left side of the body. The circulatory system is often affected. Hemorrhage is common, and body tissues may have a bluish cast from blood seepage or from poor circulation. Wounds with poor circulation and poor healing often come under the sphere of this remedy. *Lachesis* patients dislike warmth and prefer open air. A physical keynote that is frequently present is a tendency for symptoms to arise while the patient sleeps.

Clinical use: See "Insect Bites and Stings" and "Aural Hematomas" in *Skin and Ears;* "Gingivitis and Mouth Inflammation" in *Mouth, Gums, and Teeth;* "Aggression" in *Nervous System;* "Postpartum Hemorrhage" in *Reproductive System;* and "Abscesses," "Bites of Cats and Dogs," "Bites of Snakes," and "Hemorrhage" in *Therapeutic Indications by Condition.*

Lactuca virosa (Wild lettuce; Acrid lettuce)

This small remedy can increase milk flow. This is a specific use, so the patient may not show other *Lactuca* symptoms. If present, you might see great restlessness and dilated pupils. There may be some respiratory distress. If so, yawning may lessen the respiratory symptoms. The animal may also simply yawn frequently, with or without the respiratory symptoms.

Lactuca can also help some liver diseases. Here there may be irritability and confusion, and the patient may be easily provoked. The confusion may progress to stupefaction.

Curiously, according to Matthew Wood, the extremely insightful herbalist,

> Wild Lettuce is the remedy for people who have been through adversity and harshness.... It usually results from prolonged emotional suffering, resulting in emotional deadness or coldness. The *Lactuca* patient has been through rough, de-humanizing, deadening experiences. They are not, however, completely deadened— that would call for Wormwood or Sagebrush.... This is really a great remedy for negative thinking in general, people who say, "Oh, but that would never work."[1]

I list this as it reminds me of many unfortunate animals' lives. If you see liver disease in an animal who has come from an abusive home, consider *Lactuca.*

Clinical use: See "Inadequate Milk Flow" in *Reproductive System* and "Liver Disorders" in *Therapeutic Indications by Condition.*

Lathyrus (Chickpea)

This remedy is almost a specific for poliomyelitis in humans. It can be helpful in animals who develop paralyses that are similar to polio. The paralysis is usually painless and the reflexes are almost always increased. *Lathyrus* conditions tend to arise in cold damp weather. Some practitioners believe the remedy is usually indicated for males and rarely for females.

Clinical use: See "Degenerative Myelopathy" and "Coonhound Paralysis" in *Nervous System*.

Ledum palustre (Marsh tea; Wild rosemary)

Ledum is generally the first choice for any puncture wound. Though there are many other indications, our use of the remedy usually centers around a puncture of some sort. It is said to be capable of preventing tetanus if administered in time. The wounded parts may twitch, and they are often cold when *Ledum* is indicated, though warmth increases the discomfort. There also may be skin itching that is worse at night in a warm bed. The itching may concentrate on the feet and lower legs. These animals may be angry and irritable, and they may prefer to be left alone (they are as cold mentally as they are physically).

Clinical use: See "Itching" and "Insect Bites and Stings" in *Skin and Ears,* "Injuries to the Eyes" in *Eyes,* "Injuries to the Testicles" in *Reproductive System,* and "Bites of Cats and Dogs," "Bites of Snakes," and "Fleas" in *Therapeutic Indications by Condition*.

Lilium tigrinum (Tiger lily)

This is a remedy state with great mental strain and anguish. The patient is usually female, and she is very restless, fretful, and hurried. She may constantly move about in an attempt to alleviate her anguish. There are usually erotic tendencies that may be expressed by masturbation or by constant licking of the genitals. When this remedy is indicated, the female genitalia are often affected.

Clinical use: See "Discharge from the Vulva" in *Reproductive System*.

Lycopodium clavatum (Club moss; Wolf's claw)

Lycopodium is one of the major remedies in the *materia medica*. It is usually indicated in chronic disease, however, so the indications in this book are not too common. Like *Sulphur,* this is a very deep remedy, and it can cause an aggravation if repeated too frequently, especially at the beginning of treatment.

Lycopodium animals have a great sense of hierarchy. They are very subservient to those whom they understand to be above them, while they may be bullies to those beneath their level. Thus they often behave nicely for their guardians, but they may pick on other animals in the house. They often dislike children for the same reason. There is often a fear of strangers, particularly men. The *Lycopodium* personality generally prefers to have company in the same house or in the same room, but does not wish to interact with the company. These animals may be extremely fastidious.

A physical keynote is the appearance of digestive and urinary symptoms in the same animal, though not necessarily at the same time. Flatulence is another common symptom when this remedy is needed. These animals may be chilly or warm. They also age rapidly, thus you may see gray hairs on a relatively young animal (especially dogs). Symptoms often appear on the right side of the body, or they move from right to left.

Clinical use: See "Diarrhea" and "Bloat" in *Digestive System*, "Cystitis" in *Urinary System*, "Runts and Dwarfishness" in *Reproductive System*, and "Drug Reactions" and "Fear" in *Therapeutic Indications by Condition*.

Lyssin (Hydrophobinum) (Rabies)

This remedy is a nosode; it is made from the saliva of a rabid dog. It has the energy of rabies, but it is not infectious. As a nosode, this remedy is a prescription item. It is best to leave this remedy to experienced homeopathic prescribers. I do list some indications, but this is more for general information and for veterinarians. Many people recommend giving *Lyssin* after a rabies vaccination to prevent the induction of disease from the vaccine (vaccinosis). This is a false hope. We do not have any certainty that the *Lyssin* will protect the animal from vaccinosis, though it probably does no harm. It possibly protects some animals and not others. If you must vaccinate, it is worth a try, but don't assume that you can eliminate the damage with this remedy. Choose instead not to vaccinate whenever possible. In the years since publishing the first edition, I have found that a remedy made from the rabies vaccine is far superior to *Lyssin* for negating rabies vaccine damage, but this should be administered by an experienced veterinary homeopath.

Clinical use: See "Aggression" in *Nervous System* and "Bites of Cats and Dogs" and "Fear" in *Therapeutic Indications by Condition*.

Magnesia carbonica (Magnesium carbonate)

This remedy state includes a sense of numbness and prostration as a consequence of mental and physical shock. It also has an affinity to pregnancy, which can bring about this state as well. The remedy thus may be useful for weak kittens and puppies, the only indication I have listed for the remedy in this book. The animal may be restless and anxious and may have a sour smell. Milk may worsen the condition.

Clinical use: See "Weak Kittens or Puppies" in *Reproductive System*.

Magnesia phosphorica (Magnesium phosphate)

Mag phos is often indicated when there are spasms and cramping. Many women, for example, find this remedy helpful for menstrual cramps. The cramping may be intense, causing the animal to cry out. Cramping usually occurs in sudden, violent spells. Warmth may alleviate the pains. This remedy is very useful for many stomach and abdominal complaints when there is bloating and cramping.

Clinical use: See "Bloat" in *Digestive System*, "Urethral Obstruction and Catheterization" in *Urinary System*, and "Eclampsia" in *Reproductive System*.

Medorrhinum (Gonorrheal nosode)

As with other nosodes, this remedy is best used by experienced homeopaths. It is very sycotic, so it may be indicated similarly to *Thuja*. It is good for many urogenital inflammatory conditions, especially very chronic ones. These patients often have a strong sex drive, even if neutered.

Clinical use: See "Discharge from the Sheath" and "Hypersexual Behavior" in the "Male" section of *Reproductive System*.

Medusa (Jellyfish)

Like the stinging, swollen reaction to a jellyfish sting, this remedy can help with some allergic reactions. It is similar to *Apis*, but there will usually be more stinging pains, so affected animals will likely paw at their swollen faces or other swollen areas. They may be anxious as well. Some "nettle-rash" skin inflammations (hives) may also respond to *Medusa*. It is also one of many remedies that can stimulate lactation.

Clinical use: See "Inadequate Milk Flow" in *Reproductive System* and "Allergic Reactions" in *Therapeutic Indications by Condition*.

Mercurius (Mercury; Quicksilver)

There are many remedies made from different mercury compounds, and while they are each distinct remedies, there is much overlap. *Mercurius vivus* and *Mercurius solubilis* are essentially the same remedy, and these are both indicated when most texts say simply *"Mercurius."* Some animals may be more sensitive to one or the other, so if you believe *Merc* is your remedy and *Merc sol* does not help, try *Merc v* (or vice versa). You may also try *Merc corr* or another mercury remedy. *Mercurius corrosivus* is a distinct remedy with its own symptom pattern, but there are great similarities with *Mercurius.* If your companion is a male, *Mercurius corrosivus* may work better; *Mercurius (vivus* or *solubilis)* is preferred for females. If the condition is primarily right-sided, *Mercurius iodatus flavus* may yield better results, while *Mercurius iodatus ruber* may do the same for left-sided complaints that fit the *Mercurius* picture. *Mercurius* is very similar to *Silicea;* the great similarity causes these remedies to be discordant, and occasionally we see severe problems when these remedies are given in succession. It is a good rule of thumb never to use these remedies one after the other. If you have given one and wish to give the other, give *Sulphur* or *Hepar sulph* in between.

The *Mercurius* picture is one of great physical disorder. There is often severe inflammation of the mucous membranes, especially in the mouth and the digestive tract. The urogenital systems are also greatly affected. Wherever the inflammation centers, there are discharges that are usually foul. They will often be yellow-green, thick, and slimy. Wounds or inflamed lesions are almost always moist, and they are often ulcerated or decayed at the edges. Salivation is generally profuse when *Mercurius* is indicated. See the discussion of the remedy in the mouth chapter for more details on mercury's use as a drug and its impact upon mucous membranes, especially the gums.

Animals that need this remedy tend to be strong-willed; they are often irritable if they are disciplined or otherwise corrected. They may bite, for example, if they are moved from a favorite chair. As their disease worsens, they may become morose, weary, and confused. Mercury is used for thermometers; the *Mercurius* patient is like a thermometer in that he is as affected by cold as by warm. These animals do not tolerate either temperature extreme.

The lower digestive tract is frequently affected when this remedy is needed. The patient will strain throughout and long after passing stools. He may pass a normal bowel movement, then pass several small ones in an attempt to relieve the urging to stool. There is often blood in the stool. The urinary bladder is also frequently affected, with much urging and straining, sometimes along with rectal urging.

Clinical use: See "Hotspots" in *Skin and Ears;* "Gingivitis and Mouth Inflammation," "Ranula," and "Abscessed and Decaying Teeth" in *Mouth, Gums, and Teeth;* "Diarrhea" in *Digestive System;* "Sneezing and Nasal Discharge" in *Respiratory System, Nose, and Sinuses;* "Conjunctivitis," "Hypopyon," and "Corneal Ulcers" in *Eyes;* "Cystitis" and "Decreasing Kidney Function" in *Urinary System;* "Aggression" in *Nervous System;* "Discharge from the Sheath," "Paraphimosis and Phimosis," "Orchitis," "Discharge from the Vulva," and "Bad Milk" in *Reproductive System;* and "Abscesses" and "Bites of Snakes" in *Therapeutic Indications by Condition.*

Mercurius corrosivus (Mercuric chloride)

This remedy is very similar to *Mercurius,* above. While *Merc corr* is a separate remedy with its own indications, for acute purposes it is often used for the same conditions as *Mercurius. Merc corr* is more often indicated in males. The symptoms may be more intense when *Merc corr* is needed (as compared to *Mercurius*)—thus the rectal straining is often stronger, for example. If there is diarrhea, there are often white particles of tissue in the diarrhea when *Merc corr* is the correct remedy.

Clinical use: See the indications for *Mercurius,* and see "Gingivitis and Mouth Inflammation" in *Mouth, Gums, and Teeth* and "Sneezing and Nasal Discharge" in *Respiratory System, Nose, and Sinuses.*

Mezereum (Spurge olive)

The focus of *Mezereum's* affinity is in the skin and the bones. The skin is often itchy when this remedy is indicated. The animal scratches and scratches, but there is often no sign of skin disorder—that is, there are no scabs or other eruptions other than some redness caused by the scratching. Bone pains also may respond to *Mezereum,* especially in the long bones. Behaviorally, these animals may keep to themselves, though they may want to be in the same room with their guardian. They may be quite irritable. *Mezereum* symptoms usually worsen at night. The itching is worse from warmth, but the bone pains are worse from cold and dampness. Many *Mezereum* symptoms arise as a result of vaccination.

Clinical use: See "Itching" in *Skin and Ears;* "Ranula" and "Decaying Teeth" in *Mouth, Gums, and Teeth;* and "Panosteitis" in *Musculoskeletal System.*

Millefolium (Yarrow)

Both the herb and the homeopathic remedy have an affinity to blood. *Millefolium* is useful for many hemorrhagic conditions when the blood is bright red, fluid, and profuse. Hemorrhage may occur following violent exercise.

Clinical use: See "Aural Hematomas" in *Skin and Ears;* "Nosebleed" in *Respiratory System, Nose, and Sinuses;* "Injuries to the Eyes" in *Eyes;* "Postpartum Hemorrhage" in *Reproductive System;* and "Hemorrhage" and "Surgery" in *Therapeutic Indications by Condition.*

Muriatic acid (Hydrochloric acid)

Inflammation and infection come under the sphere of this remedy. The mouth and gums are especially affected. There are cracks and ulcers that often bleed, and the mouth may be dry. Damp weather often worsens or brings about a *Muriatic acid* condition. As with most acid remedies, these patients are often weak and have low vitality. They may moan and "mutter" frequently.

Clinical use: See "Gingivitis and Mouth Inflammation" in *Mouth, Gums, and Teeth.*

Myrica (Wax myrtle; Bayberry)

This herb and remedy has strong affinity to the liver and heart and can be useful for some liver conditions, especially (but not only) if the heart is also affected. Jaundice is common; lack of it may call for a different remedy. Patients are despondent, dull, and drowsy, even indifferent to attention, but may also be irritable. Their muscles and tendons are often sore (according to traditional Chinese medicine, the tendons are under the liver's influence). There is often foul-smelling mucus in the throat, which is hard to cough up or detach. They are worse after sleep and in the morning, but better after eating breakfast. They are also better in the open air.

Clinical use: See "Liver Disorders" in *Therapeutic Indications by Condition.*

Myristica sebifera (Brazilian ucuuba)

Myristica's claim to homeopathic fame is in its power to expel splinters and other foreign bodies. It may also speed the body's action in discharging pus. This is a great remedy to have on hand if you work with wood or otherwise frequently tend to get splinters. I believe this remedy is underutilized for abscesses and foreign bodies.

Clinical use: See "Foxtails and Foreign Bodies" in *Skin and Ears;* "Sneezing and Nasal Discharge" in *Respiratory System, Nose, and Sinuses;* and "Abscesses" in *Therapeutic Indications by Condition.*

Natrum carbonicum (Sodium carbonate; Washing soda)

Sensitivity to summer heat, and especially to the heat of the sun, is a keynote of this remedy. Debility is common and often arises as a consequence of heat exposure. These animals are also extremely sensitive to thunderstorms. Their fear is such that they know a storm is coming long before others do. The joints are weak in these animals as well, so they may easily sprain them with the slightest exertion. Exertion is usually difficult for these individuals. Their digestion (another type of exertion) is weak as well, thus they may have diarrhea from any change in their normal diet. They may feel worse after eating, however, especially if they have to exert themselves on a full stomach.

Clinical use: See "Fear of Noises: Fear of Thunder and Lightning" and "Overheating" in *Therapeutic Indications by Condition.*

Natrum muriaticum (Sodium chloride; Table salt)

Nat mur is one of our polychrest remedies. Like *Lycopodium,* this remedy is more useful for chronic than acute illness. It is often indicated for animals that tend to be loners and do not like a lot of attention. They may actually wish for the attention, but they do not know how to accept care, so they refuse many advances. There is an element of forlornness to these individuals. Grief and pain are often an element of the animal's past, and it may have long-term residual effects.

Nat mur is made from table salt, and many of the physical symptoms in these animals remind us of salt's impact. Though some animals are obese, many are thin and withered—rather like salt-cured meat. Emaciation is common, especially in older animals—often despite a healthy or increased appetite. Constipation is common as well, and the stools will generally be dry. The mucous membranes are also generally dry in these patients. In an apparent attempt (usually unsuccessful) to counter this dryness, *Nat mur* patients are almost always thirsty. On the other hand, they may crave salty foods and fish.

The skin may be oily and itchy, with crusts in the bends of joints. Heat is usually intolerable, especially that of the sun. These animals are hot and dry enough already. Exertion is also difficult, possibly for the same reason (heat). Being near the sea also worsens these patients. The salt air adds to their "salt burden." Open air and rest may improve the symptoms.

Clinical use: See "Gingivitis and Mouth Inflammation" and "Ranula" in *Mouth, Gums, and Teeth;* "Constipation" in *Digestive System;* "Sneezing and Nasal Discharge" in *Respiratory System, Nose, and Sinuses;* "Decreasing Kidney Function" in *Urinary System;* and "Intervertebral Disc Disease" in *Musculoskeletal System.*

Natrum sulphuricum (Sodium sulfate; Glauber's salt)

Nat sulph patients are generally worse in damp weather, especially when the weather changes from dry to wet. Dry, warm, open air improves the symptoms. These animals may be rather despondent; this may stem from an old injury to the head or spine—this remedy is often indicated for central nervous system trauma. Aversion to light is common in these animals. Yellow discharges and sometimes yellow discoloration are found in animals needing *Nat sulph.* It is sometimes helpful in liver disorders that are worse in damp climates. Diarrhea is a common symptom also. The stools are watery and yellow, and they are worse in the early morning.

Clinical use: See "Diarrhea" in *Digestive System* and "Injuries to the Brain and Spinal Cord" in *Nervous System.*

Nitri spiritus dulcis (Sweet spirit of niter; Nitrous ether)

This is a remedy with few indications, but it has a reputation for success in acute kidney inflammation. These patients will be almost in a stupor. Vomiting is common, and it worsens the dull state. Obviously, these patients should be under a veterinarian's care, but the remedy may assist their recovery.

Clinical use: See "Decreasing Kidney Function" in *Urinary System.*

Nitric acid (Nitric acid)

The picture of *Nitric acid* is one of very painful inflammation; ulcers often accompany the inflammation. People report that the pain is like a splinter. Often the inflammation occurs at the junction of the skin and mucous membrane, such as at the mouth, nose, genitalia, or anus. As the disease deepens, this same type of inflammation may occur in any part of the body. The bones are commonly affected in later stages of the *Nitric acid* illness. Abscesses and discharges are common as well. The discharges are offensive (foul-smelling) and acrid, thus the skin is irritated from contact with the discharges and pus. There may be hair loss as a result of the irritation.

Whether it is because of the sharp pain or it is simply another aspect of disease, these animals tend to be quite irritable, even vicious. Although they may seem friendly enough when left alone, they readily bite and scratch if you attempt to examine or treat them. Whereas some animals only growl, or they may swat or bite without doing much damage, these animals mean business—they readily draw blood.

Nitric acid animals often crave fats and oils. They also desire salty foods and fish. They may crave or reject cheese, and they may be averse to meats other than fish. Animals that need this remedy are almost always chilly. Their symptoms (especially the pains) are much worse from touch, even slight touch.

Clinical use: See "Hotspots" in *Skin and Ears;* "Gingivitis and Mouth Inflammation" in *Mouth, Gums, and Teeth;* "Constipation" in *Digestive System;* "Discharge from the Sheath," "Paraphimosis and Phimosis," and "Discharge from the Vulva" in *Reproductive System;* and "Abscesses" in *Therapeutic Indications by Condition.*

Nux moschata (Nutmeg)

This remedy is often indicated for females and for disorders of the female genitalia. A behavioral keynote is confusion: these animals may easily become lost in familiar surroundings. They tend to stay in a dreamy state, sort of a world of their own. They may also faint easily. The mouth is often dry when *Nux moschata* is needed, though the animal is usually thirstless. The combination of drowsiness, chilliness, and thirstlessness often points to this remedy. The stomach may have a tendency to gas production and bloat when this remedy is indicated.

Clinical use: See "Bloat" in *Digestive System* and "Urinary Incontinence" in *Urinary System.*

Nux vomica (Poison nut)

Nux is one of our most valuable remedies, especially for acute conditions (not to be confused with the lesser-utilized remedy, *Nux moschata,* above, *Nux vomica* is generally called simply *Nux*). Many animals fit the *Nux* picture: too much stimulation, too many drugs (conventional medicines), poor foods, and overeating combine to produce a worn-out body and a depleted immune system. The bodily stress makes these animals irritable when they don't feel well. They may be very friendly otherwise. Sensitivity is prominent—it may be to noise, light, or smells. The animal is on edge, in a sense, rather like a person who is hungover from a hard night of drinking.

These animals often digest their foods poorly. They may develop diarrhea easily if the diet is altered. When diarrhea is present, they usually strain during bowel movements. They may vomit as well, though this is less common than diarrhea. Vomiting (i.e. bringing up vomitus) often makes them feel much better, but commonly all they do is retch.

Mornings are the worst time for *Nux* patients. They are nauseated, they may have a headache, and they are depressed and irritable at this time of day. Chilliness is almost always present when this remedy is needed. The *Nux* patient is very sensitive to cold and drafts.

Because of the pervasive use of conventional drugs, many animals benefit from *Nux* at some time in their lives. Some homeopathic practitioners start many cases with *Nux* to "clear" or counteract the impact of prior drug use. While I do not recommend this as a routine practice, it is beneficial in many cases. *Thuja* is often used similarly for prior vaccine use; the same caution applies to this remedy.

Clinical use: See "Homeopathic Remedies for Dental Care and Extractions" in *Mouth, Gums, and Teeth*; "Vomiting," "Diarrhea," "Constipation," and "Bloat" in *Digestive System*; "Cystitis" and "Urinary Obstruction and Catheterization" in *Urinary System*; "Intervertebral Disc Disease" in *Musculoskeletal System*; "Vestibular Syndrome" and "Aggression" in *Nervous System*; "Labor Pains" and "Eclampsia" in *Reproductive System*; and "Drug Reactions," "Food and Garbage Poisoning," and "Surgery" in *Therapeutic Indications by Condition*.

Oleander (Rose laurel)

This remedy is rarely indicated, but it may be needed in some cases of weakness or paralysis of the rear legs. Diarrhea is common when *Oleander* is indicated; the diarrhea is worse in hot weather and from citrus fruit (the plant from which this remedy is made is native to Florida). The diarrheic stool often contains undigested food. These animals may be ravenous along with the diarrhea.

Clinical use: See "Degenerative Myelopathy" in *Nervous System*.

Opium (Poppy)

I include this remedy because it has some strong indications, especially obstinate constipation, a history of excessive drug use, and stupor or persistent drowsiness, especially in combination with the other symptoms. A similar state may occur following a severe fright; if you have ever seen a bird that is paralyzed from fright, this is essentially the *Opium* state. When this remedy is indicated, the condition is usually painless.

Unfortunately, as I indicated in notes where I suggested this remedy, it is not legally available in the United States at present due to quirky FDA regulations. The FDA recognizes that homeopathic medicines have no material content once they have been diluted beyond 12C or 24X, yet they classify *Opium* and *Cannabis* (marijuana) as Schedule I narcotics. Thus, most doctors and veterinarians cannot even obtain these remedies. Most European homeopathic pharmacies sell these remedies, as do pharmacies in Mexico, so residents of these countries are fortunate in having these medicines available.

Clinical use: See "Constipation" in *Digestive System* and "Labor" in *Reproductive System*.

Passiflora incarnata (Passion flower)

I use this remedy for its calming properties. It is not a sedative, but it does a great job of calming frightened animals. I use it for travel, presurgery, and other stressful situations.

Clinical use: See "Euthanasia," "Fear," and "Surgery" in *Therapeutic Indications by Condition*.

Petroleum (Coal oil)

This is a deep-acting remedy, good for many skin ailments and wounds that do not heal well. There are many indications in homeopathy, but I have only listed it in the book for potential aid for urethral strictures following catheterization, which is in a similar vein to these other aspects of poor wound healing. It may be more useful in a cat (or dog) who is generally scruffy.

Clinical use: See "Urethral Obstruction and Catheterization" in *Urinary System*.

Phosphoric acid (Phosphoric acid)

This remedy is similar to *Phosphorus* (see below), but it has the greater debility seen in acid remedies. It is also similar to *China*. These animals are weak and easily exhausted. The exhaustion permeates the mind as well, so the *Phosphoric acid* patient is apathetic and indifferent along with the physical weakness and sleepiness. Strong emotions, especially grief and sadness, may initiate this state. Diarrhea is a common accompaniment to other symptoms. The stool may forcibly squirt out of the anus. Drafts and cold air worsen these animals, and they seek warmth. These debilitated animals may have severe, painful bone conditions like spondylosis and arthritis, which may arise when fairly young.

Clinical use: See "Diarrhea" in *Digestive System*, "Arthritis, Hip Dysplasia, and Spondylitis" and "Hypertrophic Osteodystrophy" in *Musculoskeletal System*, and "Bites of Snakes" in *Therapeutic Indications by Condition*.

Phosphorus (Phosphorus)

This remedy is another polychrest. It is often useful in animals that I treat. The classic *Phosphorus* individual is outgoing, friendly, loves attention, and is vocal. He is also thin, hungry, chilly, and thirsty, and he startles easily. These animals love to bask in the sun. I lived for years with a *Phosphorus* cat who fit the stereotype perfectly. He was long and lean, and even had reddish hair (many red-haired humans are *Phosphorus* individuals). And he was loud, especially around food; he was the first in the kitchen asking for food, which brought the other cats running. His vocal persistence earned him a nickname as "the speaker of the house."

Though these animals are very friendly, they will occasionally scratch or bite. This is generally a defensive move only, and it occurs when they feel threatened, as when they are at a veterinary clinic. They will be very friendly until the moment a needle touches their skin, at which time they explode. Even then, all actions are directed toward getting away rather than with the intent to harm. The explosive nature is related to their overall tendency to startle. (The element phosphorus is very explosive and reactive, especially when it contacts water.) Thunder and lightning and loud noises almost always startle these animals.

Physically, these animals tend to have problems with bleeding and anemia. Taking a large quantity of blood, as for a transfusion, will often greatly weaken a *Phosphorus* individual. Vomiting is common also, and occurs after drinking water (remember the element's reaction to water), as soon as the water warms in the stomach. These animals also will vomit after quickly eating foods, especially dry foods. The anus may remain open after these animals pass bowel movements. The third main area of physical disease is the lungs. *Phosphorus* patients commonly cough or show other signs of respiratory illness. They love cold water to drink and will eat most foods, generally having a strong appetite. Finally, *Phosphorus* also has a strong affinity to the liver and can be useful in liver inflammations.

Phosphorus is very similar to *Causticum* and is incompatible with it, so these remedies should never be given one after the other. *Phosphorus* is also similar to *Arsenicum album*, with which it is very compatible.

Clinical use: See "Aural Hematomas" in *Skin and Ears;* "Gingivitis and Mouth Inflammation," "Abscessed and Decaying Teeth," and "Homeopathic Remedies for Dental Care and Extractions" in *Mouth, Gums, and Teeth;* "Vomiting" and "Diarrhea" in *Digestive System;* "Nosebleed" and "Cough" in *Respiratory System, Nose, and Sinuses;* "Rickets" and "Legg-Calve-Perthes Disease" in *Musculoskeletal System;* "Vestibular Syndrome" in *Nervous System;* "Postpartum Hemorrhage" in *Reproductive System;* and "Abscesses," "Euthanasia," "Fear of Noises," "Hemorrhage," "Liver Disorders," and "Surgery" in *Therapeutic Indications by Condition.*

Phytolacca (Poke root)

This remedy has an affinity to glands, including (and especially) the mammary glands. The glands are often hard and inflamed, and they are usually very sore. Any motion greatly worsens the pain. The mouth may be dark red or bluish; the same is true of the inflamed mammae. *Phytolacca* conditions may follow exposure to cold damp weather. The animal that needs this remedy may become indifferent to life and refuse food despite otherwise not appearing very ill.

Clinical use: See "Mastitis" in *Reproductive System.*

Picric acid (Picric acid; Trinitrophenol)

Weakness, tiredness, and heaviness are often a complaint in these patients. They are easily exhausted, both mentally and physically, and they give up easily. Even slight exertion greatly weakens them.

Clinical use: See "Decreasing Kidney Function" in *Urinary System,* "Degenerative Myelopathy" and "Coonhound Paralysis" in *Nervous System,* and "Prostate Affections" and "Labor" in *Reproductive System.*

Plumbum metallicum (Lead)

This heavy metal is very toxic in material doses. Poisoned animals and people may develop severe colic, anemia, and a paralytic muscle weakness. The homeopathic medicine can be effective for these conditions if the remedy matches the overall condition. The *Plumbum* animal is generally weak and restless and often prefers to be alone. Depression is common. The symptoms often arise very slowly when this remedy is needed. The reflexes are usually depressed. There may be a bluish line on the gums. Many of these animals have yellow diarrhea as an accompaniment. The symptoms may originate on the right side.

Clinical use: See "Constipation" in *Digestive System* and "Degenerative Myelopathy" in *Nervous System*.

Podophyllum (May apple)

The intestines are the primary seat of this remedy's affinity. Diarrhea is the most common indication for *Podophyllum*. The diarrhea may also alternate with other symptoms, including constipation. Most conditions are worse in hot weather and in the early morning. They also arise during teething. These animals may grind their teeth at night, especially between two and four in the morning, when the symptoms often worsen.

Clinical use: See "Diarrhea" in *Digestive System*.

Psorinum (Scabies)

This remedy is a nosode. It is made from a human with a scabies mite infestation. Most nosodes are prescription remedies in the United States because they lack acute indications. Nosodes tend to have very deep effects as well, so their use is generally best left to experienced practitioners. This nosode is not as likely as others to cause problems, so it is one that I feel is acceptable for home use in a few conditions. It will be difficult to obtain, however, except from a practitioner.

Animals that need *Psorinum* are generally dirty, oily, and smelly, and they may be extremely itchy. Bathing them does not remove the odor and smell, or may do so for a very short time only. Additionally, bathing often worsens their symptoms. These patients are generally weak and chilly. They simply have poor ability to heal or to warm themselves. They are often ravenous. Offensive diarrhea may accompany other symptoms.

Clinical use: See "Mange" in *Skin and Ears* and "Retained Testicle" in *Reproductive System*.

Pulex irritans (Human flea)

Although this remedy is made from the human flea, some practitioners report that it helps reduce itching and flea populations in cats and dogs.

Clinical use: See "Fleas" in *Therapeutic Indications by Condition.*

Pulsatilla (Windflower)

Pulsatilla is another polychrest remedy. These animals are often female; they are usually sweet, loving, and nurturing—the quintessential mother. They can be clingy and needy, however, and this neediness can make them selfish. These animals are mild and easily led or influenced, rather like sheep. They are often timid.

The physical symptoms often change frequently, or they may move from one place to another. In arthritis, for example, the pain may shift about from leg to leg. Similarly, the stools may change constantly. When *Pulsatilla* animals have discharges, the discharge is typically yellow or white and very bland; it is usually thick and profuse as well. These individuals poorly tolerate rich or fatty foods. They usually have little to no thirst, and if they have a thirst it usually appears only after eating. The *Pulsatilla* animal is often chilly, but she cannot tolerate warm air and stuffy rooms, so she appears hot. She prefers to be in open air. Lying with the head low often aggravates symptoms. The symptoms are also worsened when she first moves and improve with continued motion, as with the *Rhus tox* individual. *Pulsatilla* has a great affinity to the reproductive system.

Like *Nux vomica, Pulsatilla* is often helpful in animals with a history of a lot of drug administration—though here the animal would have a completely different picture from the *Nux* patient.

Clinical use: See "Vomiting" and "Diarrhea" in *Digestive System;* "Sneezing and Nasal Discharge" and "Cough" in *Respiratory System, Nose, and Sinuses;* "Conjunctivitis" in *Eyes;* "Cystitis" and "Urinary Incontinence" in *Urinary System;* "Arthritic Conditions" in *Musculoskeletal System;* "Orchitis," "Prostate Affections," "Discharge from the Vulva," "Postpartum Hemorrhage," "Rejection of Puppies or Kittens," "Weak Kittens or Puppies," "Inadequate Milk Flow," and "To Dry up Milk Following Weaning" in *Reproductive System;* and "Drug Reactions" in *Therapeutic Indications by Condition.*

Pyrogenium (Decomposed lean beef)

As this remedy is made from putrid meat, it is useful for many conditions when there is infection that causes a putrefying reaction in the body. The main indications for the remedy are septic states, including (but not limited to) gangrene. There is often great pain when *Pyrogenium* is needed. The pain causes the animal to shift constantly in an attempt to find a more comfortable position. He thus appears extremely restless. External heat may alleviate the pains. Red streaks may accompany local inflammation. Dorothy Shepherd, a British physician, recommended this remedy as an antidote to vaccination with combination vaccines, though it is questionable whether any remedy has the capability of negating the damaging impact of vaccination. It is better to avoid the vaccines in the first place.

Clinical use: See "Abscessed and Decaying Teeth" in *Mouth, Gums, and Teeth;* "Discharge from the Vulva" and "Postpartum Infections" in *Reproductive System;* and "Abscesses" and "Vaccine Reactions" in *Therapeutic Indications by Condition.*

Rhododendron (Siberian rhododendron; Snow rose)
Animals that need this remedy are often sensitive to windy and stormy weather; they are consequently afraid of thunderstorms. The symptoms usually worsen before storms when *Rhododendron* is the indicated remedy. Arthritic pains may accompany other symptoms. Rest worsens most symptoms, while motion alleviates them.

Clinical use: See "Orchitis" in *Reproductive System* and "Fear of Noises: Fear of Thunder and Lightning" in *Therapeutic Indications by Condition.*

Rhus toxicodendron (Poison ivy)
Rhus tox is commonly employed for joint pains and other arthritic conditions. It is classically indicated for chilly animals whose pains are worse upon initial movement but better with continued motion. These animals "warm up" out of their pains, though *Rhus tox* is not the only remedy that has this symptom. These animals are similar to those needing *Arsenicum album* in their chilliness and their restlessness at night.

Itching skin eruptions and other inflammatory conditions are also amenable to this remedy, especially if they resemble a poison ivy reaction. Swelling, itching, and redness are common in animals that need *Rhus tox*. Skin eruptions may alternate with diarrhea. The symptoms that call for this remedy often appear after exposure to cold damp weather or climates. Hot bathing and warm applications usually alleviate the symptoms. Joint pains often appear or worsen after overexertion.

Clinical use: See "Itching," "Insect Bites and Stings," and "Hotspots" in *Skin and Ears*, "Conjunctivitis" and "Corneal Ulcers" in *Eyes*, "Arthritic Conditions" and "Sprains and Strains" in *Musculoskeletal System*, "Paraphimosis and Phimosis," "Orchitis," and "Postpartum Infections" in *Reproductive System*, and "Allergic Reactions" in *Therapeutic Indications by Condition*.

Ricinus communis (Castor oil plant)
The only indication I list for *Ricinus* is for increasing milk flow. Low potencies (e.g. 3X) work best. A poultice of the leaves may also help. Edgar Cayce recommended castor oil as a topical application for many conditions as a detoxing agent.

Clinical use: See "Inadequate Milk Flow" in *Reproductive System*.

Rumex crispus (Yellow dock)
Yellow dock is a liver strengthening and cleansing herb, and the homeopathic remedy can also help liver conditions. The herb is also helpful topically to soothe itchy skin and ears. The primary indication for the homeopathic medicine is for coughs that are caused by an incessant tickling sensation in the throat. Cold air worsens all symptoms when *Rumex* is indicated. A change from warm to cold or cold to warm may also worsen the condition.

Clinical use: See "Cough" in *Respiratory System, Nose, and Sinuses* and "Liver Disorders" in *Therapeutic Indications by Condition*.

Ruta graveolens (Rue)
Ruta is similar to *Rhus tox* in its application for joint pains and injuries. *Ruta*'s special affinity is to tendons, especially flexor tendons. Bone bruises and knee injuries may also call for *Ruta*. This remedy also has similar indications to *Arnica*, for sprains and other injuries where the area feels deeply bruised. The *Ruta* patient is not as sensitive to touch as those needing *Arnica*. Animals that need *Ruta* may be somewhat irritable and quarrelsome. They may also have red, irritated eyes that tear constantly. They may have great difficulty passing stools, requiring much straining. The anus may prolapse when *Ruta* patients pass bowel movements. *Ruta* conditions often arise from overexertion and injuries. Sitting, resting, and cold worsen the symptoms, while motion and warmth alleviate them.

Clinical use: See "Arthritic Conditions," "Panosteitis," "First Aid for Broken Bones," and "Sprains and Strains" in *Musculoskeletal System*, "Injuries to the Brain and Spinal Cord" in *Nervous System*, and "Postpartum Pains" in *Reproductive System*.

Sabadilla (Cevadilla seed)

These patients tend toward nervousness and timidity, and they are easily startled, often by noise. This nervousness may alternate with the physical symptoms. There is much action on mucous membranes, with hay fever and cold-like symptoms. They may be itchy also, as though being bitten by fleas. Symptoms may start on the right side and move to the left. Often they have little thirst, and they may be averse to strong-smelling foods. They prefer hot foods and warmth in general, though they are often better in open air overall. The watery eye discharge, however, often increases in open air. They may worsen at the same time each day, just before noon, or at the new and full moons. Strong odors in general may aggravate the condition.

Clinical use: See "Sneezing and Nasal Discharge" in *Respiratory System, Nose, and Sinuses* and "Conjunctivitis" in *Eyes*.

Sabal serrulata (Saw palmetto)

Like the herb from which this remedy is made, *Sabal* has a strong affinity to the prostate gland. There may be an eye inflammation when the prostate gland is affected. Undeveloped mammary glands may also respond to *Sabal*. These animals generally do not like petting or sympathy, and they may walk away or otherwise express displeasure at too much attention. They may also dribble urine or leak urine in their sleep. Cold, damp, cloudy weather, as well as sympathy, may worsen their symptoms.

Clinical use: See "Prostate Affections" in *Reproductive System*.

Sabina (Savine)

This remedy has an affinity to the uterus and the bones. Many of these animals have a tendency to spontaneous abortion, especially about one-third (three weeks for cats and dogs) into the pregnancy. There may also be a tendency to hemorrhage bright red blood. *Sabina* patients are often sad and melancholic, especially in the morning. The symptoms are generally worse at night and in warmth, especially in warm rooms, and they are better in cool open air.

Clinical use: See "Arthritic Conditions" and "Panosteitis" in *Musculoskeletal System* and "Discharge from the Vulva" and "Postpartum Infections" in *Reproductive System*.

Sarsaparilla (Wild licorice; Red-bearded sarsaparilla)

In addition to its affinity to urinary system inflammation, this remedy is sometimes helpful for skin eruptions that follow vaccination. This is not infrequent in young animals; perhaps administering *Sarsaparilla* at this time would prevent later urinary problems in some of these individuals. There may be deep cracks around the toes in these patients as well. Animals that need this remedy may be despondent and easily offended, especially when they are in pain. Their symptoms may appear in the spring during cold wet weather.

Clinical use: See "Cystitis" in *Urinary System.*

Secale cornutum (Rye ergot)

Secale is said by many to be very like *Arsenicum album,* except that the patient is warm rather than chilly. This is true regarding many symptoms, especially the intestinal ones. *Secale* differs greatly, however, in its strong affinity to the uterus. The remedy is made from ergot, a fungus that grows on rye. The compound ergotamine has been isolated from the fungus; it is effective in inducing labor. *Secale* also has this property, and it is much safer. Other effects shared by the drug and the remedy are the ability to constrict blood vessels and slow hemorrhage. Animals that need this remedy are worse from warmth and better from cold applications and cold bathing. They are often ravenous.

Clinical use: See "Discharge from the Vulva," "Retained Placenta," "Postpartum Infections," and "Rejection of Puppies or Kittens" in *Reproductive System.*

Selenium (Selenium)

This element is below sulfur in the periodic table, and the remedy *Selenium* is similar to *Sulphur,* though the latter is much better known and utilized. These animals are sluggish and debilitated, and much worse in heat, particularly in the summer. The skin and coat are generally scaly and dirty, and hair may fall out in clumps or handfuls. A deficiency of the mineral may lead to muscle weakness; the remedy may also help some animals with weakness of muscles. The remedy is also useful for some prostate conditions. Weakness is usually present when this remedy is needed. The patient is worse in the day (especially hot days) and better after sunset. He may be deeply sad.

Clinical use: See "Prostate Affections" in *Reproductive System* and "Overheating" in *Therapeutic Indications by Condition*.

Sepia (Cuttlefish ink)

The cuttlefish is a mollusc in the same family as the squid and the octopus. These animals use their ink as a screen to hide them from potential predators. *Sepia* individuals, in a sense, share this desire to hide, but they remain hidden from and indifferent to their family and friends. These animals are among the chilliest; even when the room is warm they will sit in the sun or near another heat source. *Phosphorus* animals also do this, but they are easy to distinguish from those needing *Sepia*. The latter are sad or indifferent, and they prefer to be alone much of the time.

Greenish or yellow discharges are common in *Sepia* patients, especially from the nose and the vulva. This remedy is more commonly needed for females—it has an affinity to the uterus. Cold and cold air are intolerable to these animals and may worsen their symptoms. Warmth and hard exercise alleviates the *Sepia* state.

Clinical use: See "Constipation" in *Digestive System*; "Sneezing and Nasal Discharge" in *Respiratory System, Nose, and Sinuses*; "Urinary Incontinence" in *Urinary System*; and "Discharge from the Vulva," "Postpartum Infections," and "Rejection of Puppies and Kittens" in *Reproductive System*.

Serum anguillae (Ichthyotoxinum; Eel serum)

Eel serum causes kidney shutdown, and the homeopathic remedy can assist some cases of acute kidney disease.

Clinical use: See "Decreasing Kidney Function" in *Urinary System*.

Silicea (Silica) (Pure flint)

Silicea is one of our major remedies. This is probably due in large part to its effectiveness in removing some of the impacts from heavily vaccinated animals. Here it rivals *Thuja*, the remedy best known for vaccinosis. Animals that need *Silicea* tend to have a lot of skin troubles. They cannot heal injuries easily, so they have a lot of abscesses and suppurating (discharging pus) wounds. The bones are often weak and poorly formed as well—this remedy is helpful in many bone diseases. Diseases of the feet and the nails (including hooves) often respond to *Silicea*.

These animals are pale, delicate, and weakly, though they may be beautiful in their fine lines. Their frailness and poor nutrition is often obvious at a glance. They simply have little strength, whether for healing, for exercise, or even for passing stools. They are often timid, especially in new situations. The *Silicea* state is one of great sensitivity—to new impressions, to noise, to light, and to cold. Cold is almost always intolerable, while warmth may lessen their symptoms.

Silicea is very similar to *Mercurius*, but these remedies should not be given after or before one another. See the note under *Mercurius*. See also *Equisetum*, a small remedy that is similar and may be useful in some circumstances when *Silicea* is indicated but does not work as well as hoped.

Clinical use: See "Itching" and "Mange" in *Skin and Ears;* "Abscessed and Decaying Teeth" in *Mouth, Gums, and Teeth;* "Constipation" in *Digestive System;* "Sneezing and Nasal Discharge" in *Respiratory System, Nose, and Sinuses;* "Hypopyon" in *Eyes;* "Arthritic Conditions," "Hypertrophic Osteodystrophy," "Osteochondritis Dissecans," "Rickets," and "Legg-Calve-Perthes Disease" in *Musculoskeletal System;* "Discharge from the Sheath" and "Bad Milk" in *Reproductive System;* and "Abscesses" and "Vaccine Reactions" in *Therapeutic Indications by Condition.*

Solidago (Goldenrod)

We mostly think of goldenrod for its allergenic potential, as many humans develop hay fever upon exposure to the pollen. While the remedy does have some affinity to the eyes and nose with hay fever symptoms, *Solidago*'s influence is most important in the urinary system. You may see hay fever–like symptoms, however, in a patient with urinary disorders. The eyes may be red, burning, and watery along with the nose. There may also be a loose cough. The rear legs may have blotchy redness, even swelling, with the chronic nephritis (kidney inflammation). See Chapter Eleven, on the kidneys, for symptoms pertaining to that system.

Clinical use: See "Cystitis," "Urethral Obstruction and Catheterization," and "Decreasing Kidney Function" in *Urinary System.*

Spiranthes (Lady's tresses)

This remedy has an affinity to the breasts and to milk production. It may either encourage or diminish milk flow. Low potencies will more likely stimulate flow, while higher potencies may reduce the flow. The animal may be drowsy and may yawn a lot when *Spiranthes* is needed.

Clinical use: See "Inadequate Milk Flow" and "To Dry up Milk Following Weaning" in *Reproductive System*.

Spongia tosta (Roasted sponge)

Spongia is primarily utilized for coughs and respiratory conditions, though it also plays a part in some pancreatitis cases. Dry cold winds often bring about a *Spongia* illness. These animals may be anxious and fearful, and they often have a tendency to start from sleep. They may be very thirsty and hungry as an accompaniment, and eating can lessen their symptoms, especially the coughing. Eating usually worsens the stomach pain. Exertion and excitement, along with cold winds, worsen or incite the symptoms, while calmness and warmth generally alleviate the condition.

Clinical use: See "Regurgitation and Vomiting" in *Digestive System* and "Cough" in *Respiratory System, Nose, and Sinuses*.

Staphysagria (Stavesacre; Louse wort)

When *Staphysagria* is the indicated remedy, many of the symptoms have arisen following trauma. For the acute conditions listed in this book, the trauma is generally physical, such as lacerations and catheterization. When the remedy is used in chronic diseases, the trauma is emotional. Indignation for past offenses and repressed anger well up inside until they are released as irritability, rage, or physical disease. Any strong emotions and quarrels can worsen these patients.

In most injuries that call for *Staphysagria*, the wound is quite painful. Clean-cut wounds more often indicate the remedy than torn, blunt injuries (*Arnica* or *Calendula* are for the latter).

Clinical use: See "Abscessed and Decaying Teeth" and "Homeopathic Remedies for Dental Care and Extractions" in *Mouth, Gums, and Teeth;* "Injuries to the Eyes" in *Eyes;* "Cystitis" and "Urethral Obstruction and Catheterization" in *Urinary System;* "Injuries to the Testicles" and "Prostate Affections" in *Reproductive System;* and "Cuts and Lacerations" and "Surgery" in *Therapeutic Indications by Condition*.

Stramonium (Thorn apple)

This remedy is made from a hallucinogenic plant. The hallucinogenic state in this case is often dominated by terror; the terror induces muscle-tensing anxiety that often leads to aggression. The homeopathic medicine is frequently indicated for aggression that is based upon fear and terror. The state may arise from rabies vaccination.

The physical state is one of tension—the sympathetic nervous system (fright, fight, and flight) is often primed and ready. These animals are often afraid of the dark and may stay close to the bed, cry out, or even intentionally waken their guardians during the night for no apparent reason. Bright lights and mirrors may startle and frighten them as well. They generally do not wish to be alone; their fears are too strong.

Clinical use: See "Aggression" in *Nervous System*, "Eclampsia" in *Reproductive System*, and "Fear" and "Fear of Noise" in *Therapeutic Indications by Condition*.

Strontium carbonicum (Strontium carbonate)

Many *Strontium carb* symptoms follow hemorrhage; this leads to deep weariness, including collapse. The patient may also be anxious and fearful, be afraid of the dark, and startle easily. They may also react against their fear by becoming snappish and ill-humored as a protection. Cold, darkness, motion, touch, change of weather, and hemorrhage worsen these individuals, while warmth, light, and sun improve them. Human patients feel much better soaking in a hot bath; your dog may also desire this if he is in a *Strontium carb* state. Shock and collapse following hemorrhage during surgery is the primary acute indication, though the remedy has many chronic ones.

Clinical use: See "Surgery" in *Therapeutic Indications by Condition*.

Strychninum (Strychnine)

Strychnine poisoning causes extreme muscle tension and contraction, as well as a violent spasm in response to noises. The remedy *Strychninum* is made from strychnine. It is unlikely to significantly help an accidental poisoning from strychnine, but if similar symptoms arise from other causes, the remedy may help greatly. Eclampsia is the primary cause of this condition in dogs and is one of the few indications for the remedy. *Strychninum* may also be useful in other cases of strong muscle spasm.

Muscle reflexes will almost always be extremely increased when this remedy is needed. The pupils may be dilated as well. The plants from which *Nux vomica* and *Ignatia* are made contain strychnine, so there is similarity among these three remedies.

Clinical use: See "Eclampsia" in *Reproductive System*.

Sulphur (Sulfur)

This remedy is sometimes called the king of remedies or the chief polychrest. It has perhaps the broadest application of all the remedies in our *materia medica*, though it is most useful for chronic illness. In fact, this remedy is often not recommended for acute usage or as the first remedy in a chronic case unless the symptoms clearly and absolutely call for *Sulphur*. Otherwise, it may incite an aggravation.

Nevertheless, I have given a few indications for its use, though these are often cases when other remedies fail to cure and the condition relapses. When *Sulphur* is needed, the animal often has a poor immune system that simply cannot heal conditions that other animals readily heal. In this respect, it is similar to *Silicea*. The classic *Sulphur* animal is unkempt, as he has little interest in appearance. He is generally good-natured and friendly, and he is usually very intelligent. Dennis the Menace and the absent-minded professor are stereotypic *Sulphur* human characters. The remedy is well represented among dogs and cats as well.

These animals are usually thirsty and warm. They often have sparse appetites (their minds are more important than their bodies), though some animals have large appetites. The coat in a *Sulphur* animal is usually dry and rough, and the skin is often flaky. Standing is uncomfortable, so these animals either move around or quickly lie down. In a sense, they seem lazy. The eyes and other body openings may be deeply red, with clear or whitish discharge. Bathing often worsens the symptoms. Burning is common; the skin may itch and burn, and the anus often itches and burns when this remedy is needed. These animals may therefore scoot constantly on the ground or on carpets. They are often flea- and worm-infested. In short, these animals may not look the greatest, but they are usually a joy to have around.

Clinical use: See "Mange" and "Ear Mites" in *Skin and Ears*; "Diarrhea" in *Digestive System*; "Sneezing and Nasal Discharge" in *Respiratory System, Nose, and Sinuses*; "Conjunctivitis" and "Corneal Ulcers" in *Eyes*; "Decreasing Kidney Function" in *Urinary System*; "Discharge from the Sheath" and "Runts and Dwarfishness" in *Reproductive System;* and "Abscesses," "Fever and Infections," and "Fleas" in *Therapeutic Indications by Condition.*

Sulphur iodatum (Sulfur iodide)

This remedy is similar in many ways to *Sulphur,* but the iodine component makes it even hotter. Chin acne may respond to this remedy, though this disease is best treated by an experienced homeopath. The main acute indication is for constipation. These animals are often sluggish, and they dislike exertion.

Clinical use: See "Constipation" in *Digestive System.*

Sycotic co (Neisseria mucosa and Moraxella catarrhalis)

This remedy is one of the bowel nosodes, a group of remedies first made by doctors Bach (of the flower essences) and Paterson. These remedies were made from bowel organisms, which tend to overgrow during certain illnesses. *Sycotic co* has a great affinity to the sycotic miasm, which affects mucous membranes all over the body, generally producing catarrhal (mucus) discharges. These discharges may be in the urogenital system, the bronchi, the digestive system, or the upper respiratory system. Discharges are often yellow-green and thick. Cold damp weather worsens the illness, while being at the seaside may improve it. These animals tend to be fearful, especially of the dark, being alone, and of dogs or other animals, and they can be irritable as well. This may result in occasional outbursts in an otherwise reticent animal. This remedy can be very helpful in some upper respiratory conditions.

Clinical use: See "Gingivitis and Mouth Inflammation" in *Mouth, Gums, and Teeth* and "Conjunctivitis" in *Eyes.*

Symphytum (Comfrey; Boneset)

Comfrey is an herb with great healing properties. It stimulates healing of ulcerated sores, including stomach ulcers, and it is very effective at stimulating bone healing. The homeopathic remedy is especially useful for healing fractures, including those that heal slowly or not at all (nonunions) without the remedy. *Symphytum* is also a primary remedy for eye injuries.

Clinical use: See "Injuries to the Eyes" in *Eyes* and "Osteochondritis Dissecans" and "First Aid for Broken Bones" in *Musculoskeletal System.*

Syphilinum (Syphilis)

This remedy is a nosode. It is a very deep-acting remedy, and it has much indication in animals, even though it is a nosode of a human disease (syphilis). It is especially indicated for many ulcerated and decaying conditions. The remedy should always be used under the direction of an experienced homeopathic practitioner. I list it in the book as a suggestion for homeopathic veterinarians. In the United States the remedy is available by prescription only. It is also called *Luesinum*, usually by French sources.

Clinical use: See "Gingivitis and Mouth Inflammation" and "Ranula" in *Mouth, Gums, and Teeth;* "Conjunctivitis" and "Corneal Ulcers" in *Eyes;* "Osteochondritis Dissecans" and "Panosteitis" in *Musculoskeletal System;* and "Retained Testicle" in *Reproductive System.*

Taraxicum (Dandelion)

Here the primary affinity is to the liver and stomach; the kidney is also affected. Depression is common, as is a general sick feeling. There is appetite loss and a bitter taste in the mouth, often with bitter burping. These patients may prefer to sit and not move, but they actually improve by motion and walking around. They are also better in open air.

Clinical use: See "Liver Disorders" in *Therapeutic Indications by Condition.*

Tarentula cubensis (Cuban spider venom)

This remedy is sometimes indicated for intense inflammation with great pain. The tissues become hard and develop a bluish hue, and they burn like fire. The remedy is said to prevent bubonic plague if given during incubation. It may also help prevent damage from a brown recluse spider if given soon after the bite. Do not confuse this remedy with *Tarentula hispanica,* though the latter is somewhat similar. *Tarentula cubensis* is regularly helpful in some animals who have painful, difficult deaths.

Clinical use: See "Insect Bites and Stings" in *Skin and Ears* and "Abscesses" and "Euthanasia" in *Therapeutic Indications by Condition.*

Theridion (Orange spider)

Theridion has great nerve sensitivity, both to noise and to pains. Bone pains can be especially sharp, and noises seem to penetrate deeply. The patient may be acutely sensitive to these noises. There may be stinging pains anywhere. (Many spider remedies share this burning inflammatory state.) Noise, touch, and motion (especially jarring motion, like a bumpy car ride) worsen these patients, while rest and warmth ameliorate them.

Clinical use: See "Panosteitis" in *Musculoskeletal System.*

Thiosinaminum (Mustard seed oil)

This oil can dissolve scar tissue, both topically as well as internally, the latter in homeopathic form. It may help anywhere there is scar tissue, but its primary known indications include dissolving adhesions following abdominal surgery and helping with fibrous deposits in the ear following otitis. It has helped many people with tinnitus (ringing in the ears), also from the scarring. It has also been used successfully in fibrous uterine changes that resulted in infertility in women with pelvic inflammatory disease. I have used the remedy in posturethrostomy strictures as well as in other cases where scar tissue was an issue. It is possibly also useful for cataract and tear-duct strictures, especially following inflammation or injury.

Clinical use: See "Aural Hematomas" in *Skin and Ears,* "Urethral Obstruction and Catheterization" in *Urinary System,* and "Surgery" in *Therapeutic Indications by Condition.*

Thlaspi bursa pastoris (Shepherd's purse)

Thlaspi has one primary acute indication: cystitis and urethral obstruction. It is also occasionally indicated for hemorrhage. Herbally, shepherd's purse is also used for some uterine complaints. Prolonged estrus and bleeding may respond; the animal may start the next cycle shortly following the end of the last one. Animals that need this remedy may have a tendency to walk or pace constantly.

Clinical use: See "Cystitis" and "Urethral Obstruction and Catheterization" in *Urinary System.*

Thuja occidentalis (Arbor vitae)

Thuja is one of our commonly needed remedies for vaccinosis, or disease that arises as a consequence of vaccination. Much of the damage of vaccination centers in the urogenital systems, the spinal cord, and the skin. *Thuja* also has affinity to these regions. Many animals respond favorably to a dose of *Thuja* because of prior vaccination. Generally, the remedy is used more for chronic than acute conditions, and it may help in some cases where other remedies fail to work because the vaccine influence is too strong.

These animals often have a number of warts, moles, and other skin lumps. The coat may be poor, and the hair falls out easily or may split easily. *Thuja* patients are generally chilly, and especially sensitive to cold damp conditions. They are often fearful of strangers and of new situations.

Many people use this remedy as a routine preventive against vaccine damage. The idea is that one can vaccinate an animal and then administer *Thuja* to reverse any damage while allowing the vaccine to protect against disease. This idea is incorrect. It is unlikely that the *Thuja* will reverse the vaccine damage, and the vaccines generally do more harm than good. See Chapter Sixteen, "Vaccination," for more information.

Clinical use: See "Ringworm" in *Skin and Ears;* "Ranula" and "Abscessed and Decaying Teeth" in *Mouth, Gums, and Teeth;* "Hypopyon" and "Corneal Ulcers" in *Eyes;* "Cystitis" and "Urethral Obstruction and Catheterization" in *Urinary System;* "Hypertrophic Osteodystrophy" in *Musculoskeletal System;* "Degenerative Myelopathy" and "Injuries to the Brain and Spinal Cord" in *Nervous System;* "Discharge from the Sheath," "Prostate Affections," and "Weak Kittens or Puppies" in *Reproductive System;* and "Drug Reactions" and Vaccine Reactions" in *Therapeutic Indications by Condition.*

Thyroidinum (Dried thyroid gland)
This remedy is mostly used supportively for the thyroid gland in low potencies, or to limit the gland in high potencies. This should only be done under the care of an experienced homeopath. Low potencies may help some cases of retained testicle or some animals who do not grow properly.

Clinical use: See "Retained Testicle" in *Reproductive System.*

Tuberculinum (Tuberculosis)
This remedy, like *Syphilinum,* is a nosode. In this case, it is made from a tuberculous bovine lung. In the United States this remedy is available by prescription only, and it should be used only under the direction of an experienced homeopathic prescriber. I list some indications as suggestions for homeopathic veterinarians. The remedy is useful in humans for attention deficit and hyperactivity disorders, and I have had some success in hyperactive animals with *Tuberculinum.*

Bacillinum may be a better choice for patients who live in humid locales, whereas *Tuberculinum* may be better suited to those in dry climates.

Clinical use: See "Legg-Calve-Perthes Disease" in *Musculoskeletal System* and "Retained Testicle" in *Reproductive System.*

Urtica urens (Stinging nettle)

When this remedy is needed, there is usually itching, burning, or stinging somewhere. The remedy has an affinity to the skin, the urinary tract, the joints, and the mammary glands. Eating shellfish often causes problems for these animals, and *Urtica* will counteract the damage. Symptoms may predominantly occur on the right side, and the body may smell like urine. Nettle tea is a good kidney tonic.

Clinical use: See "Itching" and "Burns and Scalds" in *Skin and Ears,* "Cystitis" in *Urinary System,* "Inadequate Milk Flow," "To Dry up Milk Following Weaning," and "Mastitis" in *Reproductive System,* and "Allergic Reactions" in *Therapeutic Indications by Condition.*

Uva ursi (Bearberry, Kinnick kinnick)

This low-growing shrub has beautiful red berries; the plant is a great urinary tonic and anti-inflammatory, though it should only be used short-term in herbal form as it can irritate the bladder. Urine often contains mucus and blood and may contain large clots. If blood clots obstruct urine flow, consider this remedy. The urine often has a pungent strong odor.

Clinical use: See "Cystitis" and "Urethral Obstruction and Catheterization" in *Urinary System.*

Vaccin atténué bilié (BCG)

This remedy is made from Bacillus Calmette-Guérin, an attenuated form of the tuberculosis organism that has been used for vaccination against tuberculosis. It is also commonly included in killed vaccines as an immune-system stimulant. The homeopathic remedy is related to *Tuberculinum.* The only indication I know is for Legg-Calve-Perthes disease.

Animals that need this remedy will appear similar to those needing *Calcarea phosphorica* or *Silicea.* They will be chilly, thin, weakly, and poorly developed. They may fatigue easily, and they will probably be sensitive to noises. Digestion is poor in these animals; they may bloat easily after foods, and the slow transit time creates chronic constipation. They may have a rough dry cough and a persistent eye inflammation. The glands in the throat may be swollen. Symptoms may predominate on the left side. They will generally be worse from exercise and at the end of the day, and better from eating and stretching. In short, these are animals that came into the world weak and frail.

This remedy is rare. It is available to licensed health care practitioners from Boiron Laboratories in France, though it cannot be shipped to the United States due to FDA regulations. The remedy *BCG* is available at Helios, however, and it is essentially the same.

Clinical use: See "Legg-Calve-Perthes Disease" in *Musculoskeletal System*.

Veratrum album (White hellebore)

Veratrum is similar in many ways to *Arsenicum album*, but the symptoms are generally more intense when *Veratrum* is needed. Vomiting and diarrhea—often sudden and violent—predominate in this remedy state. The animal is often weak, cold, and collapsed as well. He may be cold to the touch, especially on his nose, ears, and feet. The nails may be bluish from the cold. Obviously, this animal needs veterinary care, but the *Veratrum* may pull him out of a tailspin.

Drinking water, even the slightest exertion, and wet cold weather worsen the symptoms, while warmth and rest alleviate the condition. Eating meat may improve the condition as well if the animal is not too ill. These patients are generally weak, but if not, they may be irritable.

Clinical use: See "Vomiting" and "Diarrhea" in *Digestive System* and "Food and Garbage Poisoning" in *Therapeutic Indications by Condition*.

Veratrum viride (Green hellebore; American white hellebore; Indian poke)

This remedy is related to *Veratrum album*. Many symptoms are similar. This remedy, however, has a tendency toward vascular congestion and intense heat conditions. Spasms and twitching are common as well. Prostration may follow the congestion. The pupils are often dilated, and there is an intense headache. All symptoms worsen if the patient attempts to rise from a recumbent position.

Clinical use: See "Overheating" in *Therapeutic Indications by Condition*.

Vespa crabro (European hornet)

Similarly to *Apis*, the honeybee venom, *Vespa* can be useful in allergic reactions or reactions that look like allergic ones. The patient is intensely itchy all over, especially around the affected area. Heat worsens and cold water ameliorates the itching and burning. Vinegar applications also help. The eyes may be bright red, itchy, and swollen (chemotic). They may also be glassy and bloodshot. The throat and mouth may be swollen, affecting vocalization and/or breathing. Nausea and vomiting may accompany the reaction, and the patient may be dizzy. There may be urinary urging with burning pains, also usually accompanying an allergic reaction. Bite wounds tend to be red and hot, like a sting.

Clinical use: See "Insect Bites and Stings" in *Skin and Ears* and "Bites of Cats and Dogs" in *Therapeutic Indications by Condition*.

Vipera (Common viper)

This remedy is made from a snake venom, and it is sometimes employed against the effects of snakebites. The wounds are extremely painful. There may also be an increase in reflexes, followed by a paresis (partial paralysis) in the rear legs. The patient must keep the legs elevated, as they are extremely painful if they hang down. There may be blood in the urine and kidney malfunction as well.

Clinical use: See "Bites of Snakes" in *Therapeutic Indications by Condition*.

Yohimbinum (Yohimbine)

The herb yohimbine has stimulatory effects on the male genitalia and the male sex drive. The homeopathic remedy is occasionally useful to calm oversexed male dogs who frequently mount humans and animals.

Clinical use: See "Hypersexual Behavior" in *Reproductive System*.

APPENDIX

GLOSSARY

HOMEOPATHIC AND HOLISTIC ORGANIZATIONS

HOMEOPATHIC SUPPLIERS

NOTES

SUGGESTED READING AND REFERENCE BOOKS

GLOSSARY

Acute. A condition that has arisen rapidly. Acute conditions are generally more intense than chronic conditions, though the term refers more to the time factor than to the intensity. There are four time-related classifications of illness: peracute, acute, subacute, and chronic (listed in order, with peracute being the most rapid and chronic being the slowest-moving). As used in homeopathic parlance, an acute disease is one that moves rapidly through the body and is relatively self-limiting. It is also possible to have an acute manifestation of a chronic illness, wherein the slow, insidious progress suddenly intensifies and moves into a more rapid progression. See also *chronic*, below; Chapter Two, "The Nature of Disease"; and Chapter Five, "Using Homeopathy at Home."

Aggravation. Sometimes, within a short time of administration of a homeopathic medicine, the patient experiences a brief intensification of symptoms. This usually occurs primarily in the physical symptoms, and often the patient feels emotionally and psychologically better despite the intensification. It is also called a healing crisis. See Chapter Three, "The Nature of Cure."

Allopathy. *(allos* = "other" + *pathos* = "disease")* The treatment of disease by opposing the body's efforts—treatment by contraries. Allopathic doctors treat the disease rather than the individual. We generally use the term to refer to the Western medical school that dominates medicine today. We sometimes also refer to this as conventional medicine. See Chapter One, "Introduction to Homeopathy."

Autoimmune. Disease that occurs as a consequence of the inability of the immune system to differentiate self from nonself. The result is that the immune system may attack components of its own body. The damage that follows is recognized as autoimmune disease. Examples include allergies, lupus, rheumatoid arthritis, most thyroid illnesses, many blood diseases, inflammatory bowel disease, and so on. Essentially, a huge percentage of the illness that veterinarians and physicians see today is autoimmune.

Chemosis. An extremely inflamed eye condition. The eye is red and intensely swollen under the lids (the conjunctiva are swollen), as though from a chemical irritation. See Chapter Ten, "Eyes."

Chronic. See *acute* above. A chronic disease moves slowly and insidiously, taking weeks to years to manifest. These conditions are often autoimmune, and they generally originate from poor nutrition, vaccination, and/or toxicity. It is unreasonable to expect these illnesses to disappear in less than a few months, and sometimes it takes one to three years to reverse the damage. Chronic disease is common today, and acute diseases have become less common. Much illness that we believe is acute is actually an acute manifestation of chronic illness. A good example of this in an outbreak of cystitis (urinary bladder inflammation) or hotspots on the skin. These are almost always chronic diseases, not acute diseases. See also Chapter Two, "The Nature of Disease," and Chapter Five, "Using Homeopathy at Home."

Combination remedy. A homeopathic remedy that is made by combining several different remedies, often in different potencies, into one formula. For example, some companies market a remedy for diarrhea that has several remedies that may be helpful. The theory is that the body will choose the remedy it needs from the potpourri of remedies. Some people find combination remedies helpful for acute self-limiting conditions, but they should not be used for serious illness, and they should not be continued for more than a week or so. It is possible, though unlikely, to worsen the condition by excessive repetition of incorrect remedies.

Constitutional treatment. Different practitioners use this term in many different ways. Essentially, it refers to treating the constitution, or the state of the entire body. By this definition, any time the correct homeopathic remedy is administered, it is a constitutional prescription. Most references to constitutional treatment, however, refer to the idea that an individual has a general tendency to remain in a similar state throughout her life, thus the correct constitutional remedy will remain the same. Once this remedy is found, it will correct almost any ailment or imbalance she suffers. Thus, she may be said to be a *"Pulsatilla"* animal, for example. A dose of *Pulsatilla* will generally return this patient to health. In my experience, this occurs in some patients and not in others. Other patients move through different remedy states over time and with homeopathic treatment. Some people refer to these as layers that are removed as though one were peeling an onion. Attempting to treat a deeper layer will not succeed, as each layer must be removed in sequence according to this model. As with any model, this one is useful but not totally accurate. It is perhaps more useful to think of the different remedy states as rather interwoven. Finally, "constitutional treatment" is sometimes used interchangeably with "chronic disease treatment." In this case, the suggestion is that an individual's illness is not acute, such as a cold that arose from outside, but rather is an expression of the constitutional weakness. The animal thus needs constitutional, chronic-disease treatment for the underlying susceptibility, rather than an acute remedy for the most obvious symptoms. I often adopt this last usage in the treatment chapters. See also Chapter Five, "Using Homeopathy at Home."

Cortisone. A drug produced from adrenal tissue of slaughtered animals. It is anti-inflammatory and immunosuppressive. It is rarely used today, as it has been mostly replaced by synthetic corticosteroids like prednisone. Many practitioners still use the term erroneously when they administer any related drugs, especially by injection. For this reason I place the word in quotation marks when I use it in the book.

Cure. To permanently remove symptoms of disease, with overall improvement in all aspects of health. See Chapter Three, "The Nature of Cure." See also *palliation* and *suppression*.

Eruption. In medical parlance, a lesion on the skin or a mucous membrane, such as acne, pustules, pimples, and ulcers.

Homeopathic remedy. In general usage, we refer to homeopathic remedies as medicines that have been prepared according to homeopathic methods—succussion and dilution. Technically, a remedy is only homeopathic if it is the correct remedy for a given individual. It must be similar to the disease to fit the definition (see below under *homeopathy*). Thus the homeopathic remedy is the simillimum.

Homeopathy. *(homeo* = "like" + *pathos* = "disease")* Treating disease with small doses of substances that, in large doses, can induce symptoms similar to those of the disease. In addition, homeopathic doctors treat the entire organism (the individual), not just the disease.

Infusion. An herbal solution made by pouring boiling water over dry or fresh herbs and allowing the herbs to steep until cool. It is essentially the same as making a tea, though we allow the solution to cool before straining off the herb.

Isopathy. *(iso* = "same" + *pathos* = "disease")* An offshoot of homeopathy wherein a nosode (see below) is made from the disease and *then used to treat that same disease.* It is generally not as effective as classical homeopathy—the best response occurs when a homeopathic remedy is individually prescribed to the sick individual, not to the disease. Isopathy can help in some cases, however, such as with infectious respiratory disease outbreaks in a kennel or a barn. Here the isopathic remedy may help prevent spread of the disease. Using a remedy made from a drug or a vaccine, called Tautopathy, however, can be very effective. Sometimes this latter use is incorrectly called isopathy, although isopathy is limited to remedies made from the disease, such as from a discharge.

-itis. A suffix that indicates inflammation. Thus iritis is inflammation of the iris, appendicitis is inflammation of the appendix, and so on. Conventional practitioners tend to equate inflammation with infection, but this is incorrect. Unfortunately, this assumption results in many individuals taking antibiotics unnecessarily.

Materia medica. A textbook that describes medicines and their usage. The translation from Latin is "materials of medicine." A *materia medica* is roughly equivalent to the *Physicians' Desk Reference* (PDR). It does not specifically indicate homeopathic medicines, as conventional drugs were described in *materia medicas* until this century. Currently, however, the only *materia medicas* of which I am aware are for homeopathic remedies.

Miasm. Refers to a tendency to disease. While the word originally indicated a disease tendency that was the result of an outside force or substance, we now use the term to describe the manner in which disease affects the body. There are three primary miasmas: psora, which is a tendency to underrespond to illness; sycosis, which is a tendency to overrespond to illness (such as with warts and tumors); and syphilis, wherein the animal's immune system causes destruction to the body (such as with ulcers). Each system tends to affect certain parts of the body, though there is overlap.

Nosode. A homeopathic medicine that is made from a product of disease. *Distemperinum,* for example, was made from the mucus secretion of a dog with distemper. In this example, it is important to understand that a remedy made from a laboratory culture of the distemper virus would not be the same. It is not the infectious organism alone but the essence of the disease that is captured in the nosode. Nosodes are then used in two ways. First, they are proven (see *proving* below) to determine their scope of symptoms, and this allows them to be prescribed according to homeopathic indications. Secondly, they may be used as a preventive against the disease in another member of the species. While there is much controversy around this latter usage, I have found it generally effective *if the nosode is given at about the same time as the exposure* to the infectious organism. It does not work well if given more than a few days in advance. Administration is probably best during the incubation period—the time between exposure and the first appearance of symptoms.

-osis. A suffix that indicates an abnormal, diseased condition, but the condition is not generally inflammatory. It may also denote an increase, especially when relating to blood or immune cells. For example, a neurosis is abnormal mental functioning, vaccinosis is disease caused by vaccination, and a leukocytosis is an increase in the white blood cells.

Palliation. Palliation is temporary improvement of one or more physical symptoms without affecting the underlying disease. In acute, self-limiting conditions, the disease may then disappear under its own momentum, but in chronic conditions the disease continues to worsen. See Chapter Three, "The Nature of Cure"; see also *cure* and *suppression*.

Polychrest. A polychrest remedy has broad application. It fits a large number of cases, and in essence may be considered to represent a major type or category of individuals. These remedies tend to be overused and overrepresented in the literature, but they are still generally of greater indication than other remedies. Some of the main polychrests include *Sulphur, Lycopodium, Pulsatilla, Phosphorus, Calcarea carbonica, Arsenicum album, Natrum muriaticum, Silicea,* and *Nux vomica*—but there are many more.

Potency/potentization. The potency represents the strength of a homeopathic remedy. Each remedy can be prepared at different potencies, according to the preparation. The potency is not a representation of the material quantity of the remedy, but rather its energetic strength. Thus, the potency scale is not additive—in other words, two pellets of 6C do not equal a 12C potency. Potentization occurs when the remedy is diluted and succussed (shaken) in sequential steps. See Chapter One, "Introduction to Homeopathy," and Chapter Five, "Using Homeopathy at Home," for more information.

Proving. The testing of homeopathic medicines on healthy people to determine their usefulness. The proving identifies the characteristics of each medicine, and this information is incorporated into our *materia medicas* and repertories so that it is accessible. *Proving* is an adaptation of the German word *prufung*, which means "testing." See Chapter One, "Introduction to Homeopathy."

Purulent. Discharging or containing pus.

Repertory. A stock or collection. In homeopathic parlance, it refers to a text that catalogs symptoms and conditions and then gives a list of each remedy that has the symptom or condition as part of its picture. For example, if your companion has a tooth abscess, you would look in the teeth section of *Kent's Repertory* and find *abscess;* this would denote the remedies known to have an affiliation to tooth abscesses. Each individual listing (symptom or condition plus applicable remedies) is a rubric.

Rubric. See above, under *repertory.*

Signs. See below, under *symptom.*

Simillimum. The homeopathic remedy that is most similar to the case, thus it is the correct remedy, or the remedy that is homeopathic to the case.

Succussion. The process of strong agitation that is done after each dilution during the preparation of remedies. It is thought to be succussion that engenders the great power of remedies.

Suppression. Elimination of one or more symptoms, followed by the occurrence of a more serious symptom or state. Thus the less serious symptom was suppressed—pushed deeper into the body—and the body responded by producing a more serious condition. See Chapter Three, "The Nature of Cure." See also *cure* and *palliation.*

Symptom. Symptoms are produced by the body in response to disease. By definition, a symptom represents something else. Thus, symptoms represent the disease; they are not the disease. Some people differentiate symptoms from signs by denoting the former as subjective and the latter as objective evidence of illness. Thus, a sore throat would be a symptom and a red throat a sign. I use the more modern definition, which allows symptom and sign to be somewhat interchangeable. This is because symptoms, by the former definition, are essentially unavailable when working with animals. In homeopathic terminology, there are several classes of symptoms: characteristic; common; general; local or particular; and strange, rare, and peculiar symptoms.

Characteristic symptoms accurately portray the disease in a given individual. They do not usually include common symptoms, rather they are symptoms that individualize the case and lead to the correct remedy.

Common symptoms occur in most individuals with a similar condition, thus they are of no help in individualizing the case or choosing a remedy. For example, all dogs with canine parvovirus develop diarrhea, usually bloody.

General symptoms affect the entire body; they include the body's response to its environment. We thus consider these to be of more importance than local symptoms.

Local or particular symptoms are related to local physical effects of disease. They are the least important symptoms. These are often common symptoms.

Strange, rare, and peculiar symptoms are those that are extremely unusual or unexpected. These symptoms are often very accurate pointers to a remedy.

Vital force. Hahnemann coined this term to describe the life-giving essence in all life forms. The vital force is responsible for maintaining health and life. It is similar in some ways to Qi ("chee"), the Chinese name for the energy that flows through the body and carries out the activities of the living body. The vital force (and Qi) exists separately from the material body—it is more than just a chemical or physical process.

HOMEOPATHIC AND HOLISTIC ORGANIZATIONS

National Center for Homeopathy

101 South Whiting Street, Suite 16
Alexandria, VA 22304
Phone: 703 548 7790 / Fax: 703 548 7792
E-mail: see Web site
Web site: http://nationalcenterforhomeopathy.org

The National Center for Homeopathy supplies information about homeopathy, publishes a monthly newsletter, and maintains a list of homeopathic practitioners. They also hold a yearly conference and have been instrumental in supporting homeopathy in the United States.

Academy of Veterinary Homeopathy

PO Box 232282
Leucadia, CA 92023-2282
Phone and fax: 866 652 1590 (U.S. and Canada)
E-mail: see Web site
Web site: www.theavh.org

The Academy of Veterinary Homeopathy supports the teaching and practice of classical (Kentian-Hahnemannian) homeopathy by veterinarians. They also maintain a list of veterinarians who have been certified by their organization. The list is available on their Web site and by e-mail. The address for the AVH tends to change, so check the Web site for current information.

American Holistic Veterinary Medical Association

2218 Old Emmorton Road
Bel Air, MD 21015
Phone: 410 569 0795 / Fax: 410 569 2346
E-mail: office@ahvma.org
Web site: http://ahvma.org

The American Holistic Veterinary Medical Association supports the practice of diverse holistic methods, including (but not limited to) nutrition, chiropractic, acupuncture, and homeopathy. They maintain a list of holistic veterinarians. Mail them a stamped, self-addressed envelope to receive a copy of the list, or you may find the list on the Web site.

British Association of Homeopathic Veterinary Surgeons

Stuart Marston, B.Vet. Med.,Vet. MF Hom., MRCVS

103 Golf Drive

Nuneaton, Warks. CV11 6ND

Phone: +44 (0) 7768 322 075

Web site: www.bahvs.com

This is the British equivalent of the AVH. They also maintain a referral list of homeopathic veterinarians in the United Kingdom.

HOMEOPATHIC SUPPLIERS

These suppliers offer homeopathic medicine (remedies) as well as reference materials (books, computer software, etc.) unless otherwise indicated.

Hahnemann Laboratories, Inc. (remedies only)

1940 Fourth Street
San Rafael, CA 94901
Phone: 888 4 ARNICA (888 427 6422) / Fax: 415 451 6981
E-mail: See Web site
Web site: www.hahnemannlabs.com

Homeopathic Educational Services

Mailing address: 2124 Kittredge Street
Store address: 2036 Blake Street
Berkeley, CA 94704
Phone: 800 359 9051 / Fax: 510 649 1955
E-mail: mail@homeopathic.com
Web site: www.homeopathic.com

Homeopathy Overnight

929 Shelburne Avenue
Absecon, NJ 08201
Phone: 800 ARNICA 30 (800 276 4223) / Fax: 609 646 0347
E-mail: See Web site
Web site: www.homeopathyovernight.com

Luyties (1-800-Homeopathy)

P.O. Box 8080
Richford, VT 05476
Phone: 800- HOMEOPATHY (800 466 3672) / Fax: 877 999 0090
E-mail: info@1800homeopathy.com
Web site: http://1-800homeopathy.com

The Minimum Price Homeopathic Books (reference materials only)

250 H Street
Blaine, WA 98231
Phone: 800 663 8272 / Fax: 604 597 8304
E-mail: orders@minimum.com
Web site: www.minimum.com

Natural Health Supply

6410 Avenida Christina
Santa Fe, NM 87505
Phone: 888 689 1608 / Fax: 505 473 0336
E-mail: nhs@a2zhomeopathy.com
Web site: http://a2zhomeopathy.com

New Atlantean Holistic Books (vaccine reference materials only)

P.O. Box 9638-A
Santa Fe, NM 87504
Phone: 505 983 1856 / Fax: 505 983 1856
E-mail: global@thinktwice.com
Web site: www.thinktwice.com

Treatment Options Homeopathic Laboratories

1006 West 8th Avenue
King of Prussia, PA 19406
Phone: 800 234 8879
E-mail: info@homeopathiclaboratories.com
Web site: www.homeopathiclaboratories.com
This company supplies Standard Homeopathic Remedies

Washington Homeopathic Pharmacy

4914 Del Ray Avenue
Bethesda, MD 20814
Phone: 800 336 1695 / Fax: 301 656 1847
E-mail: See Web site
Web site: www.homeopathyworks.com

Canada

Boiron Canada

816 Guimond Boulevard
Longueuil, Quebec J4G 1T5
Phone: 800 461 2066 (Canada only), 450 442 4422
Web site: http://boiron.ca

Hemkund Remedies Inc.

Surrey, B.C.
Phone: 888 543 9022 / Fax: 604 543 9031
E-mail: admin@hemkund.ca
Web site: www.hemkund.ca/home.aspx

Standard Homeopathic Canada

P.O. Box 1019, 381-A Route 139
Sutton, Quebec J0E 2K0
Phone: 800 363 8933 / Fax: 514 538 6638
E-mail: info@standard-homeopathic.qc.ca
Web site: www.standard-homeopathic.qc.ca

United Kingdom

Note: from the United States, phone numbers must be preceded by 01144.

Ainsworths Pharmacy

38 New Cavendish Street
London W1G 8UF
Phone: 207 935 5330 / Fax: 207 486 4313
Orders: 188 344 0332 / Fax: 188 334 4602
E-mail: See Web site
Web site: www.ainsworths.com/site/default.aspx

Freeman's Homeopathic Pharmacy

18-20 Main Street, Busby
Glasgow G76 8DU
Phone: 845 225 5155 (24 hours) / Fax: 845 225 5255
From outside the UK: 141 644 1165 / Fax: 141 644 5735

E-mail: info@freemans.uk.com
Web site: www.freemans.uk.com/index2.html

Helios Homeopathic Pharmacy

97 Camden Road
Tunbridge Wells, Kent TN1 2QR
Phone: 189 253 7294 / Fax: 189 254 6850
E-mail: See Web site
Web site: www.helios.co.uk

Nelson's Homeopathic Pharmacy

Nelson's House
83 Parkside
London SW19 5LP
Phone: 208 780 4200 / Fax: 208 789 0141
E-mail: See Web site
Web site: www.nelsonshomoeopathy.co.uk

Other Countries

These Web sites list pharmacies in many countries:
www.homeopathyhome.com/services/remedies.shtml
www.drlockie.com/directory.fcm?subsite=3&section=7

NOTES

Preface

1. Richard Pitcairn, DVM, PhD. Personal communication.

Chapter One: Introduction to Homeopathy

1. Samuel Hahnemann, *Organon of the Medical Art*, trans. W. O'Reilly (Redmond, WA: Birdcage, 1996), 60. The manuscript dates to circa 1842.

2. James Kent, *Lectures on Homeopathic Philosophy* (1900; repr. Berkeley, CA: North Atlantic, 1979), 22.

3. Much of the biographical material on Hahnemann comes from Harris Coulter's monumental work on the history of medicine, *Divided Legacy: A History of the Schism in Medical Thought, Vol. II* (Washington, DC: Wehawken; Berkeley, CA: North Atlantic, 1988). I highly recommend the entire series, volumes I–IV, for a fascinating look at the development of medicine in the Western world.

4. Samuel Hahnemann, *Lesser Writings*, ed. and trans. R. E. Dudgeon (1851; repr. New Delhi: B. Jain, 1990), 511–512.

5. Richard Haehl, *Samuel Hahnemann: His Life and Work* (New Delhi: B. Jain, 1921), 37.

6. Harris Coulter, *Divided Legacy: A History of the Schism in Medical Thought, Vol. I* (Washington, DC: Wehawken, 1975), 380.

7. Hahnemann, *Lesser Writings*, 248.

8. Thomas Bradford, *Life and Letters of Hahnemann* (1895; repr. New Delhi: B. Jain, 1992).

9. Constantine Hering, *Analytical Therapeutics* (New York and Philadelphia: Boericke and Tafel, 1875), 24. Quoted in Coulter, *Divided Legacy, Vol. II*, 417.

10. *The American Heritage Dictionary* Ver. 4.0, Softkey International, 1995.

11. Harris Coulter, *Divided Legacy: A History of the Schism in Medical Thought, Vol. III* (Berkeley, CA: North Atlantic; Berkeley, CA: Homeopathic Educational Services, 1982), 306.

12. Coulter, *Divided Legacy, Vol. III*.

13. Jay Yasgur, *Yasgur's Homeopathic Dictionary* (Greenville, PA: Van Hoy, 1998), 378.

14. Hahnemann, *Organon of the Medical Art*, 236–237.

Chapter Two: The Nature of Disease

1. Harriet Beinfield and Efrem Korngold, *Between Heaven and Earth: A Guide to Chinese Medicine* (New York: Ballantine, 1991), 30–31.

2. James Kent, *Lectures on Homeopathic Philosophy* (1900; repr. Berkeley, CA: North Atlantic; Berkeley, CA: Homeopathic Educational Services, 1979).

3. Philip Incao, "Nurture your Child," interview by Noelle Denke, *Lilipoh* 3, no. 11 (Winter/Spring 1998): 25.

4. Steven Jay Gould, *The Flamingo's Smile: Reflections in Natural History* (New York: Norton, 1985), 160.

5. *The American Heritage Dictionary* Ver. 4.0, Softkey International, 1995.

6. Samuel Hahnemann, *Organon of Medicine*, trans. Jost Kunzli et al. (London: Victor Gollancz, 1992).

7. Louis Pasteur, quoted in Laurie Garrett, *The Coming Plague* (New York: Farrar, Straus and Giroux, 1994), 192.

8. Francis M. Pottenger Jr., *Pottenger's Cats: A Study in Nutrition* (San Diego: Price-Pottenger Nutrition Foundation, 1995).

9. Dorothy Shepherd, *Magic of the Minimum Dose* (New Delhi: B. Jain, 1997), 211.

10. Kent, *Lectures on Homeopathic Philosophy*; George Vithoulkas, *A New Model for Health and Disease* (Berkeley, CA: North Atlantic; Mill Valley, CA: Health and Habitat, 1991); George Vithoulkas, *The Science of Homeopathy* (New York: Grove, 1980); Harris Coulter, *Vaccination, Social Violence, and Criminality* (Berkeley, CA: North Atlantic; Washington, DC: Center for Empirical Medicine, 1990); Martin Miles, *Homeopathy and Human Evolution* (London: Winter, 1992).

Chapter Four: Where to Start When You Have a Sick Companion

1. Stuart Close, *The Genius of Homeopathy* (1924; repr. New Delhi: B. Jain, 1996).

2. John Anderson, "The Poisons in Pet Food," *Alternative Medicine* 23 (1998): 82.

3. "Antibiotics: Single Largest Class of Drugs Causing Liver Injury," *Science Daily*, December 8, 2008, http://www.sciencedaily.com.

Chapter Six: Skin and Ears

1. J. Munoz and R. K. Bergman, "Some Histamine Sensitizing Properties of Soluble Preparations of the Histamine Sensitizing Factor (HSF) from

Bordetella pertussis," Journal of Immunology 97, no.1 (1966): 120–125.

2. Richard Pitcairn, DVM, PhD, and Susan Pitcairn, *Natural Health for Dogs and Cats* (Emmaus, PA: Rodale, 1995), 302.

3. M. L. Tyler and John Weir, *Acute Conditions, Injuries, etc.* (London: British Homeopathic Association, 1982), 28.

4. Pitcairn and Pitcairn, *Natural Health for Dogs and Cats*, 264.

Chapter Seven: Mouth, Gums, and Teeth

1. A. C. Guyton and J. E. Hall, *Textbook of Medical Physiology* (Philadelphia: Saunders, 1996), 818.

2. Richard Pitcairn, DVM, PhD, personal communication. The concept of feline gingivitis as a form of scurvy originated with Dr. Pitcairn, though I have expanded upon the idea.

3. John H. Clarke, *Dictionary of Practical Materia Medica* (1900; repr. New Delhi: B. Jain, 1991), 789.

Chapter Eight: Digestive System

1. Francis M. Pottenger Jr., *Pottenger's Cats: A Study in Nutrition* (Lemon Grove, CA: Price-Pottenger Nutrition Foundation, 1995).

Chapter Eleven: Urinary System

1. Michael Lieb and William Monroe, *Practical Small Animal Internal Medicine* (Philadelphia: W. B. Saunders, 1996), 312.

2. K. C. Bovee, "Management of Chronic Renal Disease," in *Renal Disease in Dogs and Cats*, ed. A. R. Michell (Oxford: Blackwell Scientific, 1988), 151.

3. Farley Mowat, *People of the Deer* (New York: Pyramid, 1968).

Chapter Thirteen: Nervous System

1. Lou Klein, lecture, National Center for Homeopathy Annual Conference, San Diego, 1998.

Chapter Fifteen: Therapeutic Indications by Condition

1. Harris Coulter, *Vaccination, Social Violence, and Criminality* (Berkeley, CA: North Atlantic; Washington, DC: Center for Empirical Medicine, 1990).

2. See Judith Reichenberg Ullman and Robert Ullman, *Ritalin-free Kids* (Rocklin, CA: Prima, 1996), for information on homeopathic treatment of attention deficit hyperactivity disorder in children and adults.

3. Jean Dodds, DVM, "More Bumps on the Vaccine Road," lecture and pro-
ceedings of the American Holistic Veterinary Medical Association
annual conference, Snowmass, CO, 1995.

Chapter Sixteen: Vaccination

1. Niels Pedersen et al., "Evaluation of a Commercial Feline Leukemia
Virus Vaccine for Immunogenicity and Efficacy," *Feline Practice* 15
(1985): 7–20; R. Sharpee et al., "Feline Leukemia Vaccine: Evaluation of
Safety and Efficacy against Persistent Viremia and Tumor
Development," *Compendium on Continuing Education for the Practicing
Veterinarian* 8 (1986): 267–268; Alfred Legendre et al., "Efficacy of a
Feline Leukemia Virus Vaccine in a Natural Exposure Challenge,"
Journal of Veterinary Internal Medicine 4 (1990): 92–98.

2. Roy Pollock and Janet Scarlett, "Randomized Blind Trial of a
Commercial FeLV Vaccine," *Journal of the American Veterinary Medical
Association* 196 (1990): 611–616; Janet Scarlett and Roy Pollock, "Year
Two of Follow-up Evaluation of a Commercial Feline Leukemia Virus
Vaccine," *Journal of the American Veterinary Medical Association* 199
(1991): 1431–1432.

3. Tom Phillips and Ron Schultz, "Canine and Feline Vaccines," in *Current
Veterinary Therapy XI,* ed. R. Kirk and J. Bonagura (Philadelphia:
Saunders, 1992), 205.

4. Ron Schultz, "Theory and Practice of Immunization," paper presented
at the annual meeting of the American Holistic Veterinary Medical
Association, Snowmass, CO, September 1995, 92–104.

5. Neil Miller, *Vaccines: Are They Really Safe and Effective?* (Santa Fe, NM:
New Atlantean, 1994).

6. Schultz, "Theory and Practice of Immunization," 92–104.

7. Christopher Day, "Isopathic Prevention of Kennel Cough—Is
Vaccination Justified?," *International Journal of Veterinary Homeopathy* 2,
no. 2 (1987).

8. Samantha McCormick, *Vaccine Skepticism: Adverse Effects and
Alternatives,* http://www.gentlebirth.org/archives/immnza1.html 1995;
with thanks to Frans Vermeulen, who published this quote in his book,
Monera (Haarlem, Netherlands: Emryss, 2005).

9. Proceso Ortega, *Notes on the Miasms* (New Delhi: National
Homeopathic Pharmacy, 1980), 46.

10. Viera Scheibner, *Vaccination: The Medical Assault on the Immune System* (Maryborough, Australia: Australian Print Group, 1993).

11. Miller, *Vaccines,* 36.

12. Scheibner, *Vaccination,* 49; J. Cherry et al., "Report of the Task Force on Pertussis and Pertussis Immunisation," *Pediatrics* Supplement 1988, 939–984.

13. Viera Scheibner, *Dangers and Ineffectiveness of Vaccinations,* videocassette, 1995.

14. Compton Burnett, *Vaccinosis and Its Cure by Thuja* (New Delhi: B. Jain, 1990), 16–17.

15. Samuel Hahnemann, *Organon of Medicine,* trans. Jost Kunzli et al. (London: Victor Gollancz, 1992), 33.

16. C. K. Csiza et al., "Pathogenesis of Feline Panleukopenia Virus in Susceptible Newborn Kittens: II. Pathology and Immunofluorescence," *Infection and Immunity* 3, no. 6 (1971): 838–846.

17. Michael Lappin, "Parenteral Administration of FVRCP Vaccines Induces Antibodies against Feline Renal Tissues," American College of Veterinary Internal Medicine Forum, Dallas, 2002.

18. Clarence Fraser, ed. *The Merck Veterinary Manual* (Rahway, NJ: Merck & Co., 1986).

19. Philip Fox, DVM, paper presented at the American College of Veterinary Internal Medicine Forum, Dallas, 2002.

20. Dee Blanco, DVM, personal communication; Don Hamilton, DVM, personal observation.

21. Arthur Young, DVM, personal communication.

22. Scheibner, *Vaccination,* 21.

23. Laurie Garrett, *The Coming Plague* (New York: Farrar, Straus and Giroux, 1994), 558–560.

24. H. Hogenesch, J. Azcona-Olivera, C. Scott-Moncrieff, et al., "Vaccine-induced Autoimmunity in the Dog," *Advances in Veterinary Medicine* 41 (1999): 733–744; J. C. Scott-Moncrieff, J. Azcona-Olivera, N. W. Glickman, et al., "Evaluation of Antithyroglobulin Antibodies after Routine Vaccination in Pet and Research Dogs," *Journal of the American Veterinary Medical Association* 221 (2002): 515–521.

25. "Unexpected Protein Found in Measles-Mumps Vaccine," *Washington Post* (Washington, DC), December 9, 1995.

26. Schultz, "Theory and Practice of Immunization," 92–104.

27. Day, "Isopathic prevention of Kennel Cough."

Chapter Seventeen: The Bigger Picture

1. Chief Seattle (Seathl): this quote I understand to be a paraphrase of Seattle's words, although there is controversy. There is a question, for example, of whether or not he saw buffaloes, since he was a Northwest native. I suspect it carries the gist of Seattle's concerns, though, as well as that of Native Americans in general. The speech was translated twice to get into English, then modified yet further. I use it because it still rings true for me.

2. John C. Van Dyke, *The Desert* (1901; repr. Layton, UT: Gibbs-Smith, 1980), 62.

3. Paul Shepard, *The Tender Carnivore and the Sacred Game* (Athens, GA: University of Georgia Press, 1973), 260.

4. Ibid., 99–100.

5. Judy Martin, "The Long Walk," presentation at Fort Union National Monument, Watrous, NM, July 18, 2009.

6. Shepard, *The Tender Carnivore and the Sacred Game*, 122.

7. Ibid., 277.

8. Martin, "The Long Walk."

9. Barry Lopez, *Of Wolves and Men* (New York: Scribner's, 1978), 2.

Chapter Eighteen: Materia Medica

1. Quoted in Frans Vermeulen, *Synoptic Materia Medica II* (Haarlem, Netherlands: Emryss, 1998).

SUGGESTED READING AND
REFERENCE BOOKS

Homeopathic Home Care Guidebooks

Animal Care

Day, Christopher. *The Homeopathic Treatment of Small Animals.* London: Wigmore, 1984. Though short on detail, this book has a lot of good information from an experienced British veterinary homeopath.

Saxton, John, and Peter Gregory. *Textbook of Veterinary Homeopathy.* Beaconsfield, UK: Beaconsfield, 2005. Peter and John's book is a good reference for homeopathic principles; it also contains a practical section with remedy guidelines.

Human Home Care

The following three books are all very good. I suggest you browse each one to see which style you like. Or purchase more than one; each has its strong points.

Castro, Miranda. *The Complete Homeopathy Handbook.* New York: St. Martin's, 1991.

Cummings, Stephen, MD, and Dana Ullman, MPH. *Everybody's Guide to Homeopathic Medicines.* New York: J. P. Tarcher/Putnam, 1997.

Panos, Maesimund, and Jane Heimlich. *Homeopathic Medicine at Home.* Los Angeles: J. P. Tarcher, 1980.

Homeopathic Reference Books

Boericke, William, MD. *Pocket Manual of Materia Medica with Repertory.* 1927. Reprint, Santa Rosa, CA: Boericke and Tafel, 1999. This is an inexpensive book with good remedy descriptions. A good place to start with a *materia medica.* See also Phatak.

Clarke, John, MD. *A Dictionary of Practical Materia Medica.* 3 vols. 1900. Reprint, Essex, UK: C. W. Daniel and New Delhi: B. Jain, 1991. This is an excellent *materia medica* from a master of the past century. Dr. Clarke gives great information on remedy sources as well as very good remedy descriptions.

Kent, James, MD. *Repertory of The Homeopathic Materia Medica.* Reprint, New Delhi: B. Jain, 1986. All modern repertories are based upon Kent. This book is inexpensive and a great place to start; many practitioners still use Kent's repertory as their primary resource.

Phatak, S. R. *Materia Medica of Homeopathic Medicines.* New Delhi: Indian Books and Periodicals Syndicate, 1977. This *materia medica* is small and inexpensive and based upon Boericke, with Dr. Phatak's additional hints. A good introductory *materia medica.*

Phatak, S. R. *A Concise Repertory of Homeopathic Medicines.* 1982. Reprint, New Delhi: B. Jain, 1991. Dr. Phatak's personal repertory is based upon many years of practice. This is a wonderful book for acute symptoms, though it has great information for practitioners as well.

Tyler, Margaret. *Homeopathic Drug Pictures.* 1952. Reprint, Essex, UK: C. W. Daniel, 1989. Dr. Tyler provides excellent pictures of remedies and highlights from the provings. Very good overall descriptions of remedies.

Vermeulen, Frans. *Concordant Materia Medica.* Haarlem, Netherlands: Emryss, 2000. This *materia medica,* though expensive, is a great compilation from several authors, beginning with Boericke.

Yasgur, Jay. *Yasgur's Homeopathic Dictionary and Holistic Health Reference.* Greenville, PA: Van Hoy, 1998. An indispensable resource that assists in understanding the older medical terms encountered in homeopathic study.

Homeopathic Theory and Principles

Close, Stuart. *The Genius of Homeopathy.* Reprint, New Delhi: B. Jain, 1996. Dr Close practiced and taught in the early 1900s. This book is based upon numerous lectures. It has a lot of very insightful information, and it provides a good overview of the homeopathic method.

De Schepper, Luc. *Hahnemann Revisited.* Santa Fe, NM: Full of Life, 2001. De Schepper has several books, all good, on classical homeopathy. They are a bit dogmatic and rigid, even opinionated; still the info is generally good.

Dhawale, M. L. *Principles and Practice of Homeopathy.* Mumbai: Institute of Clinical Research, 2001. A very good overview of homeopathic principles.

Hahnemann, Samuel. *Organon of the Medical Art.* Wendy O'Reilley, ed.; Steven Decker, trans. Redmond, WA: Birdcage, 1996. See next entry.

———. *Organon of Medicine.* Jost Kunzli, MD, et al., trans. London: Gollancz, 1989. Hahnemann's *Organon* is the bible of homeopathic medicine. The O'Reilley edition is the easiest and clearest one, and although it is more expensive, it is a beautiful book. The Kunzli edition is also very good.

There are other editions by Boericke, but these are harder to read because of the translation.

Kent, James, MD. *Lectures on Homeopathic Philosophy.* 1900. Reprint, Berkeley, CA: North Atlantic, 1979. A wonderful series of essays on the homeopathic healing art.

Roberts, Herbert. *The Principles and Art of Cure by Homeopathy.* 1942. Reprint, New Delhi: B. Jain, 1990. Very good introduction to homeopathic therapeutics.

Sankaran, Rajan. *The Spirit of Homeopathy.* Berkeley, CA: Homeopathic Educational Services, YEAR. All of Sankaran's books are interesting, though somewhat hard to read. *The Spirit of Homeopathy* is an interesting overview of homeopathic practice, but Rajan has moved on from there. Sankaran is a modern homeopath from India whose ideas have had a great impact upon the homeopathic world. His work is somewhat controversial (some homeopaths believe he strays from Hahnemann, while others feel he has greatly expanded upon Hahnemann's ideas), but he gives a very good explanation of disease and the homeopathic approach, and the book is very interesting to read—and very thought-provoking. His other books are best for advanced practitioners.

Vithoulkas, George. *The Science of Homeopathy.* New York: Grove, 1980. Excellent overview of homeopathic medicine by one of the modern masters.

Whitmont, Edward, MD. *The Alchemy of Healing.* Berkeley, CA: North Atlantic, 1993. Compelling treatise on the fundamental nature of disease and healing. The author was a homeopath as well as a Jungian scholar and psychotherapist. My copy is well worn.

History of Homeopathy and Medicine

Coulter, Harris. *Divided Legacy: A History of the Schism in Medical Thought* (4 volumes). Berkeley, CA: North Atlantic, 1975, 1977, 1981, 1994. This four-volume set covers the history of medicine, emphasizing the divergence into rationalist and empirical pathways. Volume III covers the conflict between homeopathy and allopathy in the nineteenth century. Fascinating reading.

Winston, Julian. *The Faces of Homoeopathy: An Illustrated History of the First 200 Years.* Tawa, New Zealand: Great Auk, 1999. This new book covers the history of homeopathy in the United States, with many pictures of the great homeopathic masters. It should be very interesting reading, as the author is a leading authority on the subject.

General Animal Care

Frazier, Anitra, with Norma Ecroate. *The Natural Cat: The Comprehensive Guide to Optimum Care.* New York: Plume, 2008. An excellent book on holistic cat care from a woman who really knows cats.

Frost, April, and Rondi Lightmark. *Beyond Obedience: Training with Awareness for You and Your Dog.* New York: Harmony, 1998. This book approaches training from a perspective that animals have intrinsic value; the training is thus done with respect for the animal.

Levy, Juliette de Bairacli. *The Complete Herbal Book for the Dog and Cat.* London: Faber and Faber, 1991. See the next entry.

———. *Cats Naturally.* London: Faber and Faber, 1991. These books are very interesting compilations of the author's many years of wisdom from treating animals using herbal and folk remedies.

McKinnon, Helen. *It's for the Animals "Cook" Book.* Clinton, NJ: CSA, 1998. A very good introduction to preparing foods at home. The author's approach is simple and effective. She also gives general information on holistic animal care. The book is sometimes available and sometimes not: 888 339 4382, www.itsfortheanimals.com.

Pitcairn, Richard, DVM, PhD, and Susan Pitcairn. *Dr. Pitcairn's Complete Guide to Natural Health for Dogs and Cats.* Emmaus, PA: Rodale, 2005. The best overall book on holistic animal care. Dr. Pitcairn covers everything from herbs and homeopathy to diet, vaccination, and general care.

Schoen, Allen. *Love, Miracles, and Animal Healing.* New York: Simon and Schuster, 1996. An inspiring story of the author's transition into holistic medicine. The book also gives recommendations for holistic home treatment.

Schwartz, Cheryl. *Four Paws, Five Directions: A Guide to Chinese Medicine for Cats and Dogs.* Berkeley, CA: Celestial Arts, 2004. A wonderful introduction to Chinese medicine, with generous instructions for home treatment with acupressure and herbs.

Nutrition

Balch, Phyllis A. *Prescription for Natural Healing.* Garden City Park, NY: Avery, 2006. This book has a great encyclopedia of common illnesses and recommended supplements. Very good.

Pitchford, Paul. *Healing with Whole Foods: Asian Traditions and Modern Nutrition.* Berkeley, CA: North Atlantic, 2003. My favorite nutrition book. The author combines Chinese medical and Western approaches to nutrition.

Vaccination

Coulter, Harris. *Vaccination, Social Violence, and Criminality.* Berkeley, CA: North Atlantic, 1990. Dr. Coulter presents a compelling hypothesis linking vaccination-induced brain damage to many modern ailments, including attention deficit/hyperactivity disorder, autism, and violent behavior.

James, Walene. *Immunization—The Reality behind the Myth.* Santa Barbara, CA: Bergin and Garvey, 1995. A very good book that clearly explains the problems with vaccination.

Miller, Neil. *Vaccinations: Are They Really Safe and Effective?* Santa Fe, NM: New Atlantean, 1994. An excellent overview of the vaccine issue.

Neustaedter, Randall. *The Vaccine Guide.* Berkeley, CA: North Atlantic, 1996. The author examines the pros and cons of vaccination. Excellent and well-referenced.

Scheibner, Viera, PhD. *Vaccination: The Medical Assault on the Immune System.* Maryborough, Australia: Australian Print Group, 1993. The author compiled information from hundreds of articles published in conventional medical journals. Thoroughly documented and very interesting.

Herbal Medicine

Gladstar, Rosemary. A great herbalist, with books for human care. I have *Rosemary Gladstar's Family Herbal,* but this is unfortunately out of print and expensive if you can find it. She has many other books; all are very good.

Levy, Juliette de Bairacli. Any of her books.

Tilford, Greg, and Mary Wulff. *Herbs for Pets: The Natural Way to Enhance Your Pet's Life.* Irvine, CA: Bow Tie, 2009. A great herb book specifically for animals. Well researched. The 1999 edition is a hardback. Highly recommended.

Flower Essences

Though not covered in this book, flower essences are similar to homeopathic medicines (but not the same). They offer help with many emotional and behavioral problems, though not as effectively as homeopathic remedies, in my experience. They are a good adjunct to homeopathy. A few practitioners prefer not to combine flower essences with homeopathic medicines, but I have not seen any conflict.

Kaminski, Patricia, and Richard Katz. *Flower Essence Repertory.* Nevada City, CA: Flower Essence Society, 1994, 2004. The best book on flower essences, including the English essences (Bach flower remedies). The book has a section on animal care as well as a wonderful repertory and remedy description section. I have not seen the 2004 edition, but a client told me the 1994 one was better. You can occasionally find it used.

INDEX